Wolfgang Seeger

Atlas of Topographical Anatomy of the Brain and Surrounding Structures

for Neurosurgeons, Neuroradiologists, and Neuropathologists

Springer-Verlag Wien New York

Prof. Dr. med. WOLFGANG SEEGER
Medical Director of the Department of General Neurosurgery
and Chairman of Neurosurgery of the Neurosurgical Clinic,
University of Freiburg i. Br., Federal Republic of Germany

With 258 Figures

Design: Hans Joachim Böning, Wien

Library of Congress Cataloging in Publication Data. Seeger, Wolfgang. Atlas of topographical anatomy of the brain and surrounding structures for neurosurgeons, neuroradiologists, and neuropathologists. Includes bibliographical references. 1. Brain-Anatomy. 2. Anatomy, Surgical and topographical. 3. Brain-Surgery. I. Title: Atlas of topographical anatomy of the brain and surrounding structures . . . QM 455.S4. 611'.81'0246171. 77-16683

ISBN-13: 978-3-211-81851-0 e-ISBN-13: 978-3-7091-7541-5
DOI: 10.1007/978-3-7091-7541-5

Foreword

The traditional education of the neurosurgeon and the clinician working in related specialties is based on their presumed knowledge of the macroscopic anatomy of the brain as traditionally taught. Most neurosurgical textbooks, therefore, provide macroscopic views of sections of the operative site. The literature that has accumulated in recent years on the subject of microneurosurgical operations also follows this principle.

For some years, however, the customary macroscopic representation of the anatomy of the brain has been inadequate for the needs of the neurosurgeon using refined modern operative techniques. Furthermore, despite their detailed presentation, stereotactic atlases are also insufficient for neurosurgical purposes, since the magnified views of sections reproduced in them are of little assistance to the operator in achieving spatial orientation in the brain.

In this work, therefore, an attempt is made to give a spatial representation of the brain, its vessels, and the surrounding structures, whose morphological details can be reproduced within the magnification range of the surgical microscope. The considerable variability of the vessels, which has become generally known only in recent years, has also been taken into account. At the same time, recognizable large topographical associations have been stressed for didactic reasons in the case of all structures shown with considerable enlargement.

The twofold aim – microanatomical presentation on the one hand, and a simultaneous illustration of the positional relationships in connection with the overall topic of the brain on the other – is impossible to realize by means of operation photographs or photographs of organ preparations, and it was, therefore, necessary to have recourse to anatomical drawings and operation sketches by the author. Another reason for the preference for drawings is the opportunity this affords of elucidating illustrations of complex structures by preceding them with drawings of the respective brain structure, then of the arteries, veins, meninges, etc., in stages, and then in a third step combining these in a comprehensive view representing the operative site. Moreover, it is technically almost impossible to produce simultaneous contrast preparations of the arteries and veins and thus obtain a complex photographic representation of the structures of the preparation.

The manuscript and drawings were completed in the years 1974–1976 after almost two decades of neurosurgical work. The data worked out in the early stages (Chapter 1 in particular) were used by the author as the basis for teaching programmes at the University of Giessen. Chapters 2–7, dealing with the operative technical aspects, were produced after mid-1975 and used by the author as the basis for microneurosurgical teaching of his colleagues at the University of Freiburg.

My thanks are due to Doz. Dr. E. Grote, a former colleague from Giessen, who first encouraged me to publish this work. I am grateful to Prof. A. Oksche, Director of the Anatomical Institute, University of Giessen, and Prof. J. Staubesand, Director of the Anatomical Institute I, University of Freiburg, as well as to my colleagues, in particular Dr. J. Gilsbach and Dr. H. Friedrich, for valuable suggestions and advice. Prof. U. Hachmeister, Centre for Pathology, University of Giessen, and Prof. W. Sandritter, Director of the Department of General Pathology and Pathological Anatomy, Pathological Institute, University of Freiburg, provided support by making available the necessary organic material.

Mr. K. Schmidt, Senior Dissector, Anatomical Institute I, University of Freiburg, gave suggestions and help with the production of injection preparations, which were prepared by Mr. D. Knapp, cand. med., in the course of work for his doctoral thesis. The painstaking work of translating the manuscript was undertaken by Ms. S. Brinkmann, Neurological Clinic, University of Freiburg. I wish to thank my colleagues Dr. E. Gröbner, Neurosurgical Clinic, and Prof. J. Dichgans, Neurological Clinic and Department of Neurophysiology, University of Freiburg, for looking over the translation. I am grateful to the secretaries of the Neurosurgical Clinic, University of Freiburg, Ms. E. Hilsenbek, Ms. V. Kullmann, and Ms. C. Cramer, for the helpful way in which they carried out the work of typing the German and English versions of the text.

Freiburg, January 1978 Wolfgang Seeger

Contents

Introduction

The aim of this work, as already briefly explained in the foreword, is to give a spatial representation of intracranial structures which will enable the microneurosurgeon to recognize the topographic-anatomical associations and thus facilitate his orientation during the operation. The book is intended to present the problems of the neurosurgeon to the clinician in related specialities, in particular to the neuroradiologist, thus putting him in a position to carry out preoperative examinations more purposefully than has hitherto been the case.

In carrying out the conventional preoperative radiological analysis, orientation was taken, as in the anatomical atlas, from two or three standard projections. This convention inevitably led, after continual repetition of the sagittal and lateral projections in particular, to a two-dimensional conception of structures which were in fact three-dimensional. It was consequently necessary to promote spatial conception by using different oblique projections. These oblique projections were used as follows in this book: for the representation of anatomical preparations, for the simplified representation of radiological findings, and for the illustration of the operation site.

The choice of this method suggested itself for three reasons. First, modern anatomical reproductions have unfortunately deviated from the spatial representation by oblique projection known in earlier centuries (cf. for example those by Jan Kalkar, in 1543 AD, the draughtsman of Vesalius's works). Secondly, oblique projections are seldom used in neuroradiology. They have hitherto been made only to show certain structures without superimposition by other structures. Oblique projections should be used additionally, however, in order to facilitate spatial orientation by the operator and to improve the possibility of measuring the distances between certain structures before the operation. Thirdly, it should be remembered that in microsurgical operations, more than in conventional interventions, there is a danger of losing orientation in the intracranial space. The considerable enlargement shows only a small section of the operative field at one time. Furthermore, the varying oblique positions of the head of the patient used in the different operations make orientation more difficult. Today, operations in the strict lateral or sagittal position count as exceptions.

The use of oblique projections alone is nevertheless not sufficient to prevent disorientation of the operator. In the narrow, limited, microneurosurgical operative field the danger is that important neighbouring structures, which are not visible during operative preparation, may be endangered by pulling, pressure or inadvertent thermocoagulation. It was, therefore, necessary, instead of the customary method of showing the operation site, to include surrounding structures in the illustration and to give characteristic distance measurements between different structures.

The present work consists of two main parts. The first part is intended as a brief introduction to the macroscopic anatomy. The most important brain arteries have been included in a somewhat schematized form. The venous system of the brain could not be schematized meaningfully due to its extreme variability. It is, therefore, first shown in the second part, which makes use of more realistic illustrative methods. The second part of this work is concerned with the topographic-anatomical problems of the microneurosurgeon. Here a classification according to brain regions was chosen.

The various chapters of this book are to a large extent similarly arranged. Each begins with a written presentation of the topic, usually comprising several sections. This is followed by the illustrations relating to the respective chapter. At the end of the text of each chapter the relevant literature is listed.

Note:
(for Nomenclature)

If not otherwise indicated the numbers show distance measurements in millimetres.

Part I

Anatomical Principles

Chapter 1

Brain and Cerebral Arteries

(for Veins see Part II)

A. Introduction and Notes on Nomenclature

The following survey applies only to the brain. The complicated structure of this organ and the difficulties of diagnostic visualization with conventional contrast media, which only picture the cavity systems (vessel lumina and C. S. F. spaces), necessitate a representation of the surface relief designed to meet the needs of the neurosurgeon. The surrounding bony structures and large blood vessels are well known from neuroradiological practice. Preoperative neuroradiological diagnostic techniques allow only an inadequate presentation of the relationships between the surface relief of the brain and the vascular arborizations covering it.

First, in the survey only the relationships between cerebral structures and arteries will be elaborated in order to give a general schematic view. Despite their great variability, the cerebral arteries reveal an arborization pattern which is easily understandable in principle. At operation, however, knowledge of this sort is not sufficient. This extreme variability, which has attracted a great deal of interest on the part of neurosurgeons in recent years, is therefore discussed in Part II, where the variable conditions are demonstrated under microsurgical aspects. The greater variability of the veins made it seem advisable to describe them first in Part II and to dispense with a survey here, in order to prevent too stereotyped thinking, which could lead to unpleasant surprise at the operating table.

Schematic cataloguing of the arteries seemed essential in order to facilitate orientation in the subsequent illustrations. The catalogue of arteries that follows was initially drawn up with acknowledgements to Ring (1969), as well as Stephens and Stilwell (1969). The large vessel trunks have been marked with their initials. The main trunk of these vessels has been given the number 1 – e.g., A. carotis interna = c1, A. cerebri ant. = a1 (not to be confused with the numbering of the proximal and distal segments of A. cerebri ant. and media, which has found increasing use in recent years). Higher numbers – e.g., c2, c3, c4-state the respective branch in question. This principle of abbreviation must be schematic because the branch offshoots do not always occur in this order. It is, however, a help to orientation. If a branch has subbranches these are designated by numbers after the point. Thus it is possible to designate an extended region of arborization with secondary and tertiary offshoots by simple numbering. As is well known, the nomenclature of the arteries in the international literature is not uniform. The author has limited himself to the simplest possible presentation. With regard to special questions the reader is referred in particular to the work of Newton and Potts (1974).

Catalogue of Arteries

c1	*A. carotis int.*
c2	A. ophthalmica
c3	A. hypophyseos sup.
c4	Aa. temporo-polares
c5	A. chorioidea ant.
c5.1	Rr. temp. of A. chor. ant.
c5.2	Rr. perforantes
c6	Medial group of perforating arteries (ad Subst. perfor. ant.), see m2.2
a1	*A. cerebri ant.*
a2	Perforating arteries of Chiasma
a3	A. Heubneri (A. recurrens Heubneri)
a4	A. communicans ant.
a5	A. corporis callosi mediana
a6	A. frontopolaris
a6.1	A. orbitalis
a7	A. callosomarginalis

a8	Inconstant trunk of Aa. frontales intt.
a8.1	A. frontalis int. ant.
a8.2	A. frontalis int. media
a8.3	A. frontalis int. post.
a9	A. pericallosa
a10	A. paracentralis
a11	A. praecunealis
m1	*A. cerebri media, prox. trunk*
m2	Branches of prox. trunk of A. c. m.
m2.1	Aa. temporo-polares (A. temp. ant.)
m2.2	Medial group of perforating arteries (ad Subst. perfor. ant.), see c6
m2.3	Aa. lenticulostriatae
m3	A. cerebri media, distal trunk
m4	A. frontalis ascendens (A. frontoparietalis ascendens
m4.1	A. orbito-frontalis
m4.2	A. operculo-frontalis (A. candelabra)
m4.3	A. sulci centralis (Aa. sulci centralis)
m5	A. temp. media
m6	A. parietalis post. (Aa. parietales postt.)
m7	A. angularis
m8	A. temp. post. (Aa. thalamoperforantes)
p1	*A. cerebri post.*
p2 . . .	Aa. thalamoperforatae
p3	Perforating arteries to the midbrain from the proximal segment of A. cerebri post.
p4	A. quadrigemina
p5/p5.1	A. communicans post./Rami perforantes
p6	*"A. chorioidea post."* (post. chor. group) *see Figs. 26 and 111*
p6.1	A. chor. post. med.
p6.1.1	Rr. antt.
p6.1.1.1	Rr. antt., medial branches
p6.1.1.2	Rr. antt., lateral branches
p6.1.2	Rr. postt.
p6.1.2.1	Rr. postt., medial branches
p6.1.2.2	Rr. postt., lateral branches
p6.2	A. *(Aa.)* chor. post. lat. (lateral post. chor. group)
p6.2.1	Rr. antt.
p6.2.1.1	Rr. antt., medial branches
p6.2.1.2	Rr. antt., lateral branches
p6.2.2	Rr. postt.
p6.2.2.1	Rr. postt., medial branches to Fornix and Thalamus
p6.2.2.2	Rr. postt., lateral branches to Lamina affixa and *Plexus chor.*
p7	Rr. perforantes to Crus cerebri and Tegmentum mesencephali
p8	Aa. thalamogeniculatae
p9	Aa. hippocampi
p10	Aa. splenii corp. call.
p11.1	Rr. temporales anteriores (R. temp. ant.)
p11.2	Rr. temporales postt. (R. temp. post.)
p12	A. parieto-occipitalis
p13	A. calcarina
v1	*A. vertebralis*
v2	Rr. ad medullam
v3	A. cerebelli inf. post.
v3.1	A. spinalis post. (origin from A. vertebralis possible, too)
v3.1.1	A. spinalis post., R. ascendens
v3.1.1.1	A. spinalis post., R. ascendens, Rr. ad medullam
v3.1.2	A. spinalis post., R. descendens
v3.1.2.1	A. spinalis post., R. descendens, Rr. ad medullam
v3.2	R. lateralis of A. cerebelli inf. post.
v3.3	R. medialis of A. cerebelli inf. post. (A. vermicularis)
v4	A. spinalis ant.
b1	*A. basilaris*
b2	Rr. ad pontem (pontine arteries)
b2.1	Rr. ad pontem, medial group ("Aa. medianae")
b2.2	Rr. ad pontem, lateral group
b2.2.1	Rr. ad pontem, lateral group, variation of one of the arteries: A. trigemina
b2.2.2	Rr. ad pontem, lateral group, variations of one or more of these: so-called Aa. cerebellares accessoriae
b3	A. auditiva int. (ca. 50% originate from A. cerebelli inf. ant., 50% directly from A. basilaris)
b3.1	Termination of A. auditiva int. (Meatus acusticus int.)
b3.1.1	Vestibular branch to N. VII
b3.1.2	Cochlear branches
b3.1.3	Vestibulocochlear branches
b4	A. cerebelli inf. ant.
b4.1	"RL" (rostral lateral artery after Naidich and Kriecheff), see Salamon
b4.1.1	Branch to Lobulus semilunaris superior (ascending artery)
b4.1.2	Branch to Lobulus biventer (descending artery)
b4.2	"CM" (caudomedial artery after Naidich and Kriecheff) + Rr. ad pontem (+ medullam)
b4.2.1	Branches to Plexus chorioideus
b4.2.2	Medial branch to Lobulus biventer
b4.2.3	Lateral branch to Lobulus biventer
b5	A. cerebelli sup.
b5.1	A. cerebelli sup., Rr. ad pontem and mesencephalic perforating arteries
b5.2	A. cerebelli sup., R. med.
b5.3	A. cerebelli sup., R. lat.

Extradural carotid branches are not classified, but designated with their full names. Veins have not been classified since there is no uniform international nomenclature and types of course are extremely varied.

Since the work consists mainly of illustrations it will also be understood by non-English-speaking readers. It was decided to use the international Paris Nomenclature of 1955, which is also specifically recognized by the Anglo-Saxon countries*. This was not always possible, particularly for the designation of vessels, since in this regard the Paris Nomenclature is insufficient for the needs of neurosurgeons and neuroradiologists. Many structures have been named only in recent years, and the names differ with different authors. Some designations that were still included in the Basle Nomenclature of 1898 were excluded from the Paris nomenclature. The Jena Nomenclature of 1935 did not receive general recognition and has, therefore, been left out of consideration. Many anatomical terms have been in general use in clinical work for hundreds of years and, as can be seen from the special literature, even the Paris Nomenclature has not changed this. For this reason some well-known oder designations 'e.g., for the large fissures' have been kept.

In the following catalogue the Paris Nomenclature is given as an alternative to the customary designations used in the clinic, insofar as these are used in this book. In addition, for the sake of completeness, some structures that are not illustrated have been included in the catalogue.

* "Nomina anatomica" examined by the I.A.N.C. and permitted by the Fifth International Anatomical Congress Oxford 1950, printed in England by Spottiswoode, Ballantyne and Co. G. m. b. H., London and Colchester, private printing 1955, page VII.

Nomina anatomica (Paris 1955)	Nomina anatomica (Basle 1898 and earlier, selection used in this book)
Osteologia	
Ossa cranii	
Os occipitale	
Foramen magnum	For. occipitale magnum
Pars basilaris	
Sulcus sinus petrosi inferioris	
Squama occipitalis	
Clivus	
Tuberculum pharyngeum	
Condylus occipitalis	
Canalis hypoglossi	
Fossa condylaris	
Tuberculum jugulare	
Processus intrajugularis	
Protuberantia occipitalis externa (Inion)	
(Crista occipitalis externa)	
Linea nuchae suprema	
Linea nuchae superior	
Linea nuchae inferior	
Protuberantia occipitalis interna	
Sulcus sinus sagittalis superioris	Sulcus sagitt. sup.
Sulcus sinus transversi	Sulcus transversus
Sulcus sinus sigmoidei	Sulcus sigmoideus
Os sphenoidale	
Corpus	
Clivus	
Sella turcica	
Fossa hypophyseos	
Tuberculum sellae	
Dorsum sellae	
Processus clinoideus posterior	
Processus clinoideus medius	
Sulcus caroticus	
Lingula sphenoidalis	
Crista sphenoidalis	
Rostrum sphenoidale	

Nomina anatomica (Paris 1955)	Nomina anatomica (Basle 1898 and earlier, selection used in this book)
Sinus sphenoidalis	
Septum sinuum sphenoidalium	
Apertura sinus sphenoidalis	
Ala Minor	*Ala parva*
Canalis opticus	
Processus clinoideus anterior	
Fissura orbitalis superior	
Ala major	*Ala magna*
Facies cerebralis	
Facies temporalis	
Facies sphenomaxillaris	
Facies orbitalis	
Foramen rotundum	
Foramen ovale	
Foramen spinosum	
Spina ossis sphenoidalis	
Processus pterygoideus	
Os temporale	
Pars petrosa	
Processus mastoideus	
Sulcus sinus sigmoidei	Sulcus sigmoideus
Sulcus a. occipitalis	
Foramen mastoideum	
Apex (partis petrosae)	
Canalis caroticus	
Tegmen tympani	
Eminentia arcuata	
Hiatus canalis facialis	
Sulcus n. petrosi majoris	
Sulcus n. petrosi minoris	
Impressio trigemini	
Sulcus sinus petrosi superioris	Sulcus petrosus sup.
Porus acusticus internus	
Meatus acusticus internus	
Sulcus sinus petrosi inferioris	Sulcus petrosus inf.
Processus intrajugularis	
Processus styloideus	
Foramen stylomastoideum	
Pars tympanica	
Meatus acusticus	
Porus acusticus externus	
Pars squamosa	
Processus zygomaticus	
Os parietale	
Foramen parietale	
Tuber parietale	
Linea temporalis superior	
Linea temporalis inferior	
Sulcus sagittalis	
Sulcus sinus sigmoidei	Sulcus sigmoideus
Os frontale	
Squama frontalis	
Tuber frontale	
Arcus superciliaris	
Glabella	
Margo supraorbitalis	
Foramen sive Incisura orbitalis	
Incisura sive Foramen frontale	

Nomina anatomica (Paris 1955)	Nomina anatomica (Basle 1898 and earlier, selection used in this book)
Pars orbitalis	
Fossa glandulae lacrimalis	Fossa lacrimalis
Sinus frontalis	
Os ethmoidale	
Lamina cribrosa	
Crista galli	
Lamina perpendicularis	
Cellulae ethmoidales	
Os lacrimale	
Fossa sacci lacrimalis	
Os nasale	
Vomer	
Maxilla	
Canalis infraorbitalis	
Os zygomaticum	
Processus temporalis	
Processus frontalis	
Cranium	
Lamina externa	
Diploë	
Lamina interna	
Basis cranii interna	
Basis cranii externa	
Fossa crani anterior	
Fossa cranii media	
Fossa cranii posterior	
Impressiones digitatae	
Foveolae granulares	Foveolae granulares (Pacchioni)
Fossa temporalis	
Arcus zygomaticus	
Fossa infratemporalis	
Fossa pterygopalatina	
Fissura pterygopalatina	
Foramen jugulare	
Fissura sphenopetrosa	
Fissura petro-occipitalis	
Foramen lacerum	
Cavum nasi	
Septum nasi osseum	
Apertura piriformis	
Choanae	
Orbita	
Margo supraorbitalis	
Margo infraorbitalis	
Fissura orbitalis superior	
Fissura orbitalis inferior	

Nomina anatomica (Paris 1955)	Nomina anatomica (Basle 1898 and earlier, selection used in this book)
Syndesmologia	
Suturae cranii	
Sutura coronalis	
Sutura sagittalis	
Sutura lambdoidea	
Sutura occipitomastoidea	
Sutura sphenofrontalis	
Sutura spheno-ethmoidalis	
Sutura squamosa	
(Sutura frontalis)	
Sutura frontozygomatica	
Synchondroses cranii	
Synchondrosis spheno-occipitalis	
Synchondrosis sphenopetrosa	
Encephalon	
Rhombencephalon	
Myelencephalon	
Medulla oblongata	
Sulcus medianus posterior	
Fissura mediana anterior	
Pyramis (medullae oblongatae)	
Sulcus lateralis anterior	
Sulcus lateralis posterior	
Oliva	
Pedunculus cerebellaris inferior	Corpus restiforme
Tuberculum nuclei cuneati	
Ventriculus quartus	
Fossa rhomboidea	
Sulcus medianus	
Striae medullares ventriculi quarti	
Colliculus facialis	
Velum medullare posterius	
Velum medullare anterius	
Frenulum veli medullaris anterioris	
Obex	
Apertura mediana ventriculi quarti	Foramen Magendi
Apertura lateralis ventriculi quarti (?)	Foramen Luschkae (?)*
Metencephalon	
Pons	
Sulcus basilaris	
Pedunculus cerebellaris medius	Brachium pontis
Cerebellum	
Fissura horizontalis cerebelli	
Fissura prima	
Vermis	
Lingula cerebelli	
Lobulus centralis	
Culmen	
Declive	
Folium vermis	
Tuber vermis	
Pyramis (vermis)	
Uvula (vermis)	
Nodulus	

* Usually recessus without aperture.

Nomina anatomica (Paris 1955)	Nomina anatomica (Basle 1898 and earlier, selection used in this book)
Ala lobuli centralis	
Lobulus quadrangularis	Lobulus quadrangularis sup.
Lobulus simplex	Lobulus quadrangularis inf.
Lobulus semilunaris superior	
Lobulus semilunaris inferior	
Lobulus biventer	
Tonsilla cerebelli	
Flocculus	
Pedunculus flocculi	
(Isthmus rhombencephali)	
Pedunculus cerebellaris superior	Brachium conjunctivum
*Mesencephalon**	
Pedunculus cerebri	
Crus cerebri	
Fossa interpeduncularis	
Substantia perforata posterior	
Tectum mesencephali	*Lamina quadrigemina*
Colliculus superior	
Colliculus inferior	
Brachium colliculi superioris	
Brachium colliculi inferioris	
Aquaeductus cerebri	Aquaeductus (Sylvii)
Prosencephalon	
Diencephalon	
Ventriculus tertius	
Commissura posterior	
Foramen interventriculare	For. interventriculare (Monroi)
Sulcus hypothalamicus	
Adhaesio interthalamica	
Recessus opticus	
Recessus infundibuli	
Hypothalamus	
Corpus mamillare	
Tuber cinereum	
Infundibulum	
Hypophysis	
Tractus opticus	
Chiasma opticum	
Lamina terminalis	
Fasciculus mamillothalamicus	
Ansa lenticularis	
Thalamencephalon	
Thalamus	
Pulvinar	
Taenia thalami	
Stria medullaris thalami	
Metathalamus	
Corpus geniculatum mediale	
Corpus geniculatum laterale	
Epithalamus	
Corpus pineale	
Recessus pinealis	

* Trigonum lemnisci (missing in Nomina Anat. 1955).

Nomina anatomica (Paris 1955)	Nomina anatomica (Basle 1898 and earlier, selection used in this book)
Recessus suprapinealis	
Habenula	
Commissura habenularum	
Telencephalon	
Cerebrum	
Hemispherium	
Fissura longitudinalis cerebri	
Fissura transversa cerebri	
Fossa lateralis cerebri	Fissura lat. cerebri (Sylvii)
Sulcus lateralis	
Insula	
Gyri insulae	
Gyrus longus insulae	
Gyri breves insulae	
Sulcus circularis insulae	
Sulcus centralis	
Lobus frontalis	
Polus frontalis	
Sulcus praecentralis	
Gyrus praecentralis	
Gyrus frontalis superior	Gyrus front. I
Sulcus frontalis superior	
Gyrus frontalis medius	Gyrus front. II
Sulcus frontalis inferior	
Gyrus frontalis inferior	Gyrus front. III
Pars opercularis	
Pars triangularis	
Pars orbitalis	
Gyrus rectus	
Gyri orbitales	
Lobus temporalis	
Polus temporalis	
Sulci temporales transversi	
Gyri temporales transversi	
Gyrus temporalis superior	Gyrus temp. I
Sulcus temporalis superior	
Gyrus temporalis medius	Gyrus temp. II
Sulcus temporalis inferior	
Gyrus temporalis inferior	Gyrus temp. III
Lobus occipitalis	
Polus occipitalis	
Incisura praeoccipitalis	
Lobus parietalis	
Sulcus postcentralis	
Gyrus postcentralis	
Lobulus parietalis superior	
Sulcus intraparietalis	
Lobulus parietalis inferior	
Gyrus supramarginalis	
Gyrus angularis	
Sulcus corporis callosi	
Sulcus cinguli	
Sulcus collateralis	
Gyrus occipitotemporalis medialis	
Gyrus occipitotemporalis lateralis	
Gyrus cinguli	
Isthmus gyri cinguli	
Gyrus parahippocampalis, Uncus	

Nomina anatomica (Paris 1955)	Nomina anatomica (Basle 1898 and earlier, selection used in this book)
Lobulus paracentralis	
Precuneus	
Sulcus parieto-occipitalis	Fiss. parieto-occipitalis
Sulcus calcarinus	Fiss. calcarina
Cuneus	
Corpus callosum	
Splenium corporis callosi	
Genu corporis callosi	
Rostrum corporis callosi	
Induseum griseum	
Gyrus fasciolaris	
Fornix	
Crus fornicis	
Corpus fornicis	
Taenia fornicis	
Columna fornicis	
Septum pellucidum	
Cavum septi pellucidi	
Ventriculus lateralis	
Pars centralis	
Cornu anterius	
Cornu posterius	
Cornu inferius	
Nucleus caudatus	
Caput nuclei caudati	
Cada nuclei caudati	
Stria terminalis	
Lamina affixa	Lamina affixa thalami
Taenia chorioidea	
Calcar avis	
Eminentia collateralis	
Hippocampus	
Fimbria hippocampi	
Gyrus dentatus	
Commissura fornicis	
Bulbus olfactorius	
Tractus olfactorius	
Trigonum olfactorium	
Area subcallosa	
Substantia perforata anterior	
Stria olfactoria	
Limen insulae	
Sectiones telencephali	
Putamen	
Globus pallidus	
Claustrum	
Capsula externa	
Capsula interna	
Genu capsulae internae	
Crus posterius capsulae internae	
Corpus amygdaloideum	Nucleus amygdalae
Corona radiata	
Radiatio optica	
Commissura anterior	
Meninges	
Dura mater encephali	
Falx cerebri	Falx
Tentorium cerebelli	Tentorium
Falx cerebelli (hitherto not in common use in clinical practice)	

Nomina anatomica (Paris 1955)	Nomina anatomica (Basle 1898 and earlier, selection used in this book)
Diaphragma sellae	
Cisternae subarachnoideales	
Cisterna cerebellomedullaris	
Cisterna fossae lateralis cerebri	Cist. fissurae lat. (Sylvii)
Cisterna chiasmatis	
Cisterna interpeduncularis	
Granulationes arachnoideales	Granulationes arachnoideales (Pacchioni)
Pia mater encephali	
Tela chorioidea ventriculi quarti	
Plexus chorioideus ventriculi quarti	
Tela chorioidea ventriculi tertii	
Plexus chorioideus ventriculi tertii	
Plexus chorioideus ventriculi lateralis	
Lig. denticulatum	
Nervi craniales	
Nn. olfactorii	*N. I*
N. opticus	*N. II*
N. oculomotorius	*N. III*
N. trochlearis	*N. IV*
N. trigeminus	*N. V*
Portio major	
Ganglion semilunare	
Portio minor	
N. ophthalmicus	
R. tentorii	
N. lacrimalis	
N. frontalis	
N. nasociliaris	
N. maxillaris	N. V_2
N. infraorbitalis	
Ganglion pterygopalatinum	
N. mandibularis	N. V_3
N. abducens	*N. VI*
N. facialis	*N. VII*
Geniculum n. facialis	
Ganglion geniculi (vide N. intermedius)	
N. intermedius	
N. stato-acusticus (N. octavus)	*N. VIII*
Pars vestibularis (N. octavi), Ganglion vestibulare	
N. utriculoampullaris (= "N. vestib. sup.")	
N. saccularis (= "N. vestib. inf.")	
Pars cochlearis (N. octavi)	N. cochleae
N. glossopharyngeus	*N. IX*
N. vagus	*N. X*
N. accessorius	*N. XI*
Radices craniales	
Radices spinales	
N. hypoglossus	*N. XII*

B. Superficial Structures (Survey)

In Figs. 1 to 3, starting from the conventional type of anatomical presentation, the superficial structure of the brain is reproduced schematically. The conventionally described gyri can be identified only with difficulty on the surface relief of brain specimens (Fig. 4).

C. Lateral Cerebral Surface and Arteries

The course of the vessels is also difficult to classify from the relief of the gyri. There are two reasons for this:
1) the extreme variability;
2) the vessels are only partly recognizable at the surface. Long stretches of their courses run out of sight in the depths of Sulci (Fig. 5).
The dominant lateral vessel is A. cerebri media. Its proximal trunk sends off perforating arteries to the basal ganglia, which are of vital significance (Fig. 6). The angles of branching of these arteries should be noted. Beyond Substantia perforata ant., A. cerebri media runs for a short stretch over Insula (adjacent to the basal ganglia) and divides into two main trunks in the lateral insula region, A. operculo-frontalis and the distal trunk. A. operculo-frontalis is usually sturdier than the distal trunk (Figs. 7 and 8).

D. Medial Cerebral Surface and Arteries (Figs. 9 to 12)

The medial surface of the cerebral hemisphere has a more regular structure of gyri than the lateral (Fig. 9). The region of A. cerebri anterior presents similar difficulties of identification of individual vessels to those met in the region of A. cerebri media. Figs. 10 and 11 illustrate the relationships on a fixed specimen with transparent leptomeninges. In Fig. 12 the arteries are reproduced schematically.

E. Basomedial Structures (Figs. 13 to 35)

The direction of the projections in the following illustrations deviates from the conventional method of viewing – variant which can be seen in the preparation in Fig. 13 is an interruption in Isthmus gyri cinguli: Fissura calcarina divides this gyrus instead of only narrowing it. The relief in Fissura longitudinalis is flatter than at the convexity and the base. All three cerebral arteries can be recognized on this projection (Figs. 14 and 15). If the temporal lobe is removed (Figs. 16 and 17), Cisterna ambiens with Tractus opticus and Cornu inf. lie exposed medially. Cisterna fissurae lat. (Sylvii) et insulae, Cisternae basales, and Cisterna ambiens connect with one another at the anterior border of Uncus, which is dissected in Figs. 17 and 18.
Gyrus parahippocampalis pushes medially farther forward than Cornu inf. The upwardly diverging course of Crus cerebri corresponds to this, and is closely adjacent to Gyrus parahippocampalis (compare Figs. 17 and 18). In the conventional representation Crus cerebri is shown only shortly before its entry into the pons, where it narrows into Isthmus rhombencephali. A. cerebri post. (Figs. 20 and 21) rarely passes close to the border of the pons, running more often higher up around Crus cerebri. At this point both Crura cerebri are wider than the pons. This explains why the arch of A. cerebri post. is wider in the angiogram than the trunk of A. cerebelli superior, which encircles the contour of the pons. After its two terminal branches divide, the one branch, A. calcarina, may approach very close to the medial ventricle wall if a loop reaches to Fundus of Fissura calcarina. Here Calcar avis projects into the lumen of the ventricle (Fig. 22). The oblique view of the brain in Figs. 23 to 25 is intended as an aid to understanding of the arteries of Cisterna ambiens and the basal cisterns, which are reproduced in Figs. 26 to 35.

F. Structures in the Vicinity of Ventricles (Figs. 33 to 51)

In the vicinity of Commissura ant. the 3rd ventricle and Cornu ant. of the lateral ventricle are separated from each other by the sheet of fibres of Rostrum corporis callosi and the thin sheet of cortex (Area subcallosa, Fig. 36). Caput nuclei caudati and Putamen lie laterally to this. They are connected to each other rostrally. The vascular supply comes mainly through Substantia perforata ant. (Fig. 37). Capsula interna reaches its farthest medial point between the basal ganglia at the level of Foramen interventriculare (Monroi).
A median sulcus of Corpus callosum (Fig. 36) has sometimes been observed. It is caused by A. pericallosa (Fig. 37). The relationships can be seen best in the senile atrophic brain (Figs. 36 and 37). If the whole lateral ventricle is exposed (Fig. 38), Fissura chorioidea gapes wide open after removal of Plexus chorioideus. This brings the cisternal parts of Thalamus into view. Gyrus parahippocampalis can

be recognized medially to Hippocampus and in Cisterna ambiens. The general view afforded by the preparation in Fig. 38 has been included to show the views from various directions towards the structures near the ventricles reproduced in Figs. 20 to 23. Lamina terminalis has been fenestrated, Area subcallosa and parts of Gyrus cinguli removed, and Stria medialis of Trigonum olfactorium followed up as far as Corpus callosum, after detaching the thin cortical layer (Area subcallosa).

Above Commissura ant. the deep median indentation of Rostrum corporis callosi can be recognized from the front. In Fig. 40 instead of the numerous perforations of Substantia perforata ant., the vascular pattern with the perforating arteries can be seen. The connection between Substantia perforata ant. and the region of the basal ganglia can be recognized after a longitudinal incision through the basal ganglia region (Fig. 21) lateral to Tractus opticus. In Fig. 22 some of the fibres of Rostrum corporis callosi have been left in situ. The border of Cornu ant., and the transition between the ventricular surface of Nucleus caudatus into the anterior surface of Putamen situated in the white matter, can be recognized. In Fig. 42 the same preparation is shown from above. Fissura chorioidea gapes open after resection of Plexus chorioideus (arrow). The cut surfaces of Capsula interna and Putamen are visible laterally to Nucleus caudatus. Gyrus parahippocampalis is visible in the depths of Fissura chorioidea. The section of the tapetal fibres leads to gaping open of Fissura longitudinalis with exposure of parts of Lamina quadrigemina. The extraventricular part of Thalamus can be recognized. Lamina affixa thalami takes part medially in the formation of the floor of the ventricle.

Beside the courrently used horizontal sections of computerized tomography*, the consideration of frontal section planes as used by neuropathologists would also appear to be useful (see Figs. 44 to 50), combined with other section planes.

Because of the high degree of variability of vascularization in the area of Cerebellum and lower brainstem, this part of the brain is almost exclusively dealt with in Chapter 7.

A review has already been given in Fig. 3.

* Horizontal section planes are not shown because of the difficulties in comparing anatomical preparations with computer tomograms as shown by Lang, J., Schlehahn, F., Jensen, H. P., et al. (1976).

G. References

Lang, J., Schlehahn, F., Jensen, H. P., et al.: Cranio-Cerebral Topography as a Basis for Interpreting Computed Tomograms. In: Lanksch, W., Kazner, E., Cranial Computerized Tomography. Berlin–Heidelberg–New York: Springer. 1976.

Naidich, T. P., Kricheff, I. I.: In: Advances in Cerebral Angiography, edited by Salamon, G., Part I: Anatomy: The Anterior Inferior Cerebellar Artery in Profile Anatomic-Radiographic Correlation in the Lateral Projection, p. 74. Berlin–Heidelberg–New York: Springer. 1975.

Newton, Th., Potts, D. G.: Radiology of the Skull and Brain Angiography. St. Louis: The C. V. Mosby Company. 1974.

Nomina Anatomica 1955, see: World Federation of Neurology. Problem Commission of Neuroradiology in: The British Journal of Radiology **35**, Nr. 415, 1962.

Nomina Anatomica: Oxford 1950; Paris 1955. Privatdruck London and Colchester 1955.

Ring, A.: In: The Neglected Cause of Stroke. Occlusion of the Smaller Intracranial Arteries and Their Diagnosis by Cerebral Angiography. St. Louis: Warren H. Green, Inc. 1969.

Salamon, G., Raybaud, Ch., Michotey, P., Farnarier, Pn.: In: Advances in Cerebral Angiography, edited by Salamon, G., Part I, Anatomy: Anatomic and Radiographic Study of the Fissures and Sulci of the Brain, p. 10. Berlin–Heidelberg–New York: Springer. 1975.

Sobotta–Becher: Atlas der Anatomie des Menschen, Bd. 3: Zentralnervensystem, Autonomes Nervensystem, Sinnesorgane und Haut, Periphere Leitungsbahnen, 17. Aufl. München–Berlin–Wien: Urban & Schwarzenberg. 1973.

Spalteholz, W.: In: Handatlas der Anatomie des Menschen, Bd. 3: Eingeweide, Gehirn, Nerven, Sinnesorgane, 4. Aufl. Leipzig: Hirzel. 1906.

Stephens, R. B., Stilwell, D. L.: Arteries and Veins of the Human Brain. Springfield, Ill.: Ch. C Thomas. 1969.

Literature for Further Reading

Arnold, F.: Handbuch der Anatomie des Menschen, Bd. 2, S. 1–465. Freiburg i. Br.: Herder'sche Verlagshandlung. 1847. (Cited by Meyer, 1887.)

Babin, E., Megret, M.: Variations in the drainage of the basal vein. Neuroradiolgy **6**, 154–161 (1973).

Benninghoff, A.: Lehrbuch der Anatomie des Menschen, Bd. II. München–Berlin: Lehmann. 1942. (Cited by Linc and others, 1955.)

Ferner, H., Kautzki, R.: Angewandte Anatomie des Gehirns und seiner Hüllen. In: Handbuch der Neurochirurgie I/1, p. 1–90. Berlin–Göttingen–Heidelberg: Springer. 1959.

Haller, A. von: Iconum anatomicarum corporis humani. Fasc. **7**, p. 37. Göttingen: Vandenhoeck. 1781. (Cited by Meyer, 1887.)

Kautzky, R., Zülch, K. J., Wende, S., Tänzer, A.: Neuroradiologie auf neuropathologischer Grundlage, 2. Aufl. Berlin–Heidelberg–New York: Springer. 1976.

Lazorthes, G.: Vascularisation et circulation cérébrales **I**, 323 (1961). Paris: Masson et Cie.

Luschka, H. von: Die Anatomie des Menschen, Vol. 3, Part 2, Der Kopf, p. 494. Tübingen, 1867. (Cited by Meyer, 1887.)

Wackenheim, A., Braun, J. P.: Roentgendiagnosis of the Veins of the Posterior Fossa. Berlin–Heidelberg–New York: Springer. 1976.

Warwick, R., Williams, P. L.: Gray's Anatomy, pp. 288, 987. Philadelphia: W. B. Saunders. 1973.

Winslow, J. B.: Exposition anatomique de la structure du corps humain, **4**, p. 244, § 297. Amsterdam, 1776. (Cited by Meyer, 1887.)

Zinn, J. G.: Descriptio anatomica oculi humani, 2nd ed., ed. Wrisberg, H. A., p. 194. Göttingen: Vandenhoeck. 1780. (Cited by Meyer, 1887.)

Zuckerkandl, E.: Med. Jb. (Wien), p. 343, 1876. (Cited by Meyer, 1887.)

Zuckerkandl, E.: Atlas der topographischen Anatomie des Menschen. Wien: Braumüller. 1904. (Cited by Linc and others, 1955.)

H. Illustrations
(Figs. 1 to 52)

Fig. 1. Schematic representation of supratentorial brain structures from basal direction (according to Spalteholz, 1906, with modifications and additions)

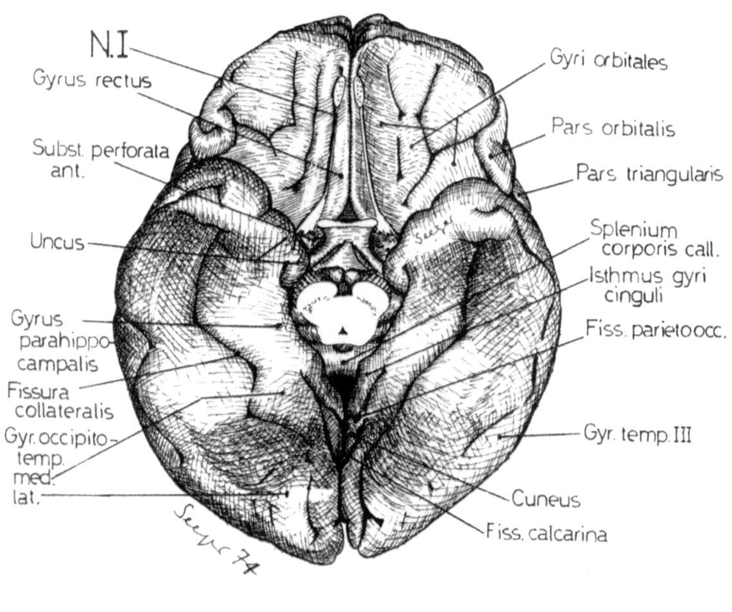
N.I
Gyrus rectus
Subst. perforata ant.
Uncus
Gyrus parahippocampalis
Fissura collateralis
Gyr. occipito-temp. med.
lat.
Gyri orbitales
Pars orbitalis
Pars triangularis
Splenium corporis call.
Isthmus gyri cinguli
Fiss. parietoocc.
Gyr. temp. III
Cuneus
Fiss. calcarina

Fig. 2. Cerebrum, lateral surface *A* and medial surface *B*

Fx Almost constant gyrus (part of Area subcallosa) running parallel to base in the neighbourhood of Gyrus cinguli (not included in the anatomical nomenclature)

F 1–3 Gyri frontales I–III
op Pars opercularis
tr Pars triangularis
or Pars orbitalis
T 1–3 Gyri temporales I–III

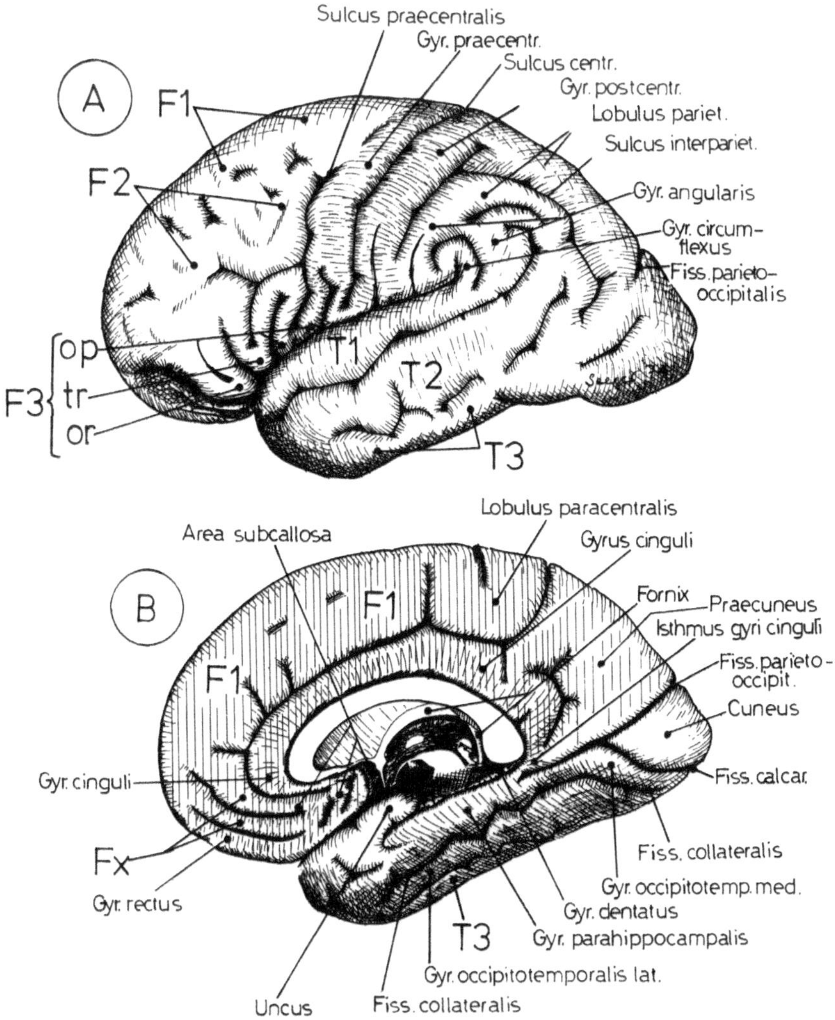
Sulcus praecentralis
Gyr. praecentr.
Sulcus centr.
Gyr. postcentr.
Lobulus pariet.
Sulcus interpariet.
Gyr. angularis
Gyr. circumflexus
Fiss. parieto-occipitalis
A
F1
F2
F3
op
tr
or
T1
T2
T3
Lobulus paracentralis
Area subcallosa
Gyrus cinguli
Fornix
Praecuneus
Isthmus gyri cinguli
Fiss. parieto-occipit.
Cuneus
Fiss. calcar.
Fiss. collateralis
Gyr. occipitotemp. med.
Gyr. dentatus
Gyr. parahippocampalis
Gyr. occipitotemporalis lat.
Fiss. collateralis
Uncus
T3
Gyr. rectus
Fx
Gyr. cinguli
B
F1
F1

Fig. 3. Outer and inner surfaces of infratentorial brain structures (according to Sobotta-Becher, 1973, modified)
A Cerebellar surface from above (adjacent to Tentorium)
B Median section
C Basal view of Cerebellum. Lower portion of Pons and Medulla oblongata resected, right tonsil removed. Flocculus stalk split at right at transition of white matter of tonsil. Cross-section through Velum medullare post.
D Dorsal view of caudal brainstem after removal of Cerebellum (left tonsil and parts of Uvula Nodulus complex left in situ).
Arrow: Velum medullare post. split open and Plexus chor. with remnants of split Pedunculus flocculi folded out

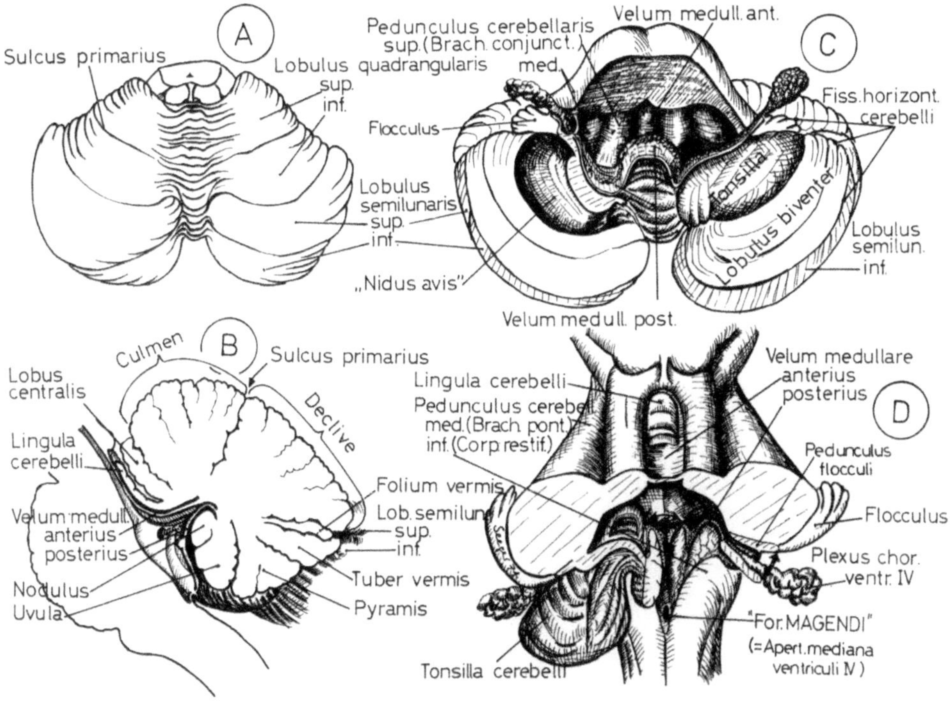
A
Sulcus primarius
Lobulus quadrangularis
sup.
inf.
Lobulus
semilunaris
sup.
inf.
„Nidus avis"
C
Pedunculus cerebellaris
sup. (Brach. conjunct.)
med.
Velum medull. ant.
Flocculus
Fiss. horizont.
cerebelli
Tonsilla
Lobulus biventer
Lobulus
semilun.
inf.
Velum medull. post.
B
Culmen
Sulcus primarius
Declive
Lobus
centralis
Lingula
cerebelli
Velum medull.
anterius
posterius
Nodulus
Uvula
Folium vermis
Lob. semilun.
sup.
inf.
Tuber vermis
Pyramis
D
Lingula cerebelli
Pedunculus cerebelli
med. (Brach. pont.)
inf. (Corp. restif.)
Velum medullare
anterius
posterius
Pedunculus
flocculi
Flocculus
Plexus chor.
ventr. IV
"For. MAGENDI"
(=Apert. mediana
ventriculi IV)
Tonsilla cerebelli

Fig. 4. Preparation of brain seen from lateral viewpoint. Midbrain section. The markedly protruding convex cerebellar surface (with the closely fitting tentorium) fits into the corresponding concavity of the undersurface of the occipital lobe. The generally accepted differentiation of the gyrus relief is almost impossible to recognize even after removal of the vessels: Differentiation of *F 1* to *F 3* almost impossible, Gyrus praecentralis split up into several areas, Gyrus supramarginalis and Gyrus angularis not concentric but ordered longitudinally. One typical example of the many possible variants of gyrus relief

 FIG. 4

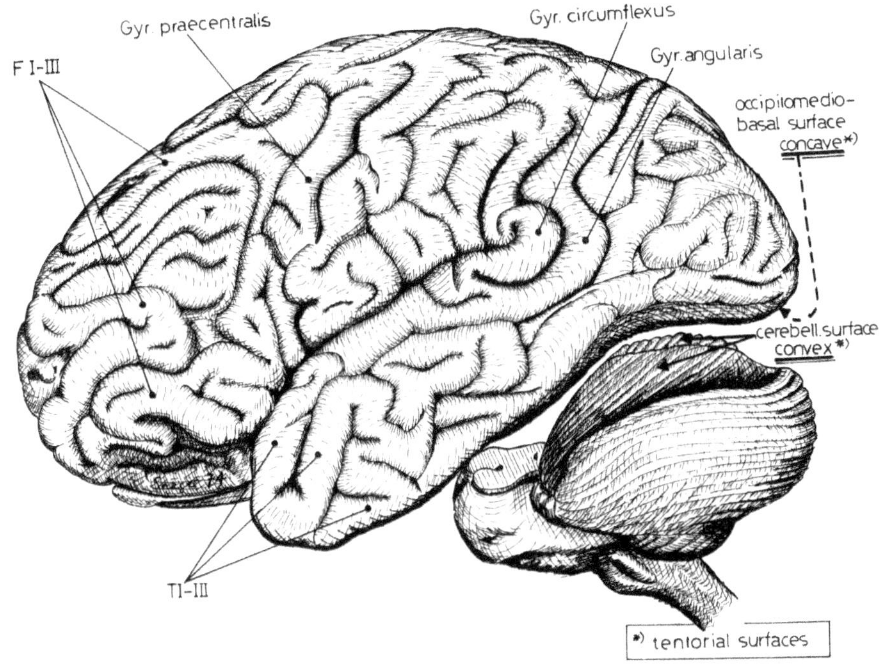
Gyr. praecentralis
Gyr. circumflexus
Gyr. angularis
F I-III
occipitomedio-
basal surface
concave*)
cerebell. surface
convex*)
TI-III
*) tentorial surfaces

Fig. 5. In contrast to angiogram, course of vessels on surface is difficult to identify. Vessels dip into sulci over long stretches of their course. Vessels of Sylvian fissure lie mainly in insularparietal region, not close to surface of temporal lobe. Typical kink in course of A. angularis at its exit from the posterior part of Fissura cerebri lat. (Sylvii) – 'angularis point of A. angularis'

Fig. 6. Slightly schematic representation of terminal arborization of carotid. Angled exit of arteries passing to Substantia perforata ant.

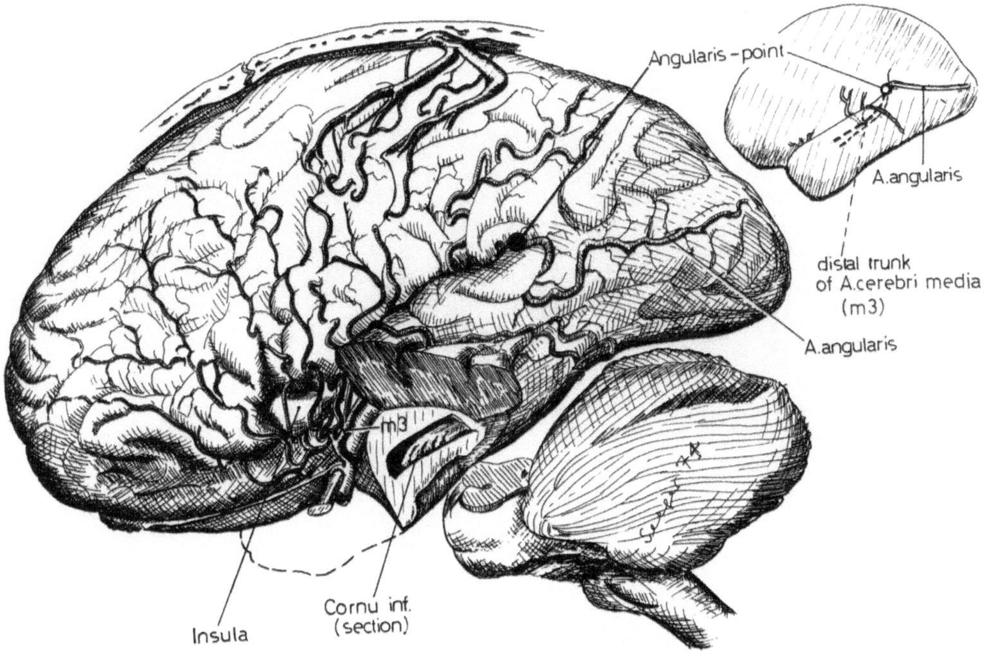
Angularis-point
A.angularis
distal trunk
of A.cerebri media
(m3)
A.angularis
m3
Insula
Cornu inf.
(section)

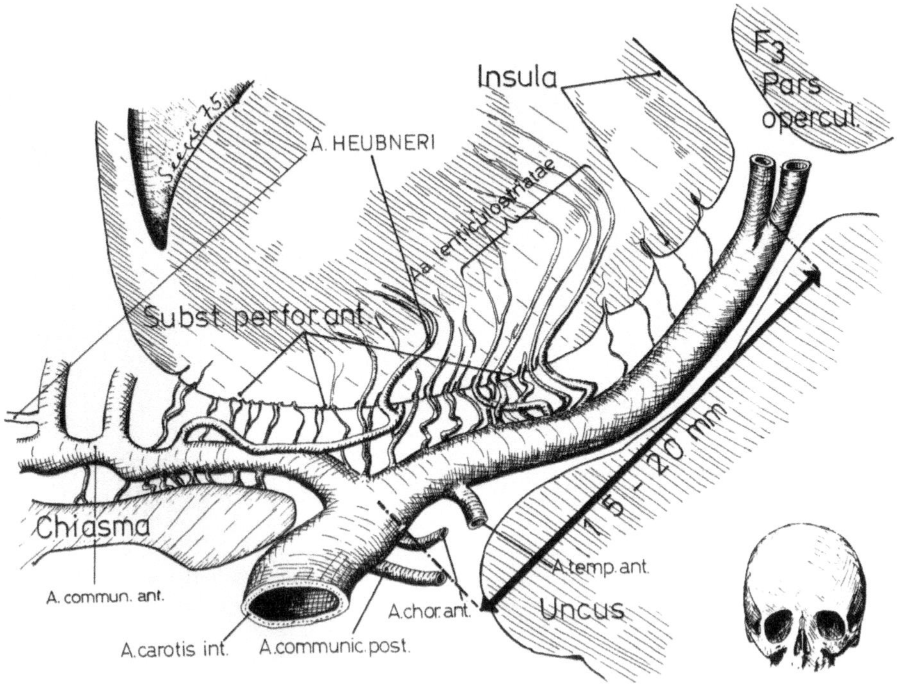
F3
Pars
opercul.
Insula
A. HEUBNERI
Aa. lenticulostriatae
Subst. perfor.ant.
15 - 20 mm
Chiasma
A.temp.ant.
A. commun. ant.
A.chor.ant.
Uncus
A.carotis int.
A.communic.post.

Fig. 7. Terminal arborization of carotid and ramification of proximal trunk of A. cerebri media on Insula. Distal branches of A. operculo-frontalis do not return to lower border of opercular gyri, but pass through the sulci to the convexity

FIG. 7

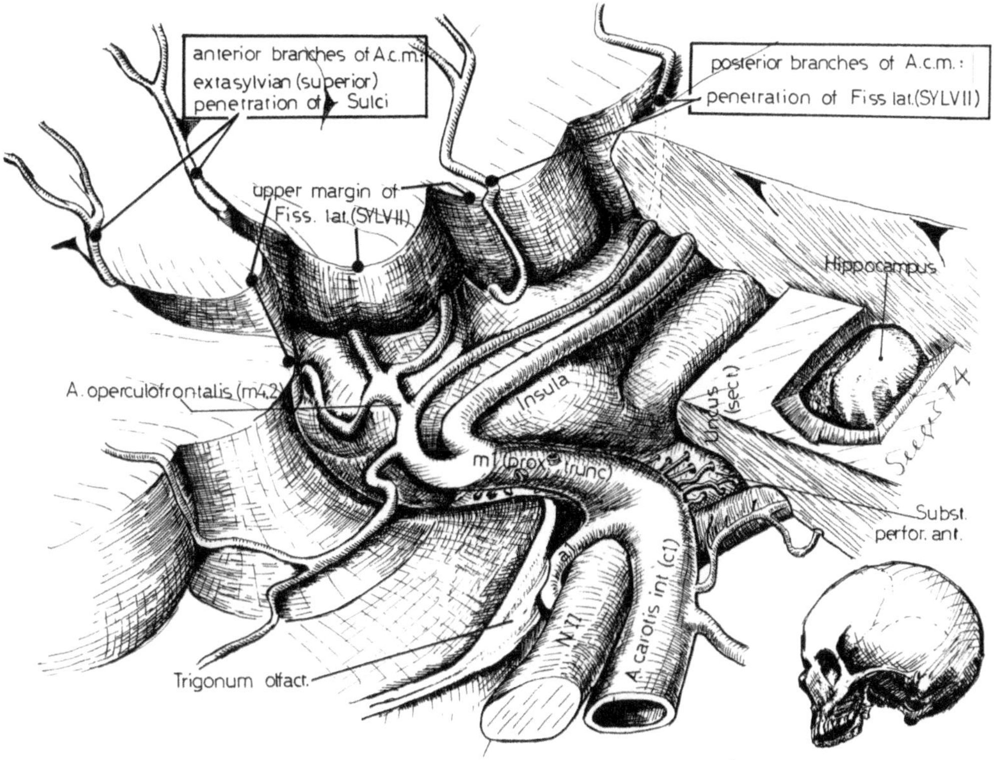
anterior branches of A.c.m.:
extasylvian (superior)
penetration of Sulci
posterior branches of A.c.m.:
penetration of Fiss lat.(SYLVII)
upper margin of
Fiss. lat.(SYLVII)
Hippocampus
A. operculofrontalis (m4.2)
Insula
Uncus (sect.)
m1 (prox. trunc)
Subst.
perfor. ant.
A. carotis int. (c1)
N. II
Trigonum olfact.

Fig. 8. Schematic representation of ramifications of A. cerebri media

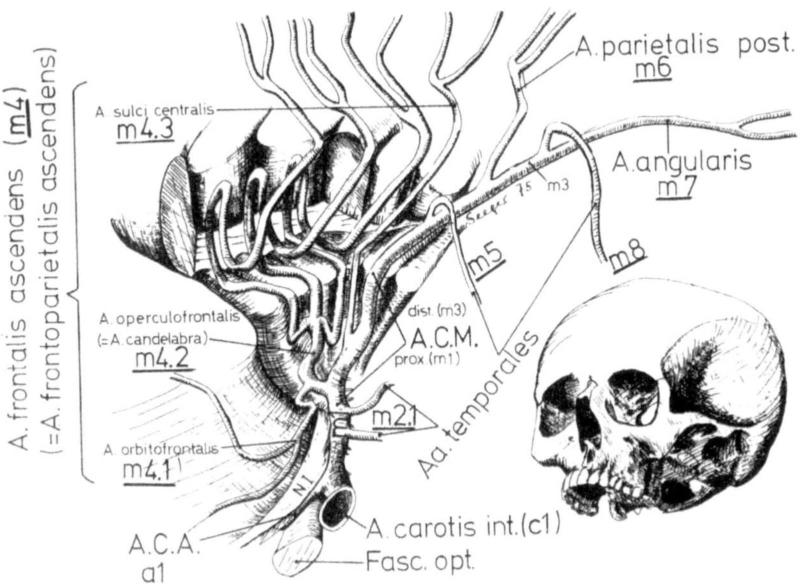
A. frontalis ascendens (m4)
(=A. frontoparietalis ascendens)
A. sulci centralis
m4.3
A. operculofrontalis
(=A. candelabra)
m4.2
A. orbitofrontalis
m4.1
A.C.A.
a1
A. parietalis post.
m6
A. angularis
m7
m3
m8
m5
dist. (m3)
A.C.M.
prox. (m1)
m2.1
Aa. temporales
A. carotis int. (c1)
Fasc. opt.

Fig. 9. Preparation showing medial surface of left hemisphere. Leptomeninges and vessels removed

Fig. 10. Preparation of Fig. 9 with leptomeninges and vessels

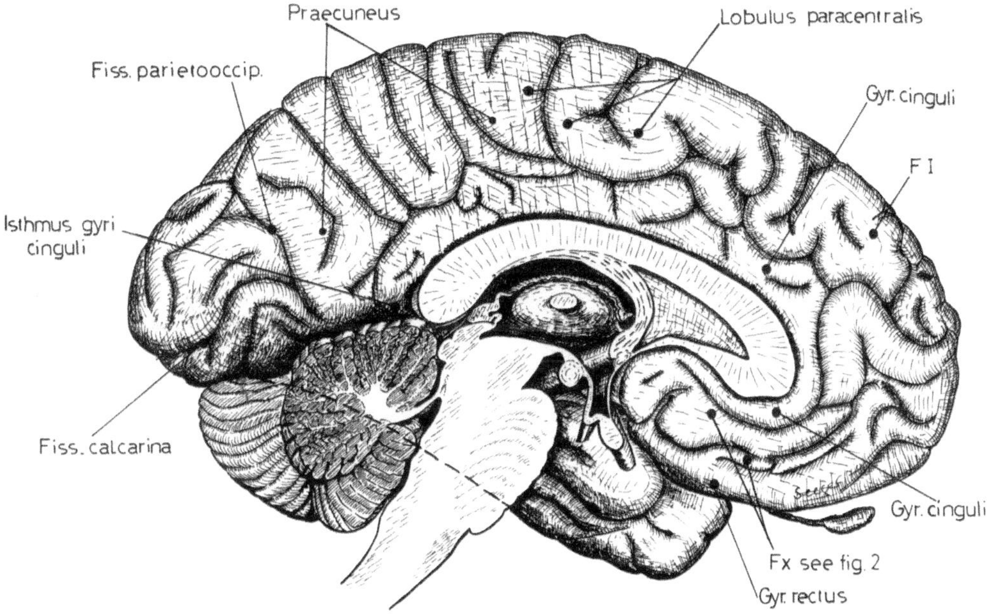
Praecuneus
Lobulus paracentralis
Fiss. parietooccip.
Gyr. cinguli
F I
Isthmus gyri cinguli
Fiss. calcarina
Gyr. cinguli
Fx see fig. 2
Gyr. rectus

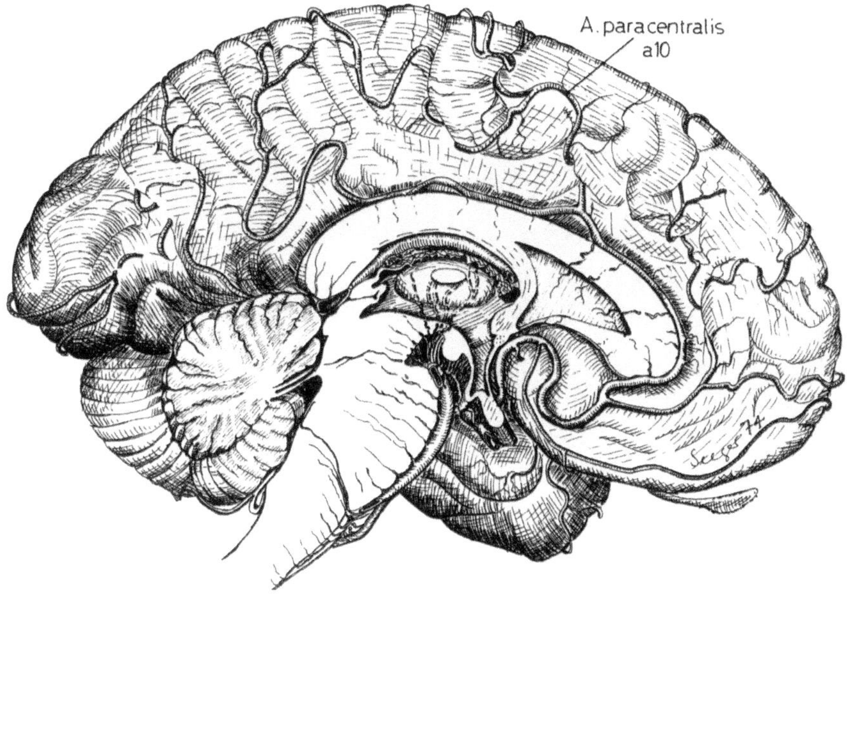
A. paracentralis
a10

Fig. 11. Nomenclature of vessels for preparation of Fig. 10

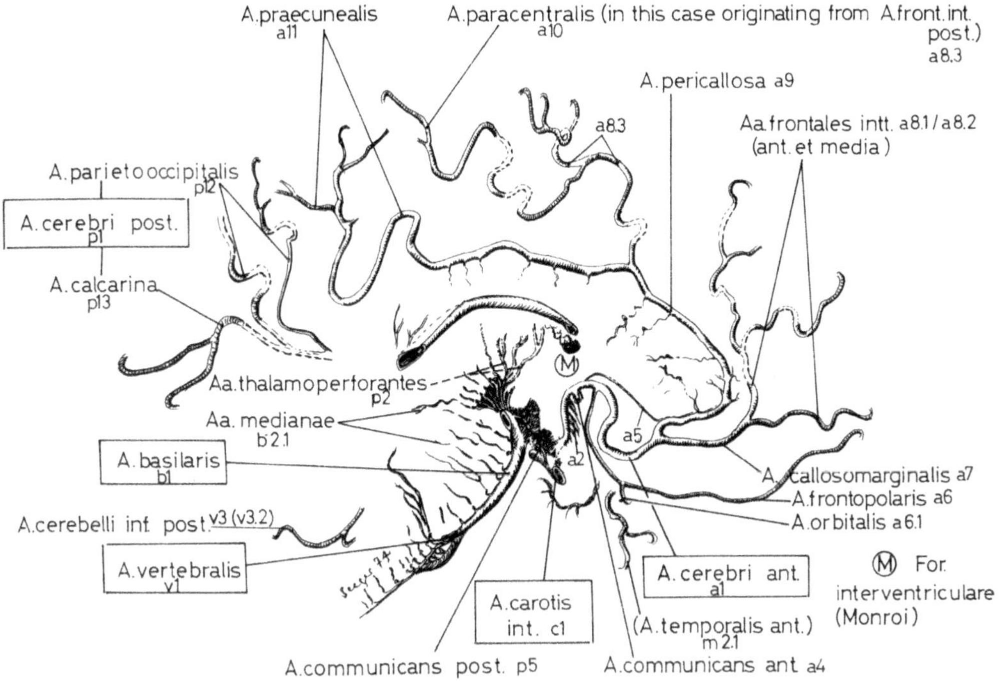
A.praecunealis a11
A.paracentralis (in this case originating from A.front.int. post.) a10 a8.3
A.pericallosa a9
a8.3
Aa.frontales intt. a8.1 / a8.2 (ant. et media)
A.parietooccipitalis p12
A.cerebri post. p1
A.calcarina p13
Aa.thalamoperforantes p2
Aa. medianae b2.1
A. basilaris b1
A.cerebelli inf. post. v3 (v3.2)
A. vertebralis v1
a5
a2
A. callosomarginalis a7
A.frontopolaris a6
A.orbitalis a6.1
A. cerebri ant. a1
M For. interventriculare (Monroi)
A.carotis int. c1
(A.temporalis ant.) m 2.1
A.communicans post. p5
A.communicans ant. a4

Fig. 12. Schematic simplification of branches of A. cerebri ant.
× A. corporis callosi mediana *(a 5)*

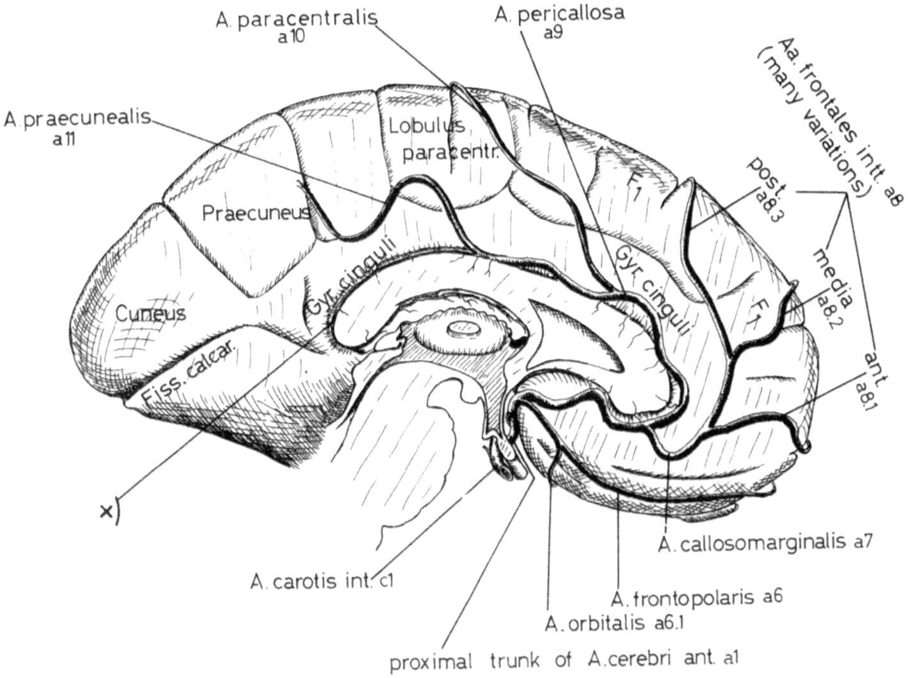
A. paracentralis
a 10
A. pericallosa
a9
Aa. frontales intt. a8
(many variations)
A. praecunealis
a 11
Lobulus
paracentr.
post.
a8.3
F1
Praecuneus
Gyr. cinguli
Gyr. cinguli
media
a8.2
Cuneus
F1
Fiss. calcar.
ant.
a8.1
x)
A. callosomarginalis a7
A. carotis int. c1
A. frontopolaris a6
A. orbitalis a6.1
proximal trunk of A. cerebri ant. a1

Fig. 13. Oblique view of left cerebral hemisphere form basomedial direction. Crus cerebri *(cc)* and Tegmentum mesencephali *(ms)* cut transversely. Tegmentum mesencephali also cut longitudinally *(ms')*. Frequent variant: Isthmus gyri cinguli interrupted by Fissura calcarina. Direct transition of Fissura collateralis into Fissura calcarina and Fissura parieto-occipitalis

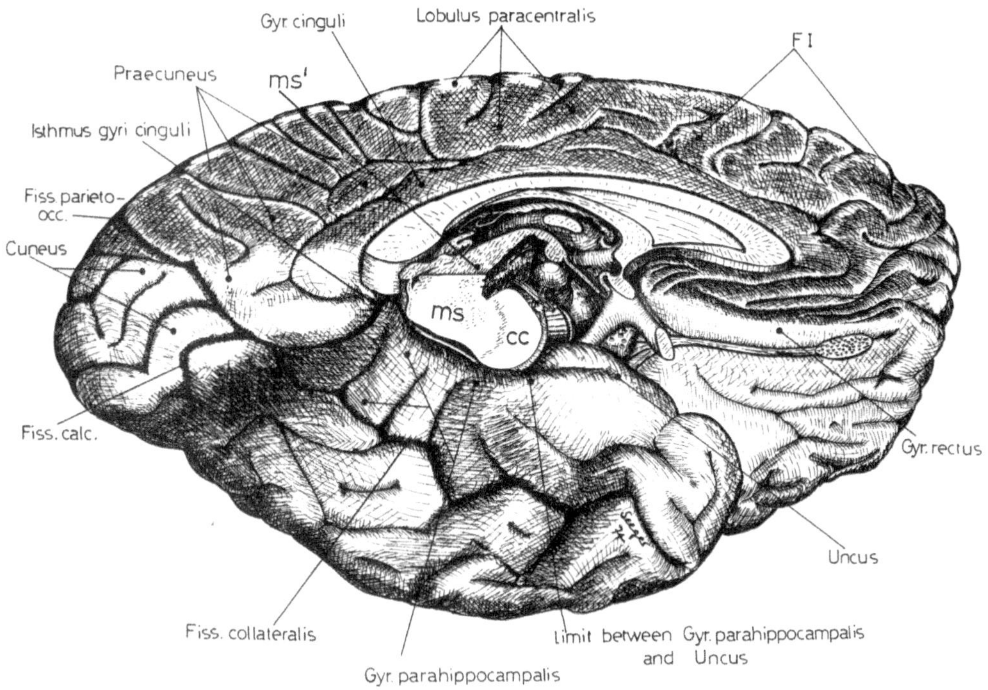
Gyr. cinguli
Lobulus paracentralis
F I
Praecuneus
ms'
Isthmus gyri cinguli
Fiss. parieto-occ.
Cuneus
ms
cc
Fiss. calc.
Gyr. rectus
Uncus
Fiss. collateralis
Limit between Gyr. parahippocampalis and Uncus
Gyr. parahippocampalis

Fig. 14. Enlarged section from Fig. 13 with vessels drawn in

FIG. 14

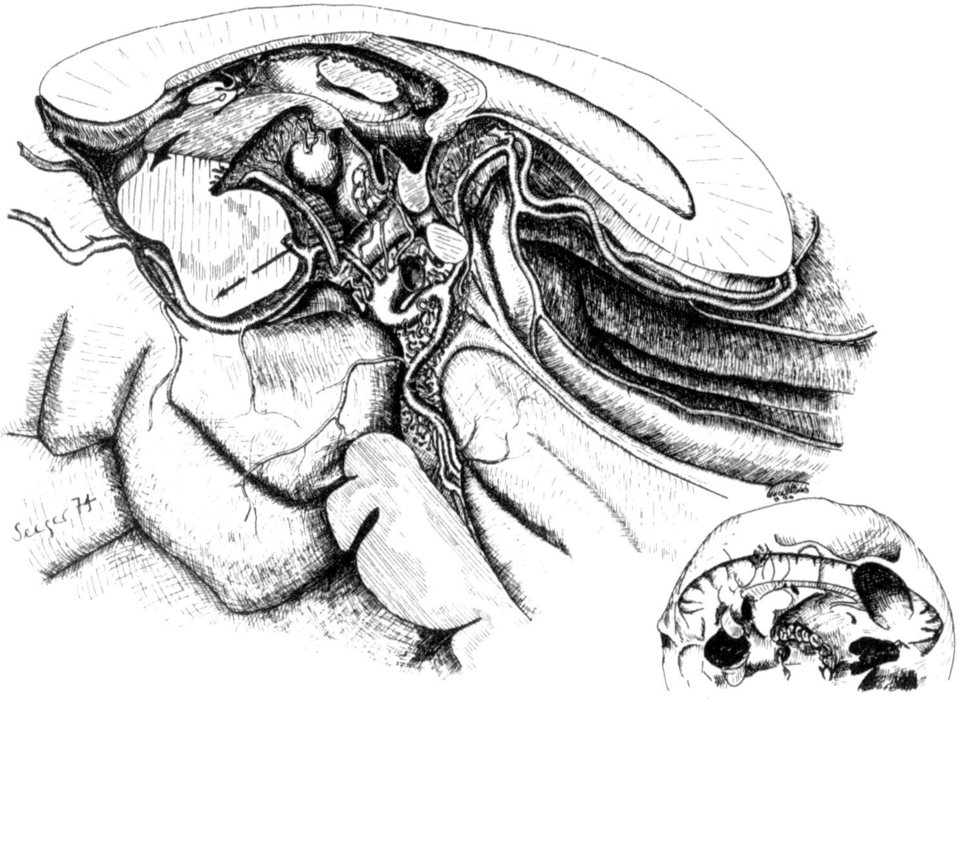

Fig. 15. Nomenclature of vessels in Fig. 14

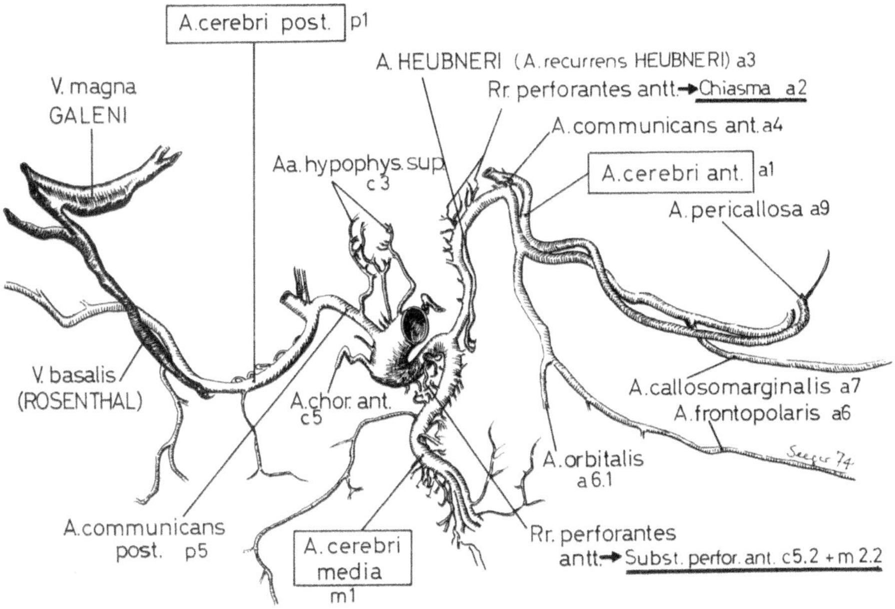
A.cerebri post. p1
A. HEUBNERI (A.recurrens HEUBNERI) a3
Rr. perforantes antt.→Chiasma a2
V. magna GALENI
A.communicans ant. a4
Aa. hypophys. sup. c3
A.cerebri ant. a1
A. pericallosa a9
V. basalis (ROSENTHAL)
A.chor. ant. c5
A.callosomarginalis a7
A.frontopolaris a6
A.orbitalis a6.1
A.communicans post. p5
A. cerebri media m1
Rr. perforantes antt.→Subst. perfor. ant. c5.2 + m 2.2
Seeger 74

Fig. 16. Basal view of left half of the whole brain

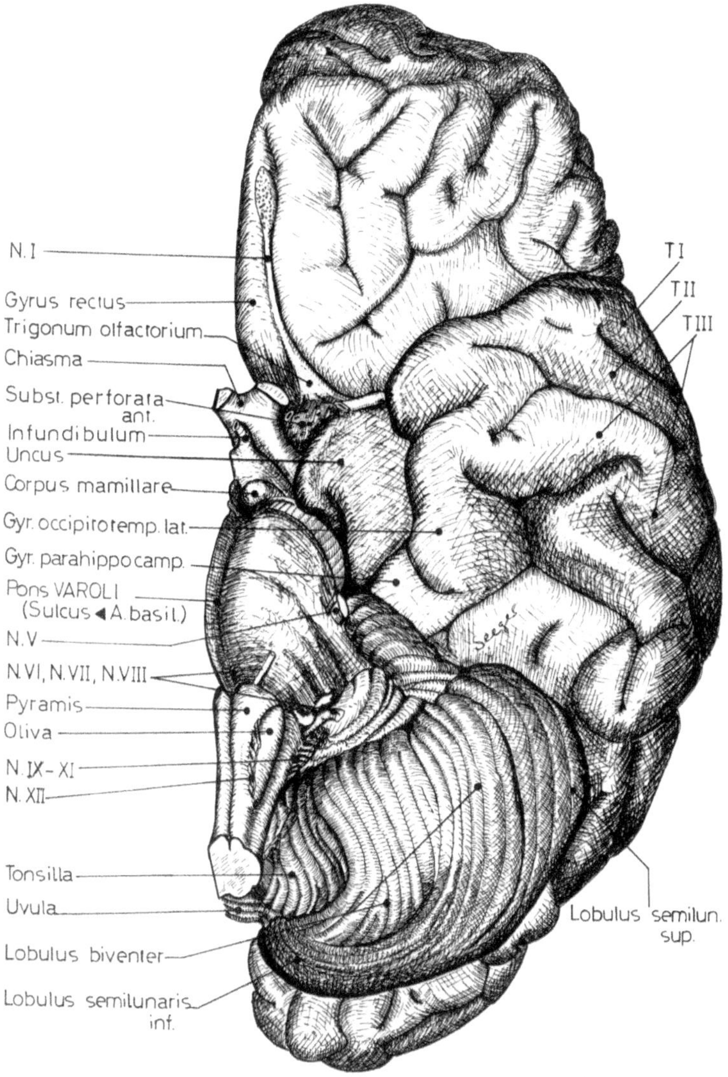
N. I
Gyrus rectus
Trigonum olfactorium
Chiasma
Subst. perforata ant.
Infundibulum
Uncus
Corpus mamillare
Gyr. occipitotemp. lat.
Gyr. parahippocamp.
Pons VAROLI (Sulcus ◄ A. basil.)
N. V
N. VI, N. VII, N. VIII
Pyramis
Oliva
N. IX – XI
N. XII
Tonsilla
Uvula
Lobulus biventer
Lobulus semilunaris inf.
T I
T II
T III
Lobulus semilun. sup.

Figs. 17 and 18. The same preparation after removal of temporal lobe. Parietal gyri take a transverse course in columnar formation in vicinity of opened Fissura lat. (Sylvii) Ⓗ Heschl's gyrus (gyri)

Fig. 17

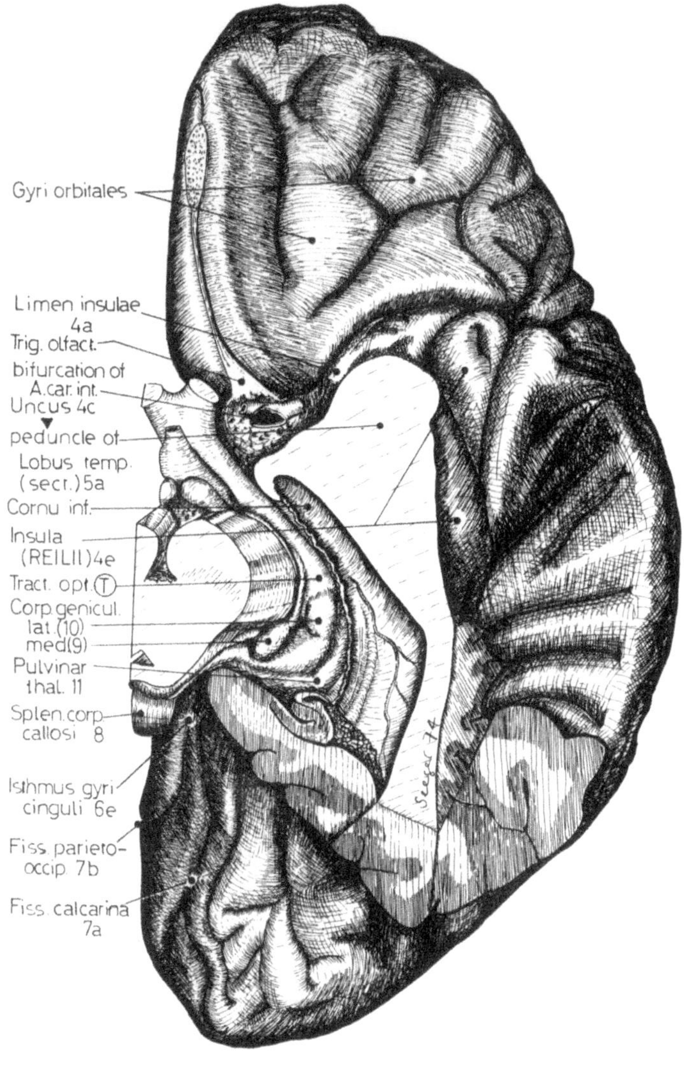
Gyri orbitales
Limen insulae 4a
Trig. olfact.
bifurcation of A.car. int.
Uncus 4c
peduncle of Lobus temp. (secr.) 5a
Cornu inf.
Insula (REILII) 4e
Tract. opt. (T)
Corp. genicul. lat. (10) med (9)
Pulvinar thal. 11
Splen. corp. callosi 8
Isthmus gyri cinguli 6e
Fiss. parieto-occip. 7b
Fiss. calcarina 7a
Seeger 74

FIG. 18

Fig. 18

FIG. 18

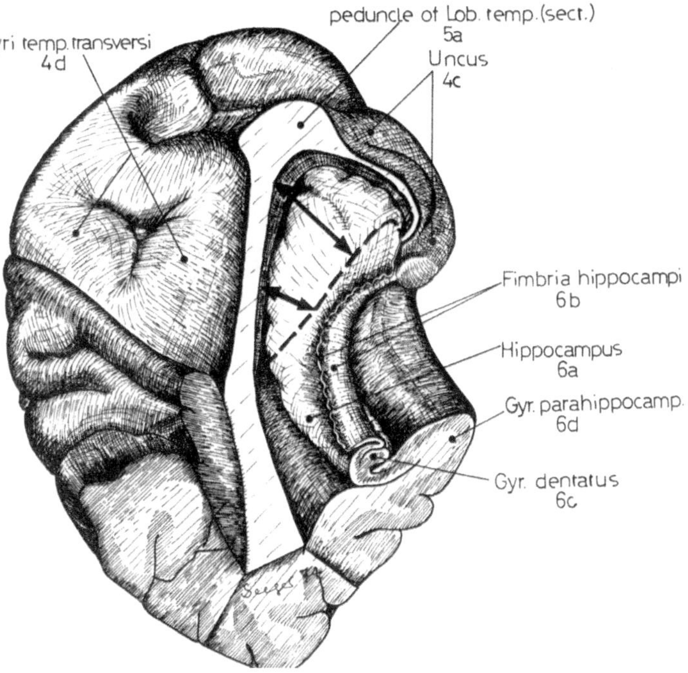
peduncle of Lob. temp. (sect.)
5a
Gyri temp. transversi
4d
Uncus
4c
Fimbria hippocampi
6b
Hippocampus
6a
Gyr. parahippocamp.
6d
Gyr. dentatus
6c

Fig. 19. Designation of structures in Figs. 17, 18, 22 and 24

1	Pars orbitalis	gyri frontalis III
2	Pars triangularis	
3	Pars opercularis	
4 a	Limit of Insula ("Limen insulae")	
4 b	Posterior border of Insula	
4 c	Anterior portion of Uncus for reception of Insula	
4 d	Middle temporal lobe region with transverse gyri	
4 e	Insula	
5 a	Connection of temporal lobe to Putamen region. Anteriorly: Uncus/Amygdala region. Neighbourhood: Tractus opticus *T*, Substantia perforata ant. *(5 b)* et Cornu inf.	
5 b	Substantia perforata ant.	
5 c	Substantia perforata post.	
5 d	Ansa peduncularis	
6 a	Hippocampus	parts of allocortex
6 b	Crus fornicis with insertion of Plexus chor. ("Fimbria fornicis")	
6 c	Gyrus dentatus	
6 d	Gyrus parahippocampalis	
6 e	Isthmus gyri cinguli	
7 a	Fissura collateralis	
7 b	Fissura calcarina	
7 b'	Calcar avis	
8	Splenium corporis callosi	
9	Brachium quadrigeminum inferius et Corpus geniculatum mediale	
10	Brachium quadrigeminum superius et Corpus geniculatum laterale	
11	Pulvinar thalami	
12 a	Stria medullaris in roof of Cornu inf.	
12 b	Taenia chorioidea	
13	Cauda nuclei caudati	
14	Colliculus sup. et inf.	
×	Section of roof of Cornu inf.	

Arrows in Fig. 18: During preparation a thin ependymal lamella was removed from the roof of Cornu inf.

Fig. 20. Preparation of Fig. 17 with vessels sketched in

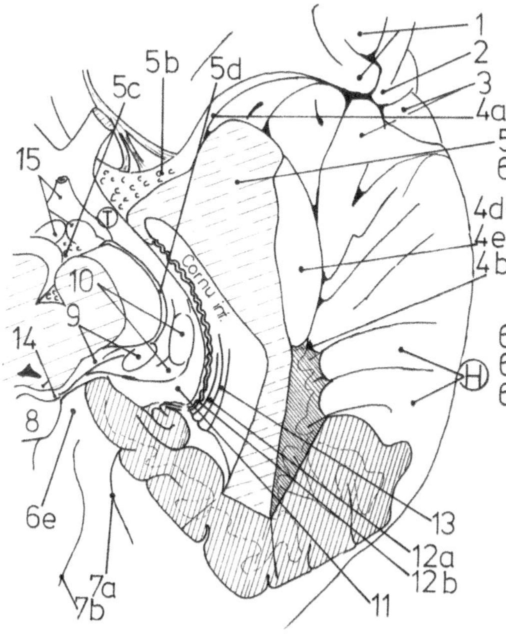
1
2
3
4a
5a
5b
5c
5d
15
T
Cornu inf.
4e
4b
10
9
14
H
8
6e
7a
7b
13
12a
12b
11

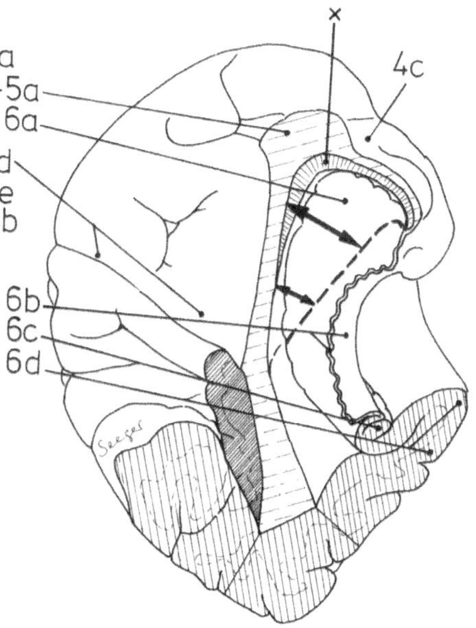
×
4c
5a
6a
4d
6b
6c
6d

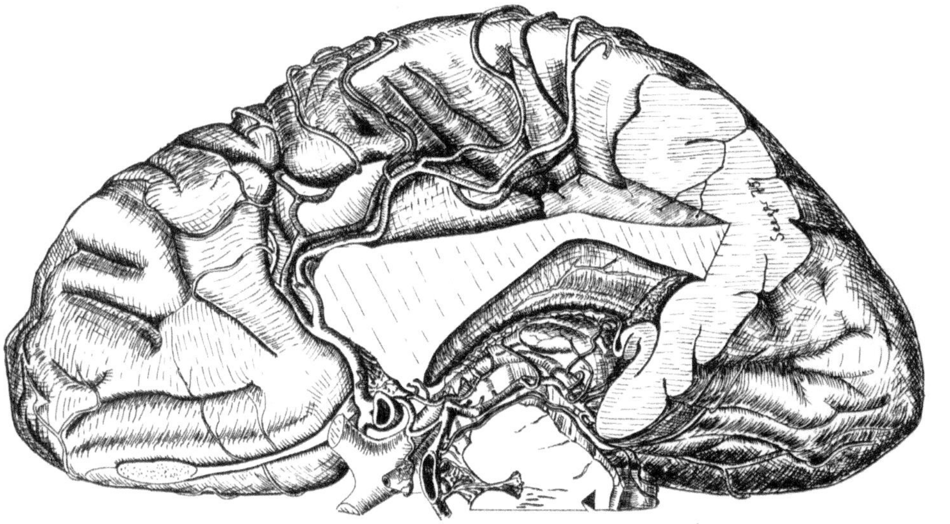

Fig. 21. Nomenclature of vessels in Fig. 20 (for abbreviations see catalogue of arteries and previous illustrations)

FIG. 21

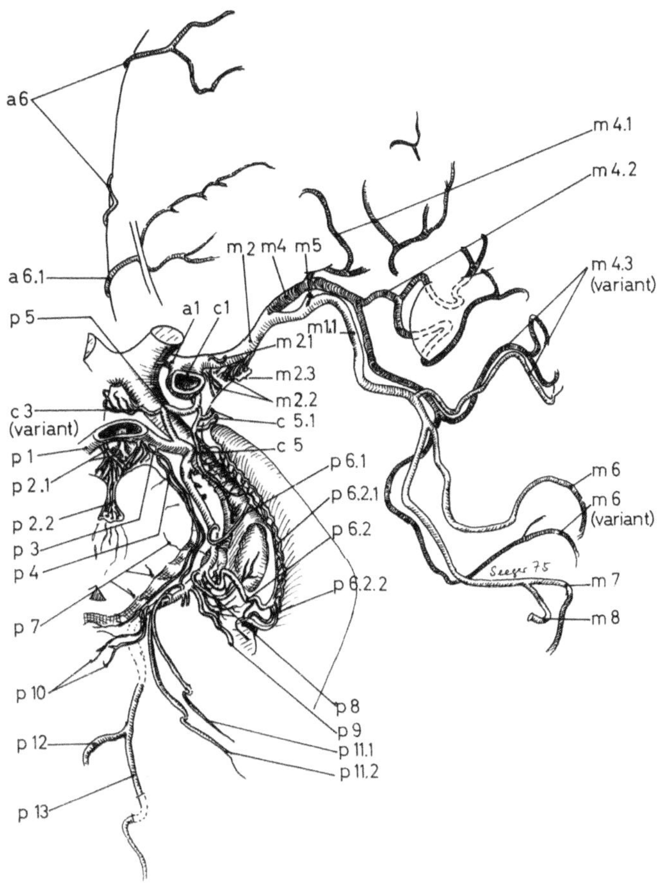

a6
m 4.1
m 4.2
m 2
m4
m5
m 4.3
(variant)
a 6.1
p 5
a1
c1
m1.1
m 2.1
m 2.3
m 2.2
c 3
(variant)
c 5.1
c 5
p 1
p 2.1
p 2.2
p 3
p 4
p 6.1
p 6.2.1
p 6.2
p 6.2.2
m 6
m 6
(variant)
m 7
m 8
p 7
p 10
p 12
p 13
p 8
p 9
p 11.1
p 11.2

Fig. 22. Enlarged section of a similar preparation to Fig. 20, contralaterally. Relationships of A. calcarina *(p 13)* in Fissura calcarina *(7 b)* to Cornu post. with Calcar avis. For designations of brain structures see Fig. 19; (for vessels structures see Fig. 21 and catalogue of arteries, pages 3–4)

FIG. 22

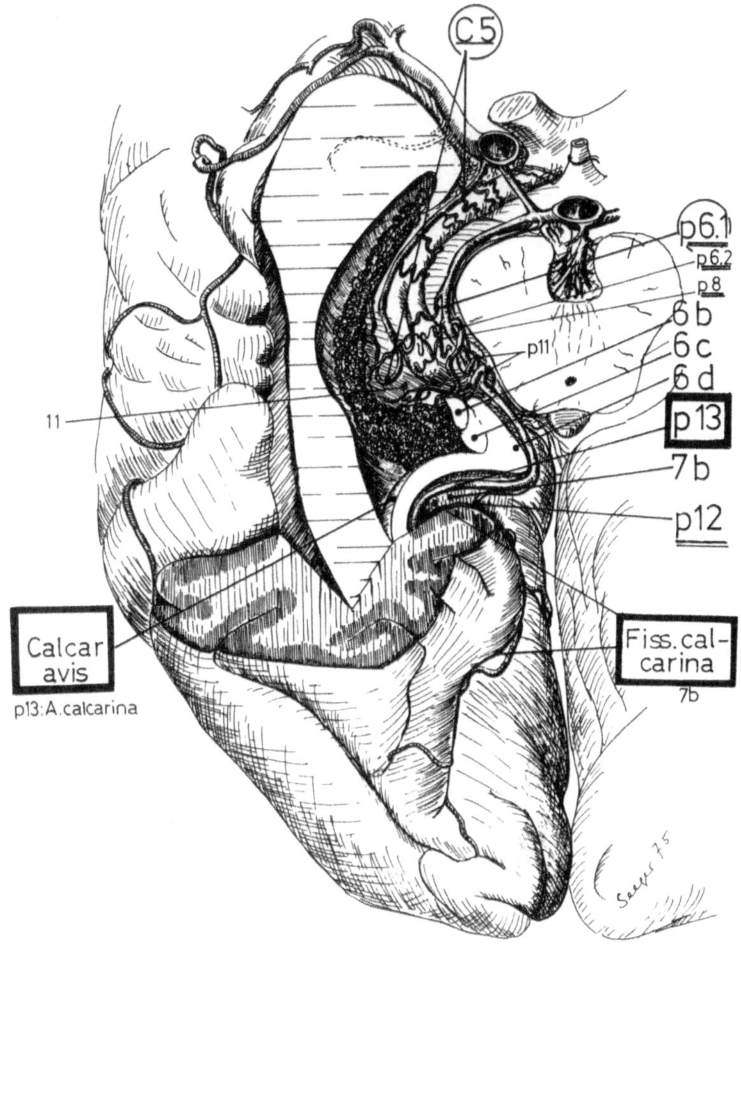

p13: A. calcarina

Fig. 23. General view of a preparation after removal of temporo-occipital region. Posterolateral view. Parieto-occipital region raised, Chiasma stretched, Medulla oblongata slightly contorted (see arrow). Lateral ventricle opened wide and Corpus callosum lifted off quadrigeminal region

Fig. 24. Designation of structures in Fig. 23

1–14 see Fig. 19

15 Tuber cinereum et Corpus mamillare

16 Gyrus cinguli

17 a Commissura fornicis

17 b Crus fornicis (section)

17 c Fissura chorioidea (after removal of Plexus chorioideus)

18 Cut surface of temporal lobe

19 Bridging gyrus with interruption of Fissura lat. (Sylvii) merging of parietal and temporal lobes in vicinity of Heschl's transverse gyrus (section)

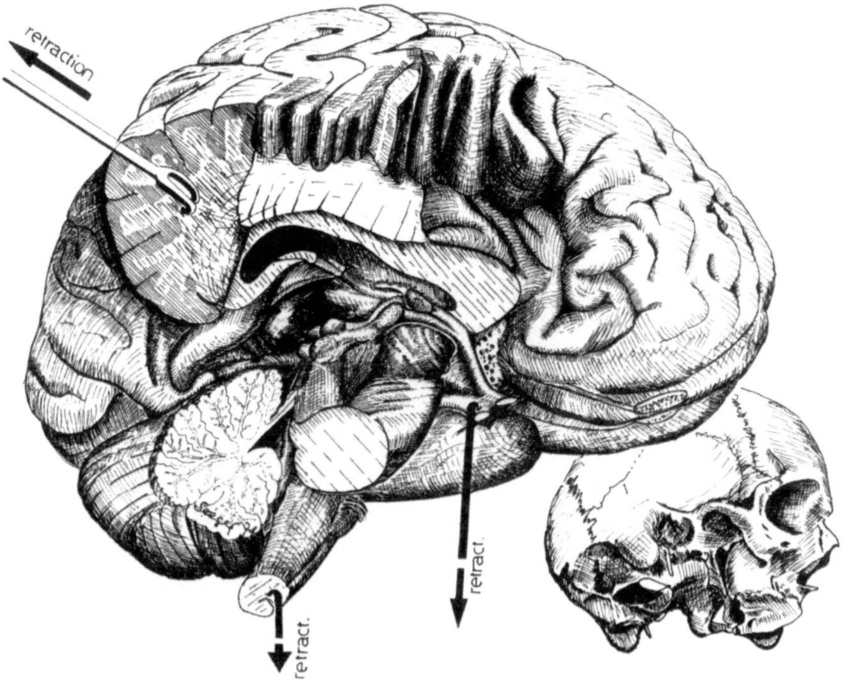
retraction
retract.
retract.

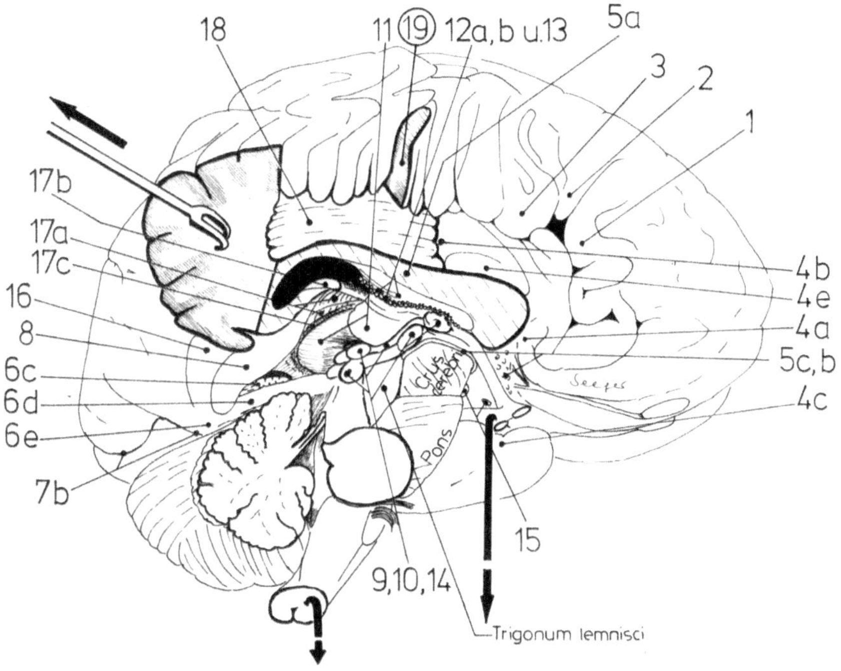
18
11
19
12a, b u.13
5a
3
2
1
17b
17a
17c
16
8
6c
6d
6e
7b
4b
4e
4a
5c, b
4c
Crus cerebri
Pons
15
9,10,14
Trigonum lemnisci

Fig. 25. Preparation of Fig. 23 with vessels sketched in

FIG. 25

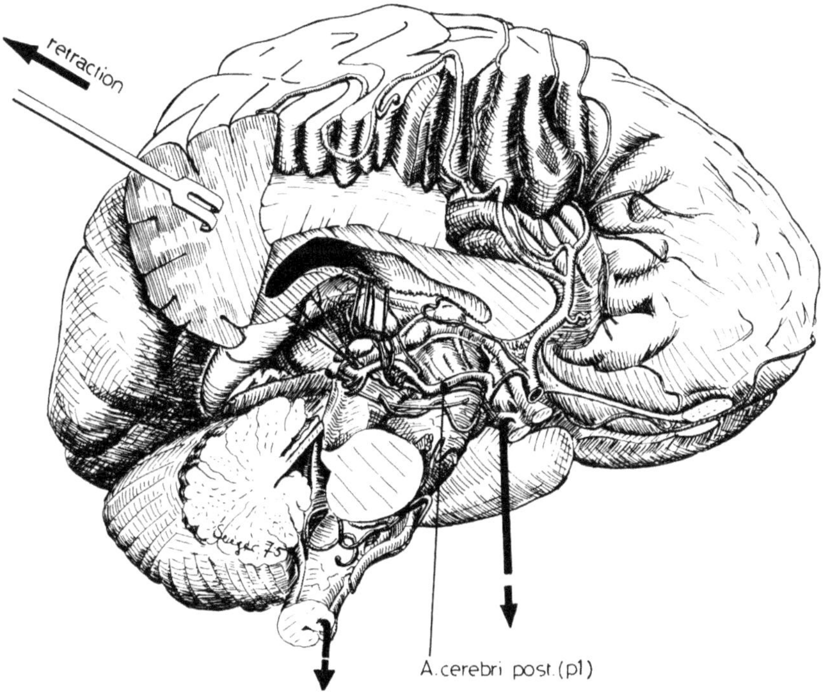

Fig. 26. Posterior choroidal group

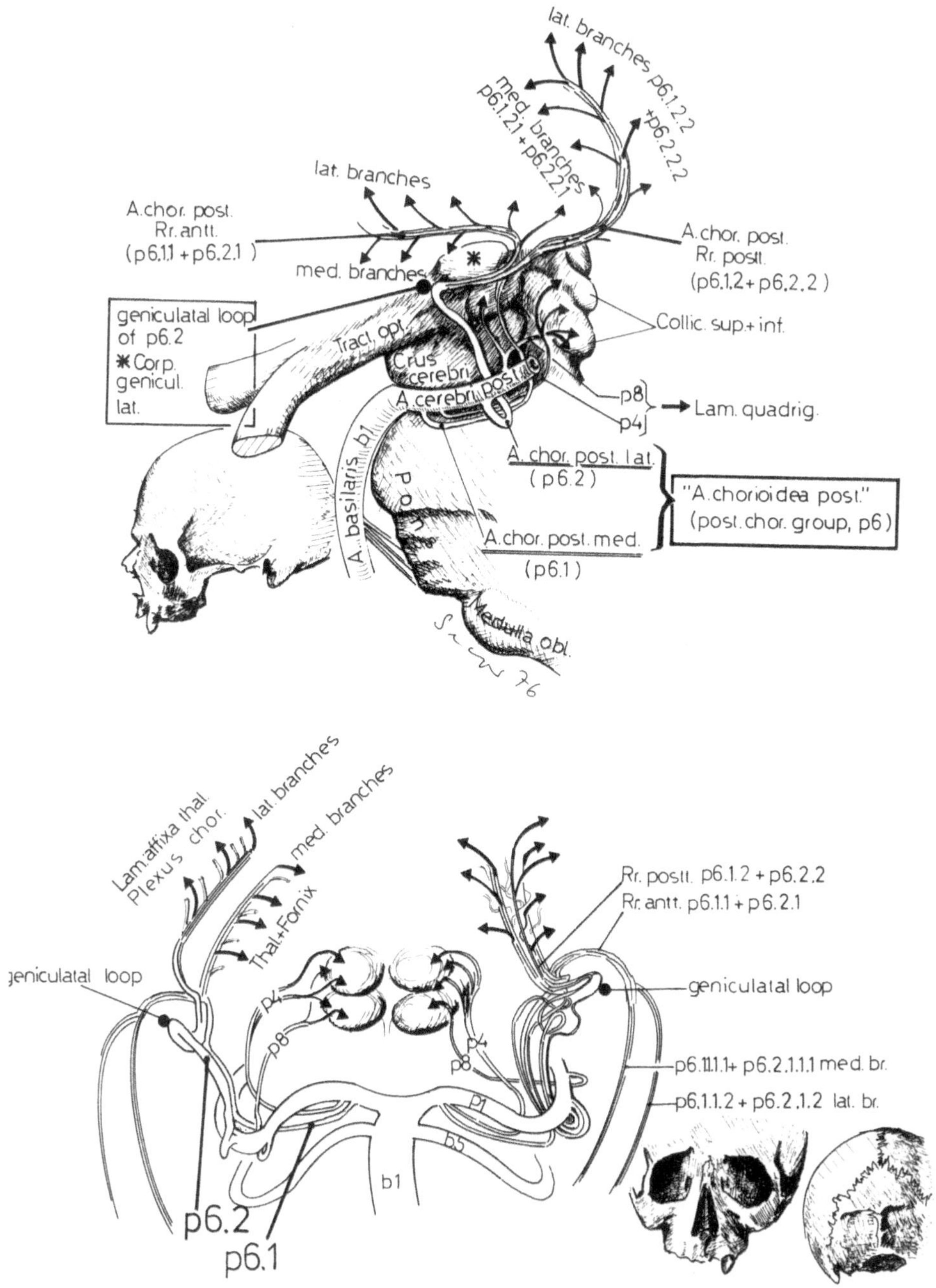
lat. branches p6.1.2.2 +p6.2.2.2
med. branches p6.1.2.1 + p6.2.2.1
lat. branches
A.chor. post. Rr. antt. (p6.1.1 + p6.2.1)
med. branches
A.chor. post. Rr. postt. (p6.1.2+ p6.2.2)
geniculatal loop of p6.2
✱Corp. genicul. lat.
Tract. opt.
Crus cerebri
Collic. sup.+ inf.
A.cerebri post.
p8
p4
Lam. quadrig.
A. basilaris b1
Pons
A. chor. post. lat. (p6.2)
"A.chorioidea post." (post. chor. group, p6)
A.chor. post. med. (p6.1)
Medulla obl.
Lam. affixa thal.
Plexus chor.
lat. branches
med. branches
Thal.+Fornix
geniculatal loop
p4
p8
Rr. postt. p6.1.2 + p6.2.2
Rr. antt. p6.1.1 + p6.2.1
geniculatal loop
p6.1.1.1+ p6.2.1.1.1 med. br.
p6.1.1.2 + p6.2.1.2 lat. br.
p1
b5
b1
p6.2
p6.1

Fig. 27. Schematic representation of vertebralis-basilaris system. For designation of vessels see catalogue of arteries, pages 3–4

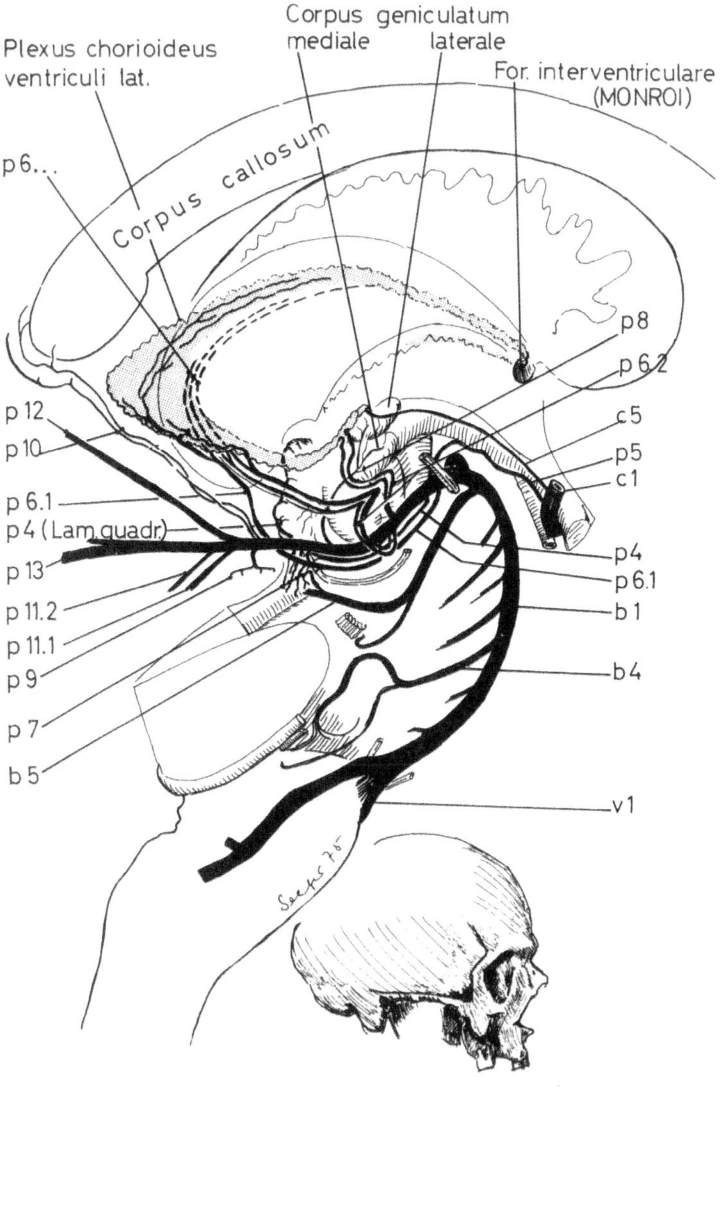
Corpus geniculatum
mediale
laterale
Plexus chorioideus
ventriculi lat.
For. interventriculare
(MONROI)
Corpus callosum
p6...
p8
p6.2
c5
p5
c1
p12
p10
p6.1
p4 (Lam.quadr.)
p13
p11.2
p11.1
p9
p7
b5
p4
p6.1
b1
b4
v1

Fig. 28. Preparation of brainstem from anterolateral view with vessels sketched in

FIG. 28

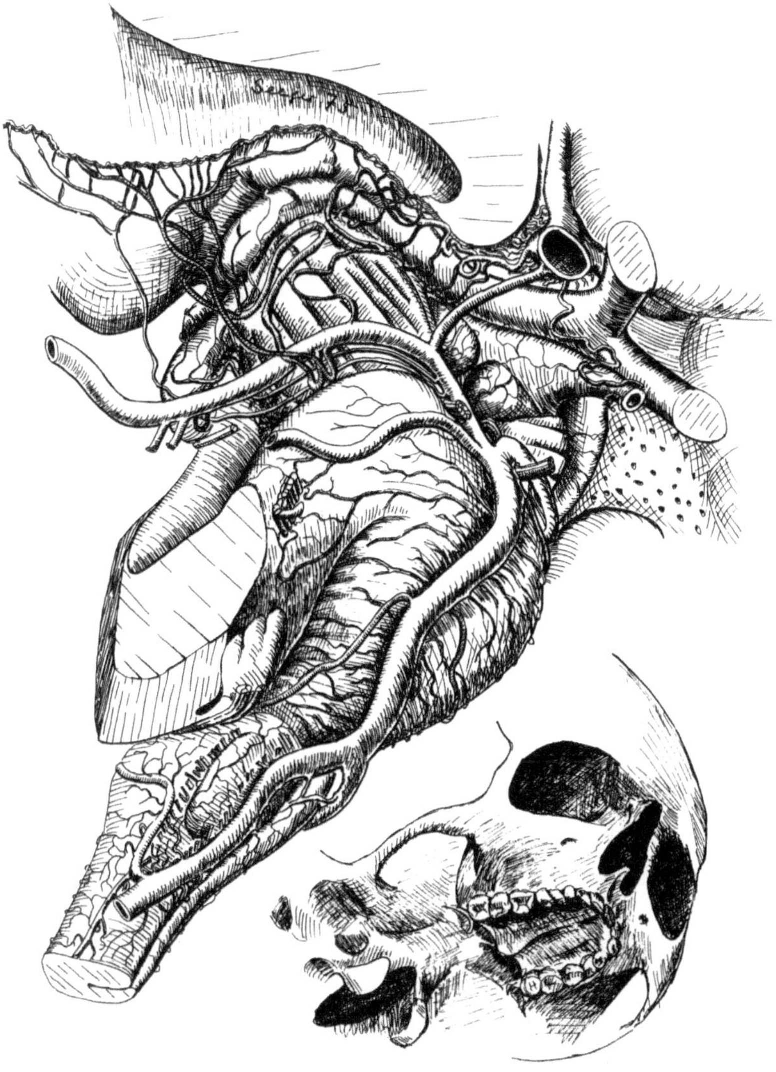

Fig. 29. Designation of vessels in Fig. 28. For explanation of abbreviations see catalogue of arteries, pages 3–4

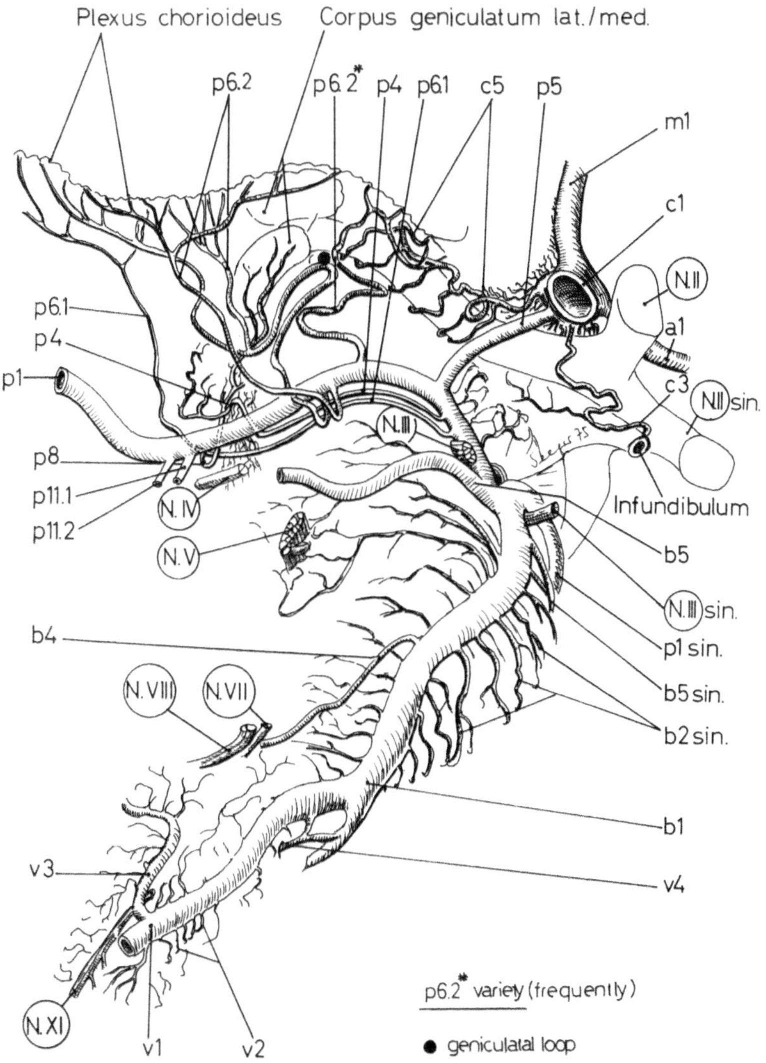
Plexus chorioideus
Corpus geniculatum lat./med.
p6.2
p6.2*
p4
p6.1
c5
p5
m1
c1
N.II
a1
c3
N.II sin.
Infundibulum
p6.1
p4
p1
p8
p11.1
p11.2
N.III
N.IV
N.V
b5
N.III sin.
p1 sin.
b5 sin.
b2 sin.
b4
N.VIII
N.VII
b1
v3
v4
N.XI
v1
v2
p6.2* variety (frequently)
geniculatal loop

Fig. 30. Resection of right occipitotemporal region. Brainstem retracted in caudal direction, left occipital pole retracted laterally (arrows)

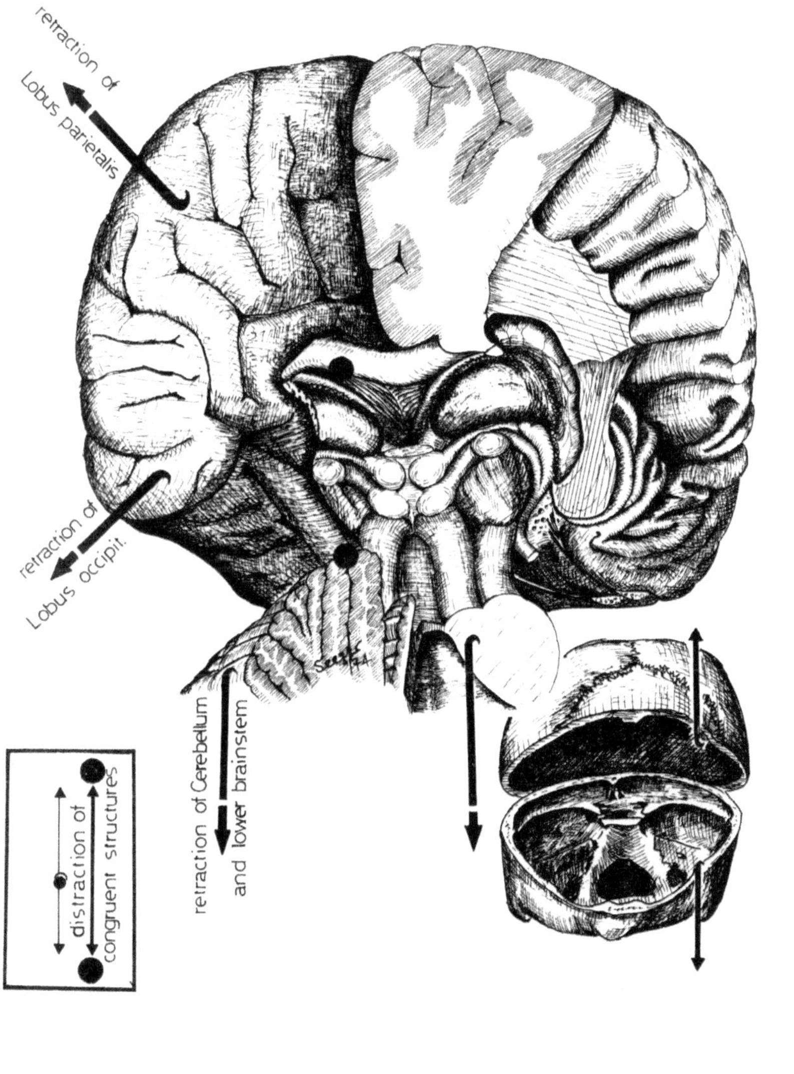
retraction of Lobus parietalis
retraction of Lobus occipit.
retraction of Cerebellum and lower brainstem
distraction of congruent structures

Fig. 31. Designation of structures in Fig. 30. For explanation see Figs. 17 and 18

1	Pars orbitalis	gyri front. III
2	Pars triangularis	
3	Pars opercularis	

4 a Limen insulae
4 b Posterior border of Insula
4 e Insula
5 a Uncus (section)
5 b Substantia perforata ant.
6 b Crus fornicis
6 c Gyrus dentatus
6 d Gyrus parahippocampalis
6 e Isthmus gyri cinguli
7 a Fissura collateralis
7 b Fissura calcarina
8 Splenium corporis callosi
9 Brachium quadrigeminum inf. et Corpus geniculatum med.
10 Brachium quadrigeminum sup. et Corpus geniculatum lat.
11 Pulvinar thalami
12 a Taenia chorioidea
12 b Stria medullaris
13 Cauda nuclei caudati
14 Colliculus sup. et inf.
17 a Commissura fornicis
17 b Crus fornicis (section)
17 e Taenia fornicis – cf. also Figs. 17–19, 23, and 24
18 Cut surface of temporal lobe

FIG. 31

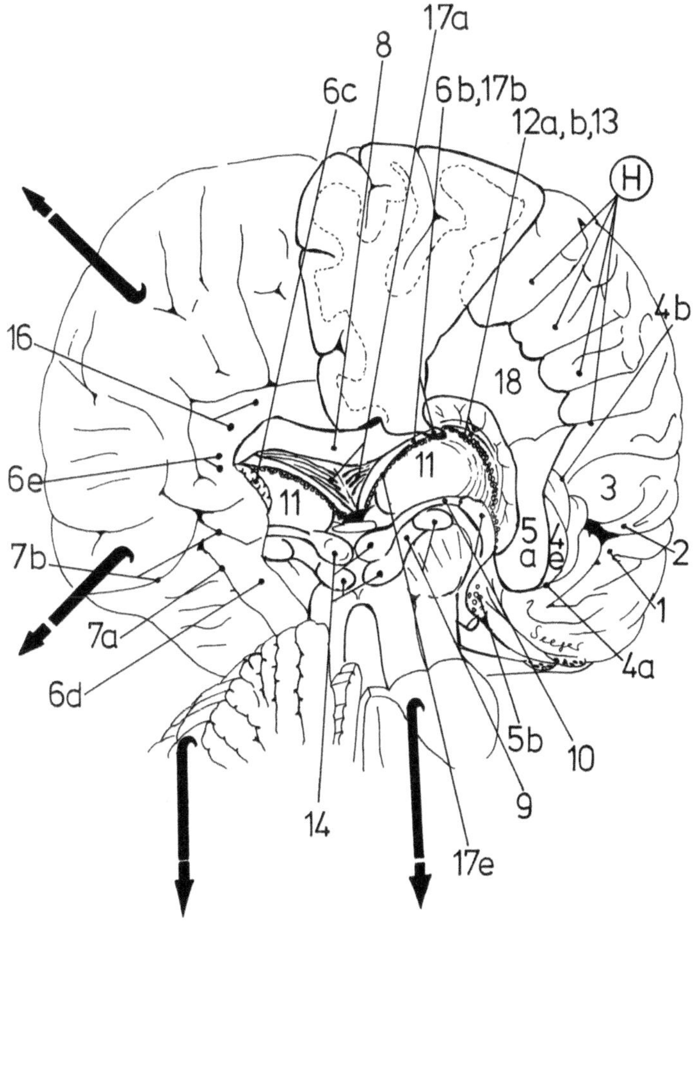
17a
8
6c
6 b,17b
12a, b,13
H
4b
16
18
11
11
6e
3
5
4
2
a
e
7b
1
7a
4a
6d
5b
10
9
14
17e

Fig. 32. Detail of preparation in Fig. 30 (midbrain cut). Widening of Commissura fornicis due to senile atrophic ventricular enlargement

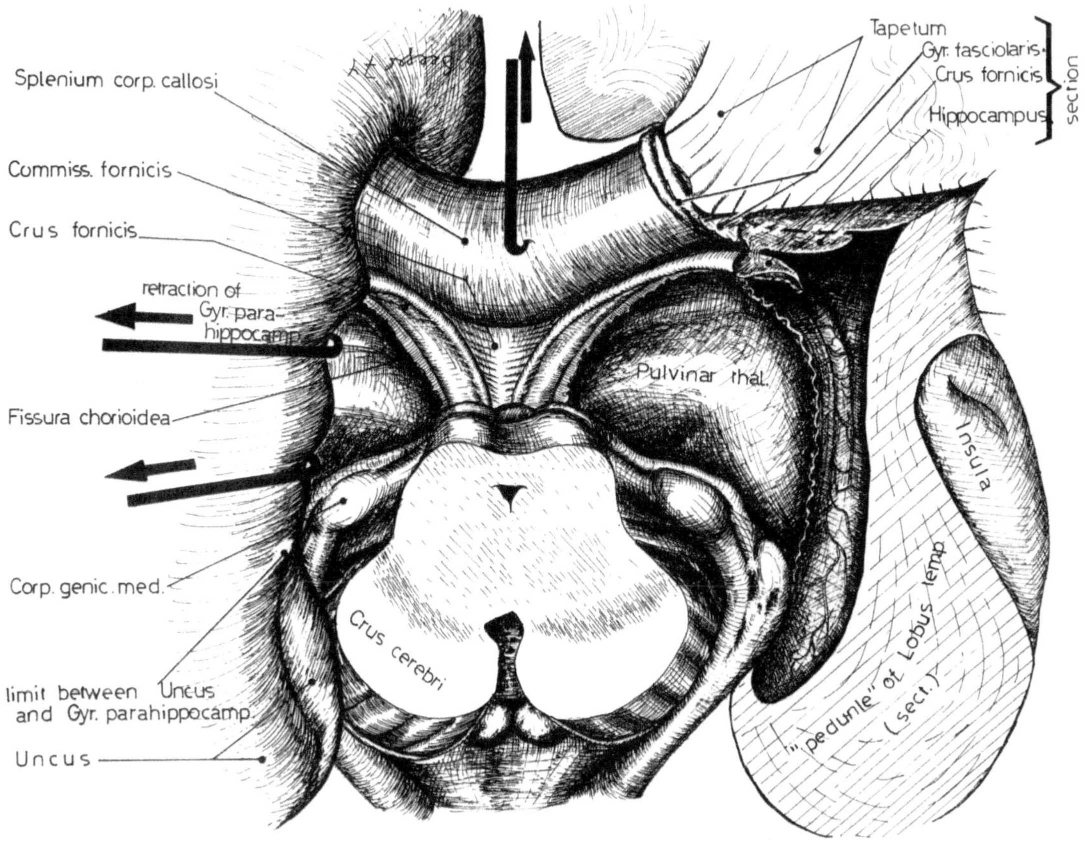
Splenium corp. callosi
Commiss. fornicis
Crus fornicis
retraction of Gyr. para-hippocamp.
Fissura chorioidea
Corp. genic. med.
limit between Uncus and Gyr. parahippocamp.
Uncus
Tapetum
Gyr. fasciolaris
Crus fornicis
Hippocampus
section
Pulvinar thal.
Insula
Crus cerebri
"pedunle" of Lobus temp. (sect.)

Fig. 33. Preparation of Fig. 32 with arteries sketched in

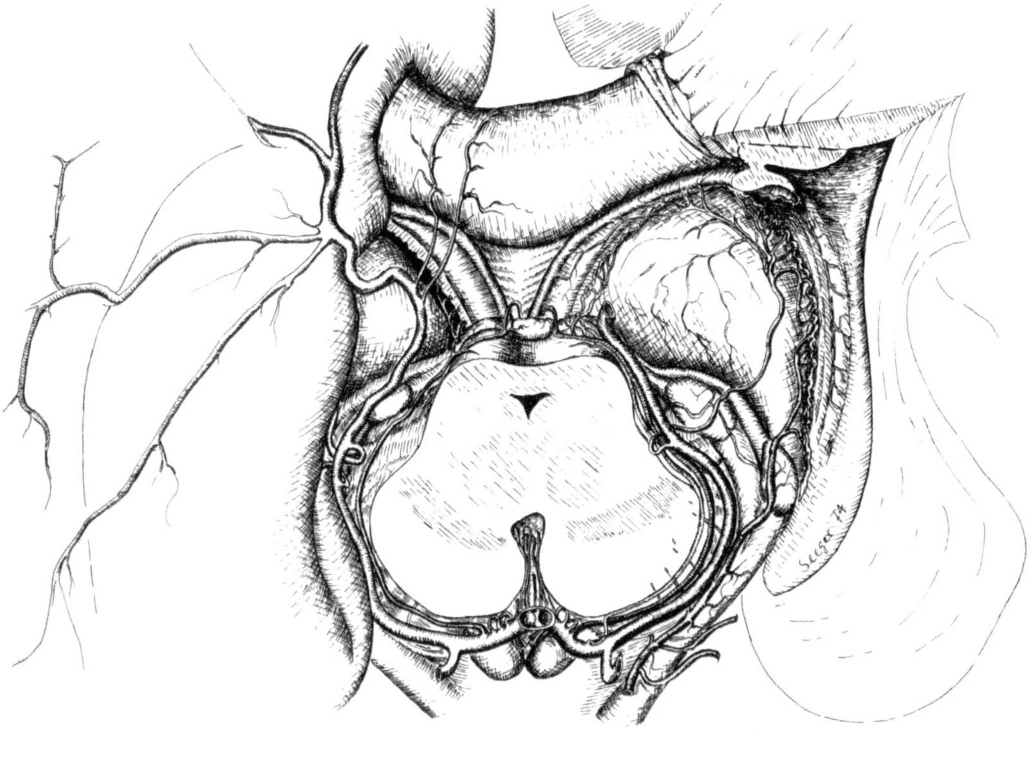
Seeger 74

Fig. 34. Designation of vessels in Fig. 33

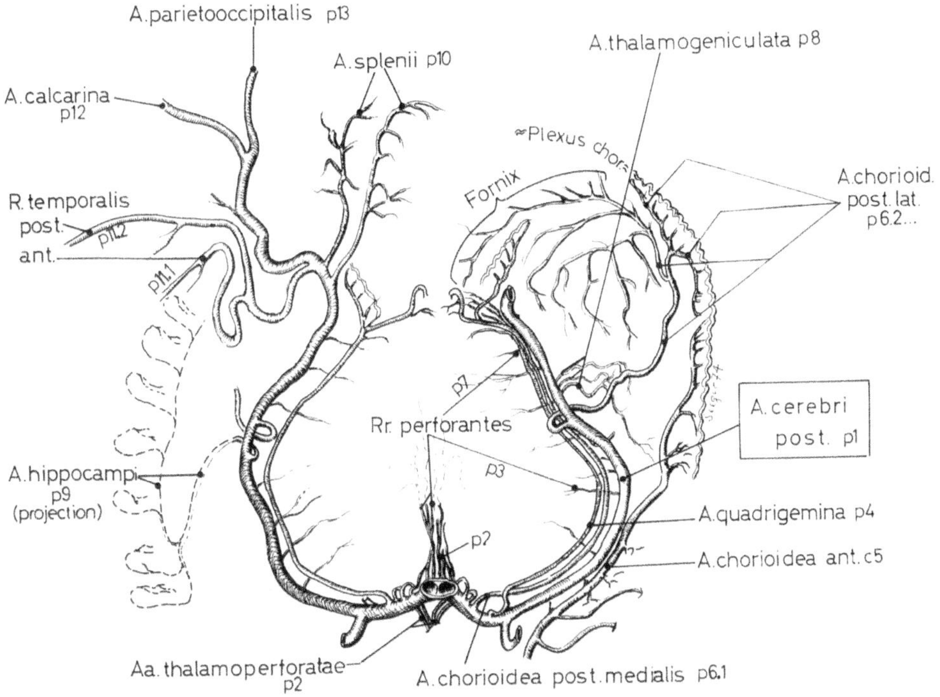
A.parietooccipitalis p13
A.splenii p10
A.thalamogeniculata p8
A.calcarina p12
Plexus chor.
Fornix
A.chorioid. post. lat. p6.2...
R. temporalis post.
p11.2
ant.
p11.1
p7
A.cerebri post. p1
Rr. perforantes
p3
A.hippocampi p9 (projection)
A.quadrigemina p4
p2
A.chorioidea ant. c5
Aa. thalamoperforatae p2
A.chorioidea post. medialis p6.1

Fig. 35. Branches of A. cerebri post. from dorsal direction. Section above Isthmus rhombencephali

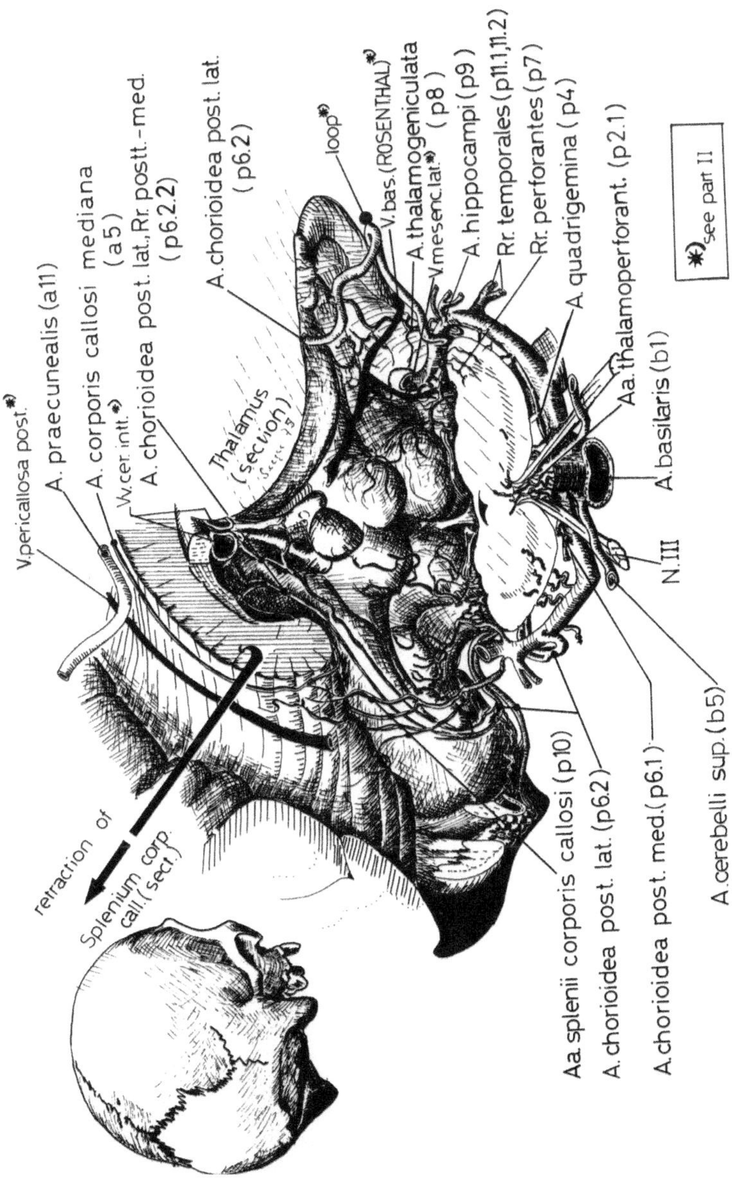

V.pericallosa post.*)
A. praecunealis (a11)
A. corporis callosi mediana (a5)
Vv.cer. intt.*)
A. chorioidea post. lat., Rr. postt.-med. (p6.2.2)
A. chorioidea post. lat. (p6.2)
Thalamus (section)
loop*)
V.bas.(ROSENTHAL)*)
A. thalamogeniculata
V.mesenc.lat.*) (p8)
A. hippocampi (p9)
Rr. temporales (p11.1,11.2)
Rr. perforantes (p7)
A. quadrigemina (p4)
Aa. thalamoperforant. (p2.1)
A. basilaris (b1)
N.III
*) see part II
retraction of
Splenium corp. call. (sect.)
Aa. splenii corporis callosi (p10)
A. chorioidea post. lat. (p6.2)
A. chorioidea post. med. (p6.1)
A. cerebelli sup. (b5)

Fig. 36. Left frontal region from medial direction. Section through basal ganglia complex. Senile atrophic brain with enlarged 3rd and lateral ventricles. At the level of Commissura ant. a narrowed zone of Pallium (consisting mainly of fibres of Rostrum corporis callosi) pushes between Fissura longitudinalis and the enlarged Cornu ant.

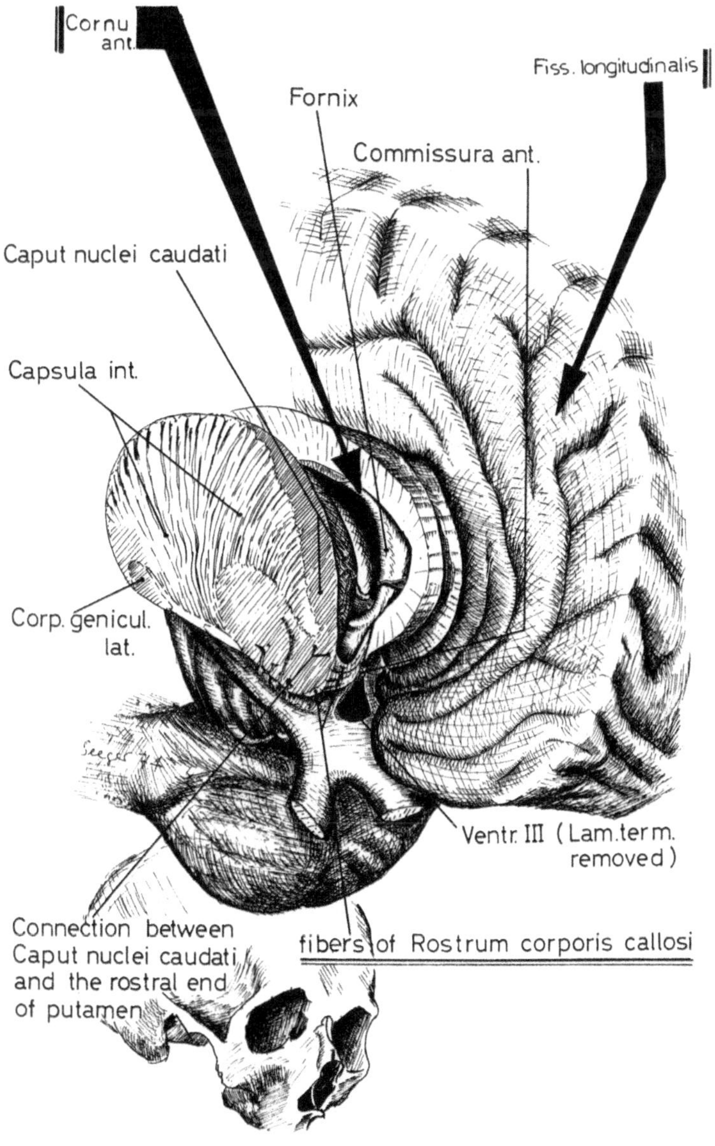
Cornu ant.
Fiss. longitudinalis
Fornix
Commissura ant.
Caput nuclei caudati
Capsula int.
Corp. genicul. lat.
Ventr. III (Lam.term. removed)
Connection between Caput nuclei caudati and the rostral end of putamen
fibers of Rostrum corporis callosi

Fig. 37. Preparation of Fig. 36 with vessels. For designation of vessels see catalogue of arteries, pages 3–4

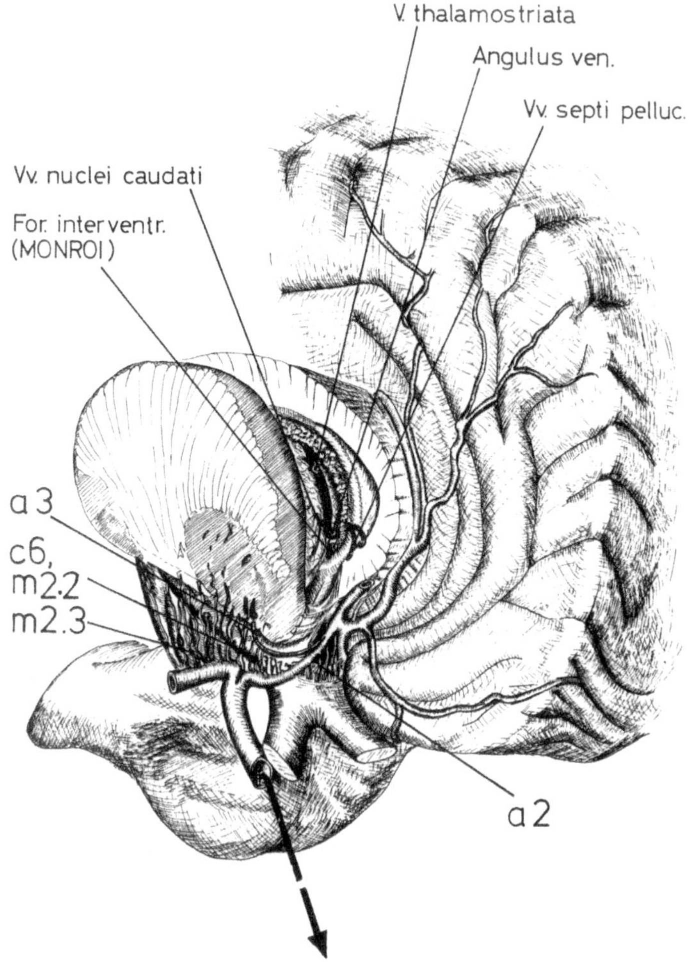
V. thalamostriata
Angulus ven.
Vv. septi pelluc.
Vv. nuclei caudati
For. interventr.
(MONROI)
a3
c6,
m2.2
m2.3
a2

Fig. 38. General view of preparation in Figs. 39 to 43. After removal of Plexus chorioideus the Fissura chorioidea gapes wide open (arrows). Below it Gyrus parahippocampalis is visible extracerebrally

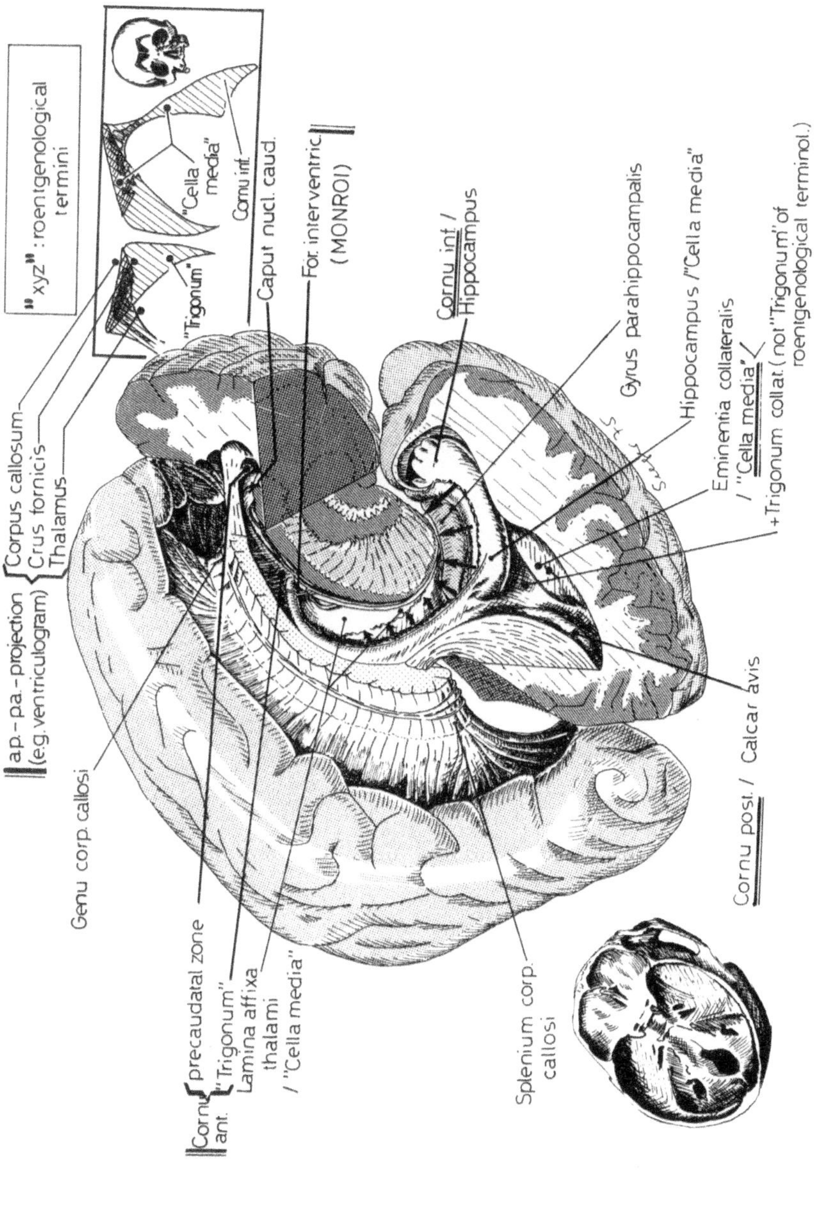
"xyz": roentgenological termini
a.p.-p.a.-projection
(e.g. ventriculogram)
Corpus callosum
Crus fornicis
Thalamus
"Trigonum"
"Cella media"
Cornu inf.
Caput nucl. caud.
For. interventric.
(MONROI)
Cornu inf. /
Hippocampus
Gyrus parahippocampalis
Hippocampus /"Cella media"
Eminentia collateralis
/ "Cella media"
+Trigonum collat. (not "Trigonum" of
roentgenological terminol.)
Cornu post. / Calcar avis
Splenium corp.
callosi
Cornu
ant.
precaudatal zone
"Trigonum"
Lamina affixa
thalami
/ "Cella media"
Genu corp. callosi

Fig. 39. Anterobasal view in direction of course of N. opticus. Lamina terminalis resected

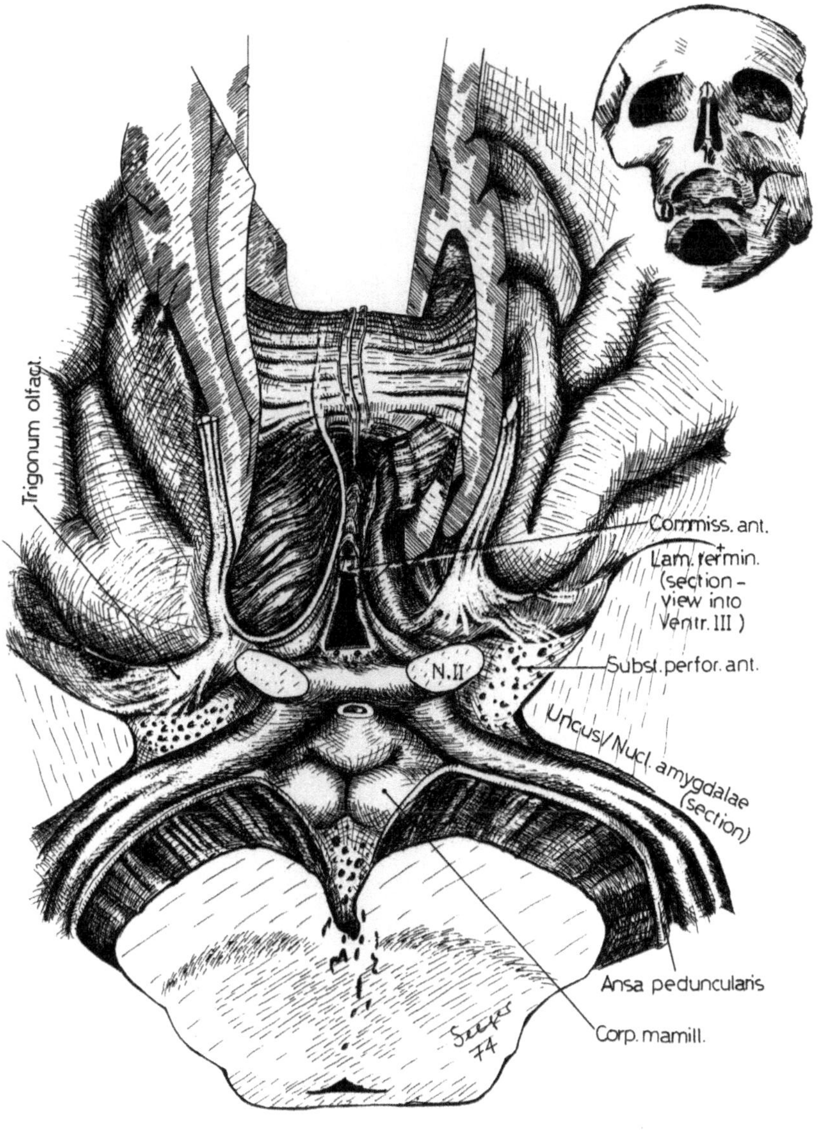
Trigonum olfact.
Commiss. ant.
+
Lam. termin.
(section -
view into
Ventr. III)
N.II
Subst. perfor. ant.
Uncus/Nucl. amygdalae
(section)
Ansa peduncularis
Corp. mamill.

Fig. 40. Preparation of Fig. 39 with vessels

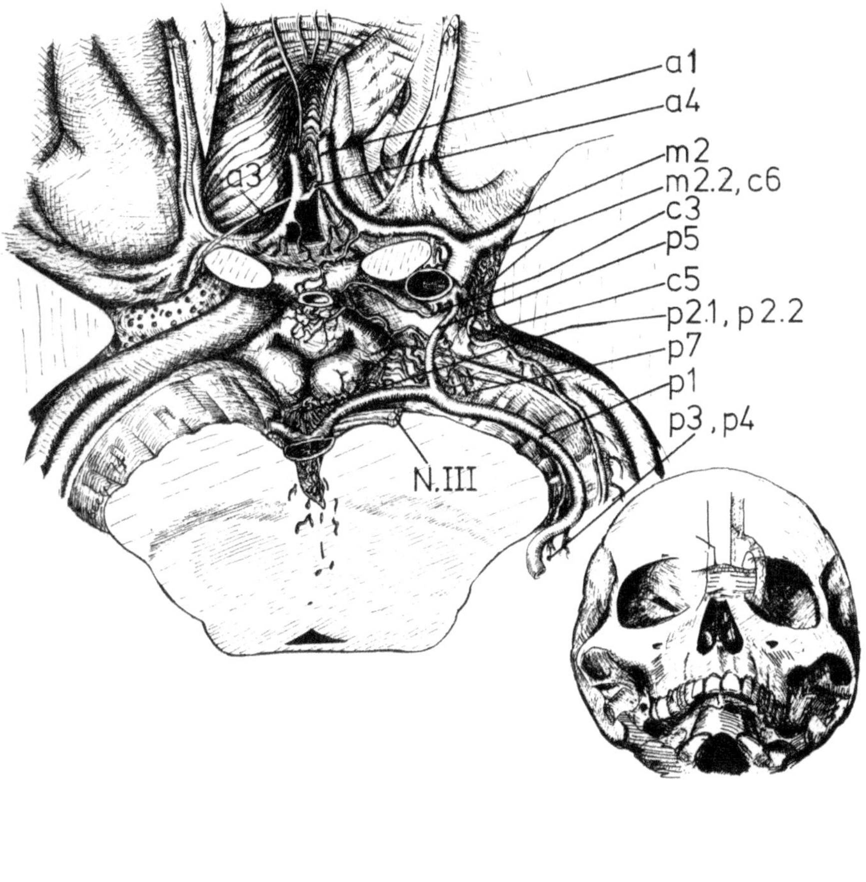
a1
a4
a3
m2
m2.2, c6
c3
p5
c5
p2.1, p 2.2
p7
p1
p3, p4
N.III

Fig. 41. Preparation of Fig. 39 after separation of right hemisphere. Vessel perforations of Substantia perforata ant. with relationship of Putamen and Globus pallidus. Merging of Caput nuclei caudati with anterior part of Putamen recognizable from cut surfaces

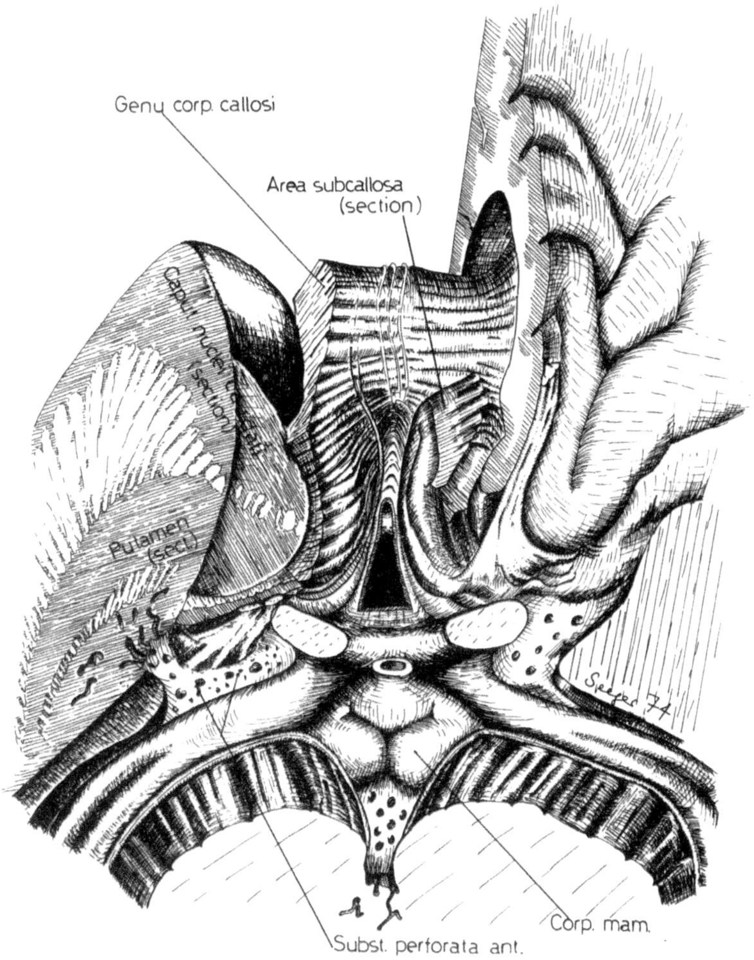
Genu corp. callosi
Area subcallosa (section)
Caput nuclei caudati (section)
Putamen (sect.)
Corp. mam.
Subst. perforata ant.
Sleeper 74

Fig. 42. View of opened anterior horn from anterosuperior direction after removal of right cerebral hemisphere at basal ganglia complex. Positional relationships between Caput nuclei caudati and Putamen

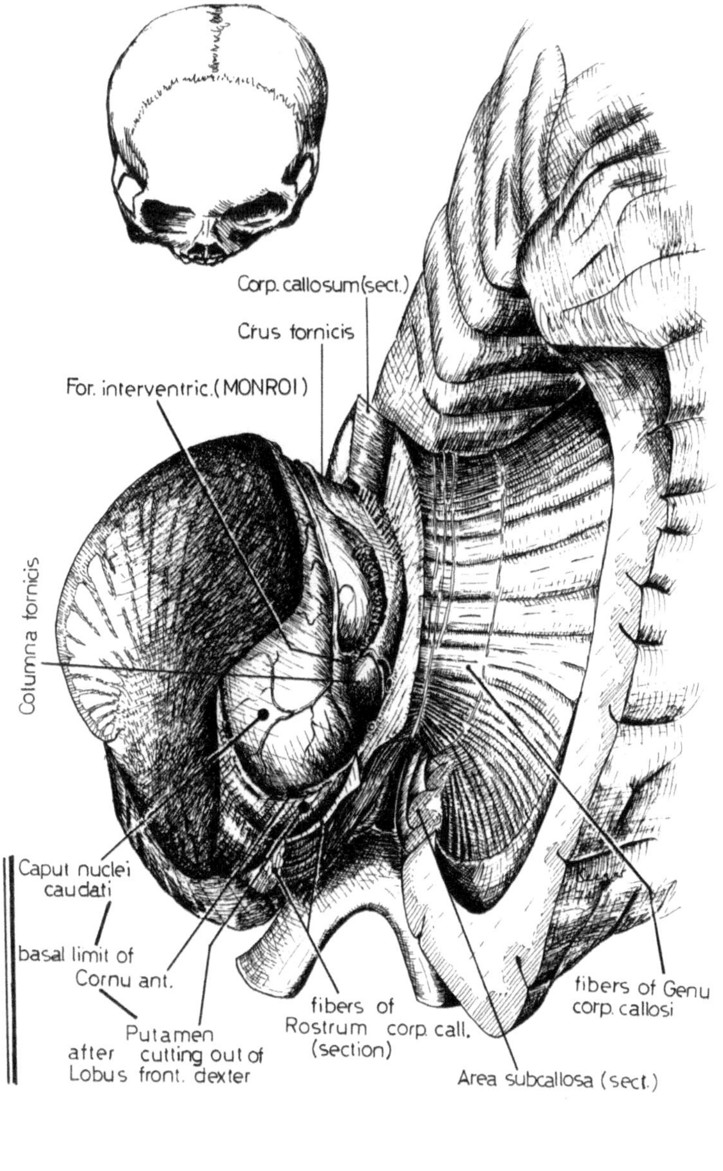
Corp. callosum(sect.)
Crus fornicis
For. interventric.(MONROI)
Columna fornicis
Caput nuclei caudati
basal limit of Cornu ant.
Putamen after cutting out of Lobus front. dexter
fibers of Rostrum corp. call. (section)
fibers of Genu corp. callosi
Area subcallosa (sect.)

Fig. 43. The same preparation from posterosuperior direction with parts of temporo-occipital region retained basally
Arrow: Fissura chorioidea gapes after removal of Plexus chor.

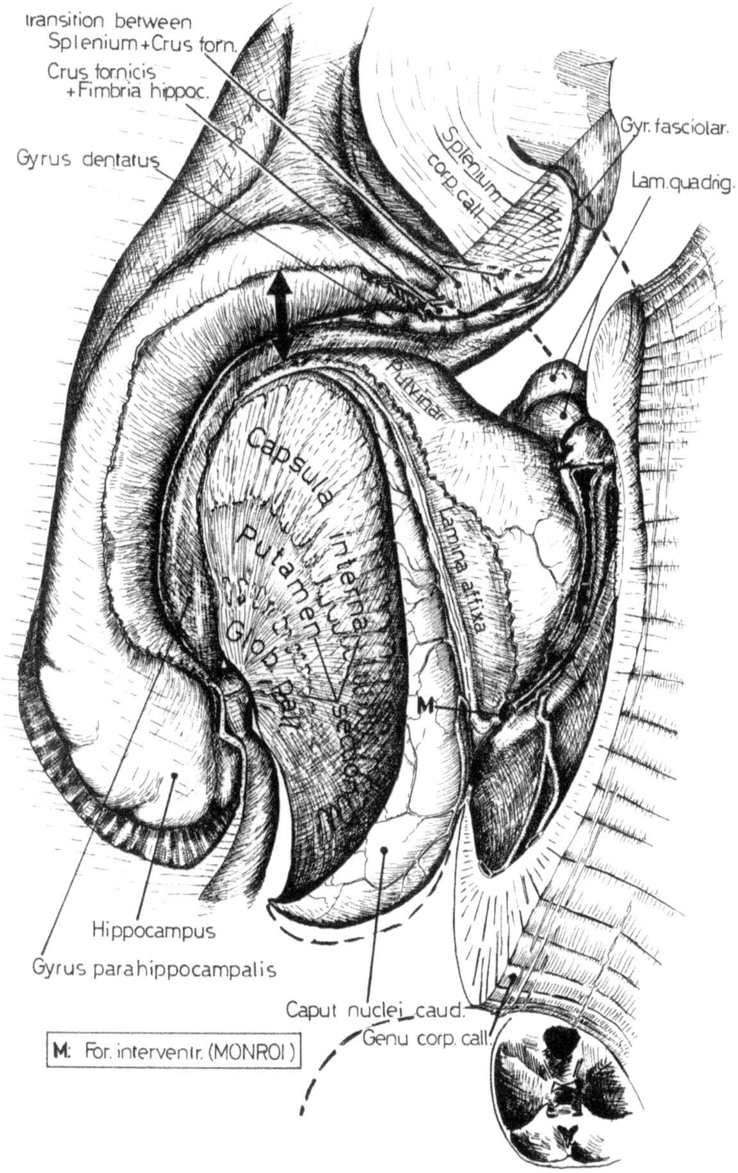
transition between
Splenium+Crus forn.
Crus fornicis
+Fimbria hippoc.
Gyrus dentatus
Splenium corp. call.
Gyr. fasciolar.
Lam. quadrig.
Pulvinar
Capsula interna
Putamen
Glob. pall.
Lamina affixa
M
Hippocampus
Gyrus parahippocampalis
Caput nuclei caud.
Genu corp. call.
M: For. interventr. (MONROI)

Figs. 44 to 46. Section planes of preparations in Figs. 47 to 50

Symbols to Figs. 44 to 50

1 a Genu corporis callosi
1 b Rostrum corporis callosi
1 c Truncus corporis callosi
1 d Splenium corporis callosi
2 White matter
3 a Caput nuclei caudati
3 b Corpus nuclei caudati
3 c Cauda nuclei caudati
4 V. thalamo-striata
5 Stria medullaris
6 a Columna fornicis
6 b Corpus fornicis
6 c Crus fornicis
6 d Fimbria hippocampi
7 a Hippocampus
7 b Gyrus parahippocampalis
8 Uncus
9 Foramen interventriculare (Monroi)
10 Lamina affixa thalami
11 Taenia chorioidea
12 Plexus chorioideus ventriculi lateralis
13 Corpus geniculatum mediale
14 Corpus geniculatum laterale
15 Tractus opticus
16 a Insula
16 b Limen insulae
16 c Substantia perforata ant.
17 Crus cerebri
18 Corpus mamillare
19 Ansa peduncularis
20 Gyrus fasciolaris/Gyrus dentatus
21 Putamen
22 Capsula externa
23 Capsula extrema
24 Claustrum
25 Capsula interna
26 Calcar avis
27 Commissura ant.
28 Nucleus amygdalae/Uncus

Fig. 44. View from medial with section planes

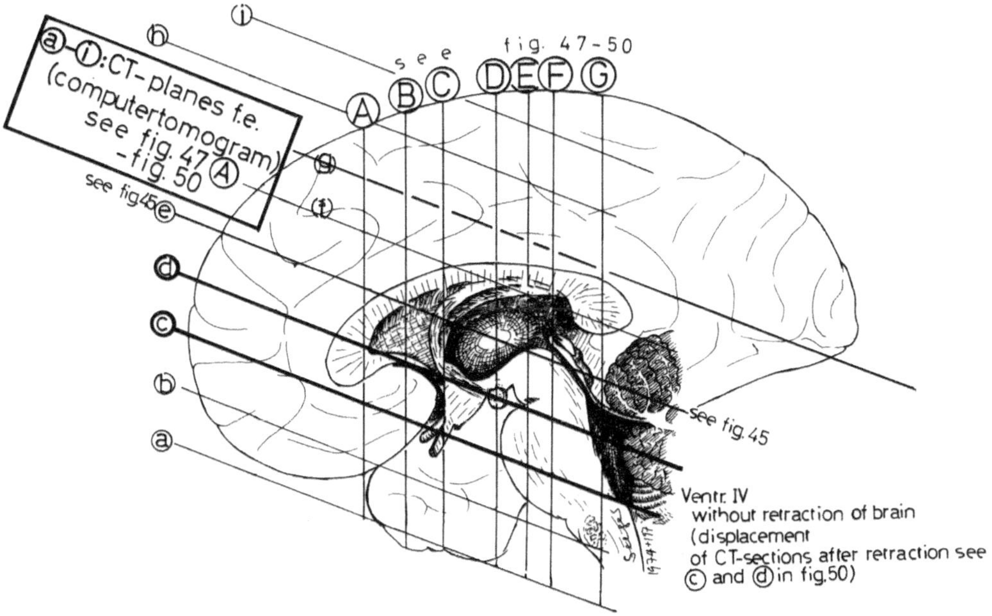

a – i: CT-planes f.e. (computertomogram) see fig. 47 A – fig. 50
see fig. 47 – 50
A B C D E F G
a b c d e f g h i
see fig. 45 e
see fig. 45
Ventr. IV
without retraction of brain
(displacement
of CT-sections after retraction see
c and d in fig. 50)

Fig. 45. Section planes in the ventricle viewed from above (left), and from laterally (right)

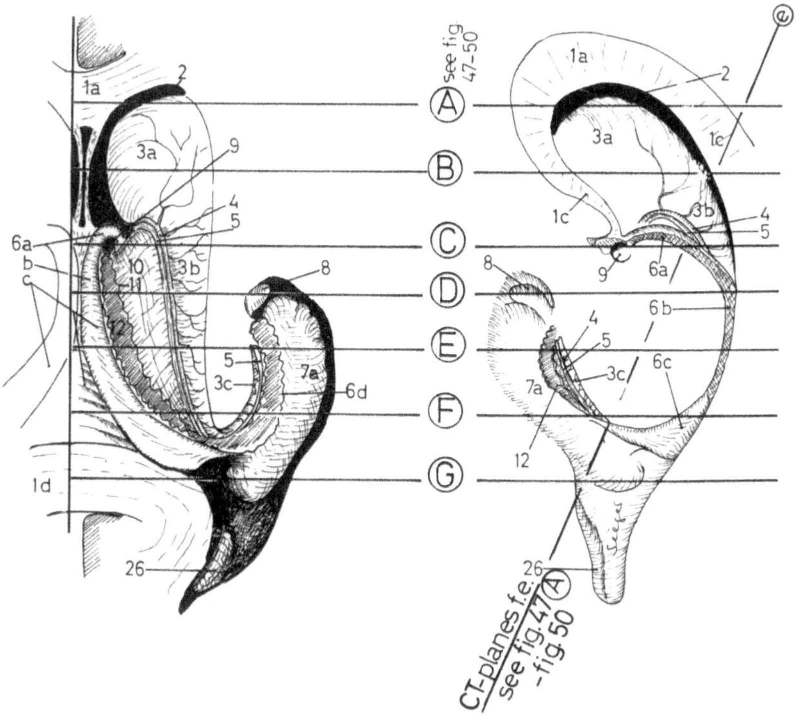
see fig 47–50
1a
2
3a
9
4
5
6a
b
c
10
11
12
3b
8
5
3c
7a
6d
1d
26
A
B
C
D
E
F
G
e
1c
3b
6a
6b
6c
7a
CT-planes f.e. see fig. 47 (A) - fig. 50

Fig. 46. Section planes from a basal view. Lobus temporalis in this preparation was removed in order to show positional relationships to deep basal structures

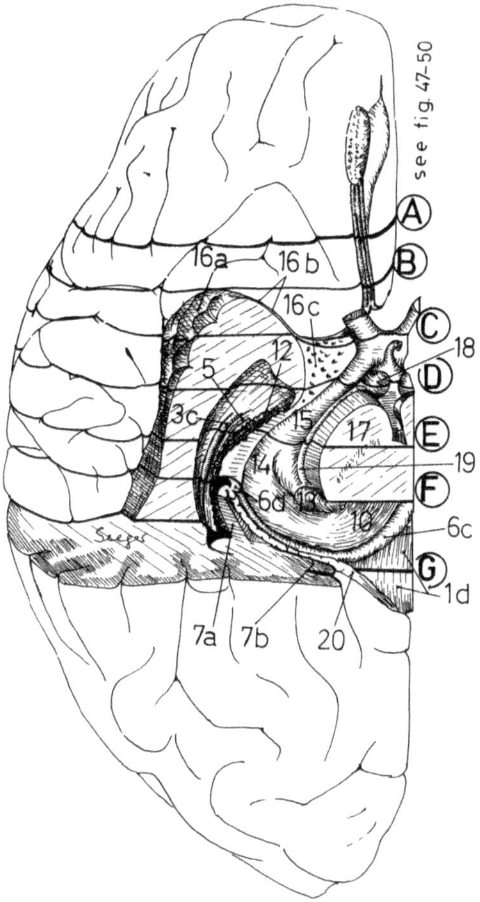
see fig. 47–50
A
B
C
D
E
F
G
16a
16b
16c
12
5
3c
15
17
18
14
19
6d
13
10
6c
1d
7a
7b
20
Seeger

Figs. 47 to 50. Series of frontal sections, positions see Figs. 44 to 46
A Distances of CT planes entered
CT sections not exactly vertical to the section planes of *A–G*, distances of CT planes 26 mm (or 13 mm). With only slight changes of the CT section plane, greatly differing structures are reached

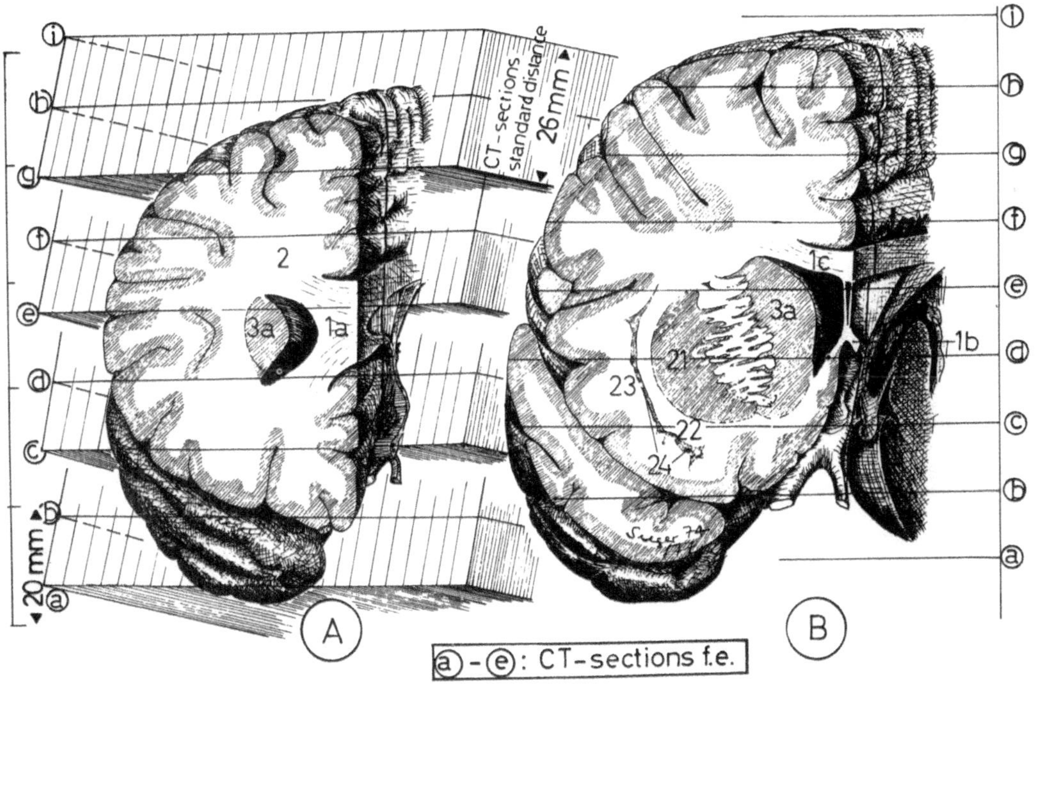

ⓐ - ⓔ: CT-sections f.e.

FIG. 48

Fig. 48

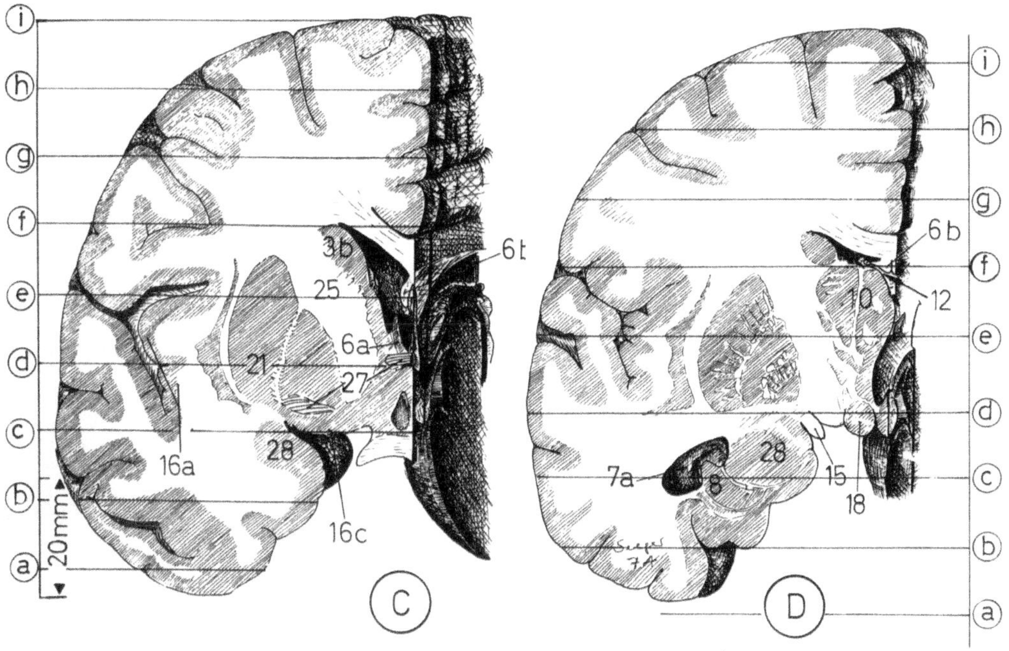
i
h
g
f
e
d
c
b
a
20mm
3b
25
6b
6a
21
27
28
16a
16c
C
6b
12
10
15
18
7a
8
28
D

Fig. 49

Fig. 50

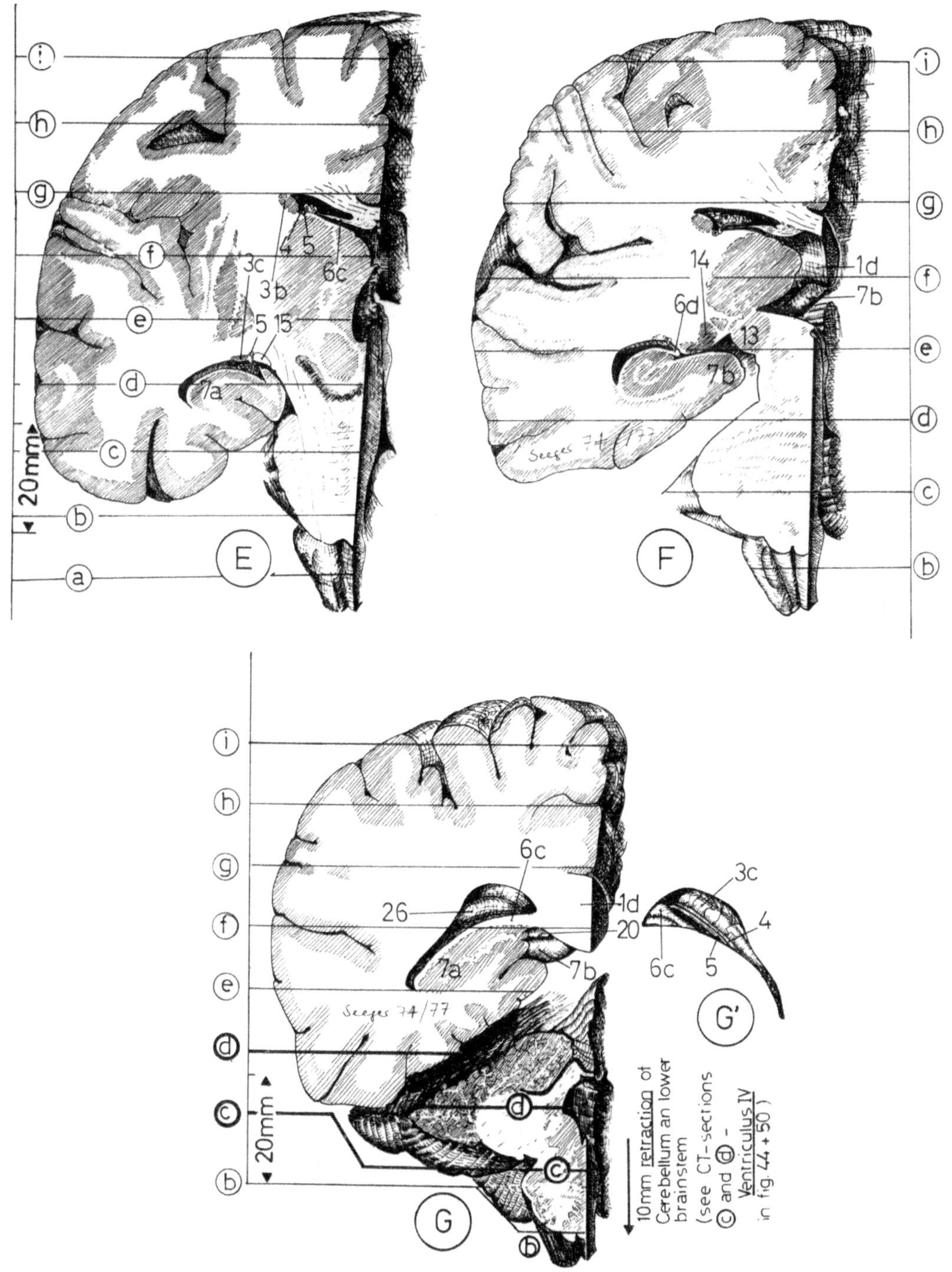
E
F
G
G'
20mm
3c
3b
4
5
6c
15
7a
14
1d
7b
6d
13
26
20
Seeger 74/77
10mm retraction of Cerebellum an lower brainstem
(see CT-sections ⓒ and ⓓ - Ventriculus IV in fig. 44 + 50)

Fig. 51. Sagittal section of anterior two-thirds of right hemisphere, and frontal section at level of posterior border of Corpus pineale

1 Commissura ant.
2 Chiasma et Recessus opticus
3 Infundibulum
4 a Corpus mamillare
4 b Columna fornicis (Pars tecta)
4 c Columna fornicis (Pars libera) + Septum pellucidum
4 d Corpus fornicis
4 e Commissura fornicis
4 f Crus fornicis
4 g Cauda nuclei caudati et Fimbria fornicis
5 Foramen interventriculare (Monroi)
6 a Massa intermedia et Thalamus
6 b Pulvinar thalami
7 Taenia thalami
8 Fissura transversa cerebri
9 Corpus pineale, Lamina quadrigemina
10 Lamina terminalis
A Oblique view from right anterior direction
B Basal view of preparation

Fig. 52. Third ventricle. Enlarged dimer-X-ventriculogram combined with air encephalography (Indian ink copy with additional cerebral structures)

For designations see also Fig. 50
11 Aquaeductus cerebri (Sylvii)
12 Recessus suprapinealis
13 a Rostrum corporis callosi
13 b Genu corporis callosi
13 c Splenium corporis callosi

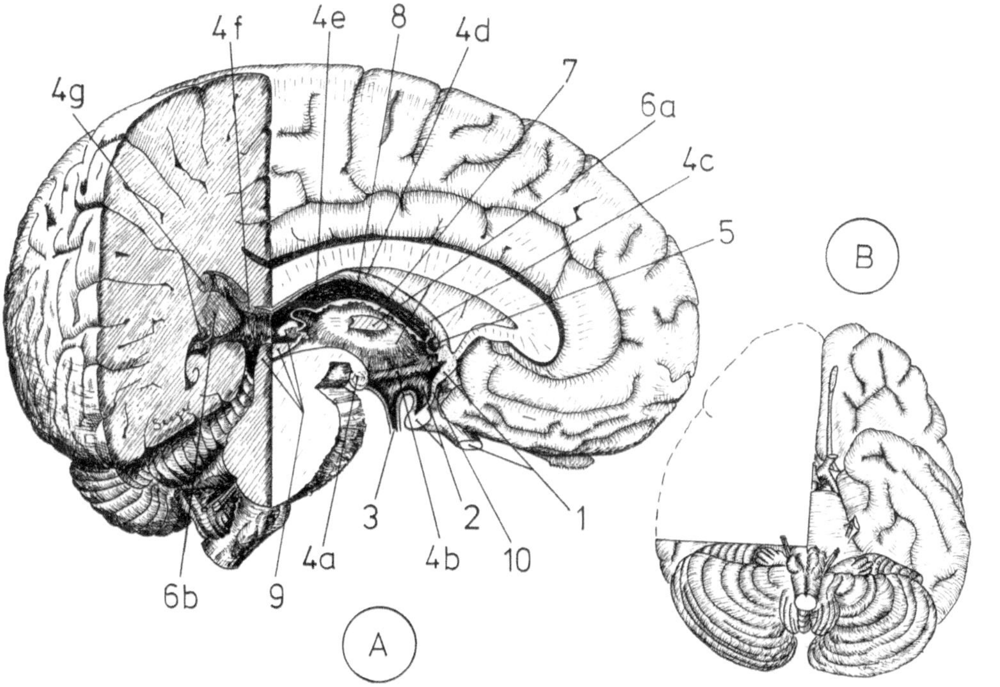
4f
4e
8
4d
4g
7
6a
4c
5
B
3
2
1
4a
4b
10
6b
9
A

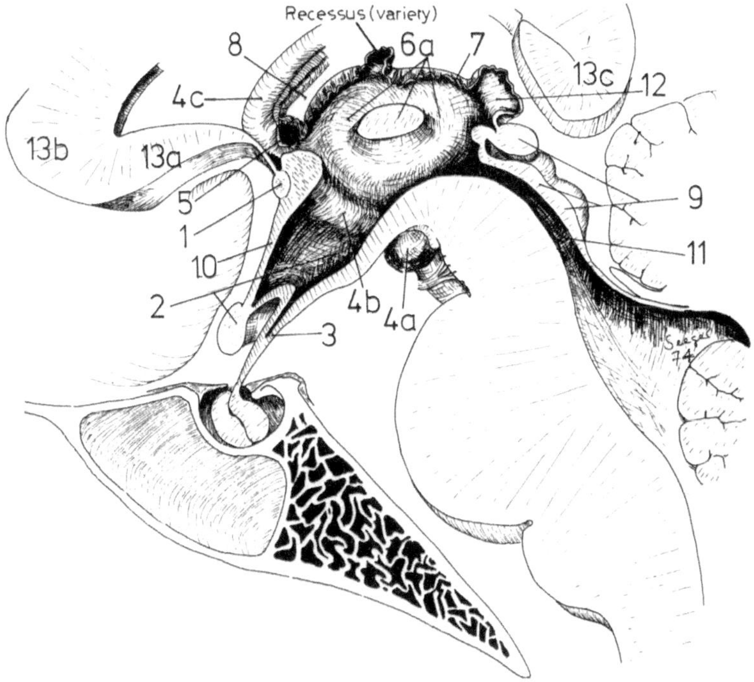
Recessus (variety)
8
6a
7
13c
12
4c
13b
13a
5
1
10
2
9
11
4b
4a
3

Part II

Topographical Anatomy of the Brain and Surrounding Structures Microneurosurgical Aspects

Chapter 2
Frontal Lobe and Upper Brainstem

A. Surface of Frontal Lobe

The limits of the frontal lobe are defined by Sulcus centralis, Fissura longitudinalis, the anterior portion of Fissura lateralis (Sylvii), the border between Gyrus rectus and Lamina terminalis, as well as the orbital gyri and Substantia perforata ant. The distance of Gyrus praecentralis from Bregma varies considerably (Fig. 53). >50 mm laterally to Bregma the precentral region closely approaches the coronal suture (Fig. 53). In the polar region of the frontal lobe at a lateral distance of 30 mm from the midline Pars orbitalis of Gyrus front. III is approached, and thus, in the dominant hemisphere, the motor speech centre (Fig. 53). Of the measurements in Fissura longitudinalis (Fig. 54) the most important is the distance of Genu corporis callosi and the knee of A. pericallosa from the frontal pole. The anterior border of Substantia perforata ant., which coincides with the base of Trigonum olfactorium and with the bifurcation of A. carotis interna (Fig. 54), is difficult to localize from the polar area because of the deep basal curvature of the orbital brain medially. The distance of the pole to the posterior edge of Lamina cribrosa (25 mm) is emphasized. Caudatum and Putamen are vaulted over Substantia perforata ant. This is the most densely vascularized zone, and it supplies these structures from a basal direction (Figs. 54 and 56).

B. Deep Brain Structures

Frontal sections at a depth of 35 to 50 mm (Fig. 55) show only tangentially cut anterior fibres of Corpus callosum without opening Cornu ant. (Fig. 55), although immediately in front of Cornu ant. numerous fine vascular cross-sections herald its proximity. Within a few millimetres at varying depth A. pericallosa and the knee of Corpus callosum appear medially, and the tip of Cornu ant. laterally. Here the anterior portion of Caudatum and Putamen, here joined together, is already visible. Caudatum and Putamen combine in the characteristic formation of "Corpus striatum" (Fig. 56). Already at a depth of <50 mm laterally the anterior portion of Insula is reached (Fig. 53), and Cornu ant. somewhat deeper. The lateral portion of Cornu ant. lies only 5 to 10 mm medially to the medial portions of Insula. In this 5-mm-wide zone lies the anterior portion of Corona radiata (Fig. 58). If in making the exposure it ist intended to conserve Insula and Cornu ant. (as at operation), it is advisable to proceed in stages, using Fissura longitudinalis, the frontal pole, and Bregma for orientation and paying attention to the distance measurements, insofar as the brain is not deformed by a space-occupying process (Figs. 58 and 59).

The border area between the basomedial extracerebral space and the ventricular system is structurally complicated (Figs. 59 to 62). Frontal sections in the zone between Genu corporis callosi and tangentially cut anterior portion of Putamen (*II* in Figs. 56 and 59) with removal of Area subcallosa, give a general view of the anterior portion of Lamina terminalis (Figs. 59–62). They show that between the floor of Cornu anterius and Fissura longitudinalis before Lamina terminalis there lies a sheet of fibres of Rostrum corporis callosi only a few millimetres wide. Putamen is a close neighbour of Cornu ant. and Fissura longitudinalis. Even with careful removal of cortical substance of Area subcallosa in the vicinity of A. communicans ant., Putamen is reached at a depth of a few millimetres. At dissection in an upward direction the lateral ventricle is also soon reached in front of Commissura ant.; Substantia perforata ant. is rolled in concavely upwards and backwards, and at the transition between Chiasma and Lamina terminalis it forms a convex margin, in a backward direction laterally and upwards, and in a forward direction medially and basally (Fig. 61, below right).

Arteries:

The distance of both carotid arteries from each other is very variable in the vicinity of the dural penetration point. In Fig. 63 a lower limit value is given: the distance of A. carotis int. from the midline may be reduced to 5 mm (see also Renn and Rhoton, 1975). The length of A. carotis int. and the direction of its course are also known to vary. The trunk of A. cerebri ant. arises either laterally to the posterior N. opticus region, laterally to Chiasma, or laterally to the anterior region of Tractus opt. (Figs. 91 and 92).

A. communicans post. and A. chorioidea ant., arising laterally and posteriorly from A. carotis int., branch out into perforating arteries variable in number and calibre, most of which penetrate into the furrow between Hypothalamus and Tractus opticus. There are various types, in which also the surface of Tractus opt. is directly perforated. Others reach Substantia perforata ant. and thus belong to Aa. lenticulostriatae. Other branches run as far as Corpora mamillaria and Substantia perforata post.

A. communicans post. and A. chorioidea ant. may mutually replace each other in the Hypothalamus-Tractus opticus furrow. The anterior medial region is supplied autonomously by A. communicans post.; A. chorioidea ant. supplies autonomously the posterolateral region between Hypothalamus and Tractus opticus, including portions of Substantia perforata ant., which is otherwise supplied from the carotid bifurcation (Fig. 68 *A* and *C*), (Mauritz, 1977). The perforating arteries arising from the carotid bifurcation and the adjoining sections of A. cerebri anterior and media, and running to Substantia perforata ant., have a somewhat more regular course. Substantia perforata ant. forms a continuous zone with the perforation zone of Chiasma opticum in front of Lamina terminalis (Figs. 60 to 62). If A. carotis int. is lightly pulled downwards and A. cerebri anterior upwards, it will be seen that the group of lateral perforating arteries passes into the deeply indrawn and upwardly convex Substantia perforata ant. The small branches become shorter medially. Finally their course winds downwards along the lower border of Lamina terminalis (lower picture, right, in Fig. 61). Heubner's artery with its transverse course is an exception (Figs. 62 and 63).
The upper hypophyseal artery arising at the back of A. carotis int. and taking course in a medial direction cannot always be exposed and is difficult to identify either with frontal or with frontomedial exposure. Its exit from A. carotis int. and the transition into the upper portion of the hypophyseal stalk are difficult to localize.
Perlmutter and Rhoton (1976) have investigated the considerable variations in the proximal and distal portions of A. cerebri anterior in the vicinity of A. communicans ant. The most important types are shown in Figs. 63 and 64. Kribs and Kleihues showed that in over 70% A. recurrens (Heubneri) arises, either at the level of A. communicans ant. or immediately above it, out of the distal segment of A. cerebri ant. Heubner's and the other perforating arteries attracted early attention due to the fact that they supply the rostral basal ganglia region (injection preparations of Ostrowski et al., 1960). The lateral perforating branches arising from A. cerebri ant. and A. cerebri media were analyzed by Kaplan in 1965. Of the variants of the anterior-communicans-ant.-complex illustrated in Fig. 63, well known through surgical intervention, the reader is referred to little-known duplications of A. communicans ant. (Fig. 63 *B, C, D, E*) and to duplications of the proximal segment of A. cerebri ant. (Fig. 63 *D*). The trifurcation of ascending A. cerebri ant. described by Perlmutter and Rhoton in 1976 was also recently mentioned in the work of Marino, who describes the varying distal pattern of the course of A. cerebri ant. in these cases.
In Fig. 65 an attempt is made to give a spatial representation of the various types of course. The variable development of right-left communications in the course of A. pericallosa is remarkable. In no case do they contain a genuine distal anastomosis of both Aa. cerebri anteriores, but only partial bilateral supply from one A. pericallosa in the distal section. Marino's type described in Fig. 65 under *A* was confirmed in a preparation by the author. The case described by Marino with triple A. pericallosa (Fig. 65 *D*) corresponds to the one described by Perlmutter and Rhoton (Fig. 64 *G*).
From the distribution patterns of Marino can be concluded that a fusion of both distal portions of A. cerebri ant. into an unpaired A. cerebri ant. and missing A. communicans ant. in Fissura longitudinalis is also possible. Such an arterial course is also conceivable – e.g., at operation of an aneurysm of A. cerebri ant.
At least the larger arteries are sheathed by arachnoidal duplicatures, which vary in extent, sacculation, development of gaps, and thickness. They may

either be opaque or so delicate that they tear away when touched with the forceps. Fig. 66 *B* shows schematically the principal extent of arachnoid membrane formations, which in stretches are split up into tougher or more delicate trabeculae. Laterally, Gyrus parahippocampalis/Uncus is always clearly demarcated from the tentorial edge. Under this, N. oculomotorius can only be followed for a short distance and emerges medially out of a likewise flat arachnoid membrane from the richly vascularized region of the lateral and posterior perforating arteries (Rr. perforantes of A. communicans post., and Aa. thalamoperforatae from the bifurcation of A. basilaris). In Fig. 66 these two membranes separate by retraction of Uncus, as at operation, whereas in situ they are in contact with each other. The lateral arachnoidal wall of Cisterna chiasmatis is perforated in several places, as is the posterior wall in front of A. basilaris. Only in the opticus-carotis region anteromedially are the arachnoid layers smoothly lined out. Between Gyri recti, the two Nn. optici and Tuberculum sellae an anterior arachnoid membrane is extended, which encloses A. carotis int. and Nn. optici, extends laterally into Fissura lat. (Sylvii), and sheathes basally the perforating arteries from A. chorioidea ant., A. communicans post. with the (at this point increasingly irregular) fragmentation of Arachnoidea. In a forward direction the membrane continues as the covering of Fissura longitudinalis. Even with wide exposure of Cisterna basalis and its neighbouring cisterns, recognition of A. basilaris with its branches may be difficult from the front in the presence of arachnoid adhesions, but from the lateral approach it can be easily identified (Fig. 66, arrow *g*).

Because of superimposition by arachnoid membranes, the dense vascular network of Aa. thalamoperforatae and the terminal portion of A. basilaris, Corpora mamillaria are almost always invisible, particularly since visualization is only possible with a mirror due to their deeply embedded position in the operative field, as stated by Sugita et al. in 1975.

Extirpation of Arachnoidea between the two Nn. optici or separation of the long, loosely coiled perforating arteries behind A. carotis int. allows a view into the suprasellar space (Fig. 68).

The conservation of these arteries is vital. Schlesinger's compilation shows a regular arterial supply system of the parenchyma of the upper brainstem in the vicinity. The larger the vessel trunks are in their extracerebral course in the vicinity of the basal cisterns, the greater is their variability (Stephens and Stilwell), and thus the possibility of unexpected postoperative neurological deficits. Support should therefore be given to the recommendation of Yaşargil that in the case of aneurysms a fine-calibre A. communicans post. with its Aa. perforantes should be dissected out of the aneurysm, in order not to endanger Hypothalamus*.

Finally it should be added that the lateral group of perforating arteries, which extends from Substantia perforata ant. to Substantia perforata post., is supplemented in a posterior direction by perforating arteries originating from A. basilaris and A. cerebri post. They may reach in a lateral direction as far as Hypothalamus. Their supply regions are often not confined to Fossa interpeduncularis, midbrain Tegmentum, and Thalamus.

Poorly vascularized or nonvascularized zones of the wall of Cisterna chiasmatis are situated

1) between the two Nn. optici
2) between N. opticus and A. carotis int.
3) behind A. carotis int. over N. oculomotorius and in front of A. cerebri post., medial to Uncus (see Fig. 66 *A* and *B*).

From these three positions Cisterna chiasmatis can be viewed without injury to the vessels. In the presence of space-occupying suprasellar lesions the approach is easier because of the widening of space by tumour, but is difficult in the presence of tough-walled arachnoid cysts and even more so of Arachnitis adhaesiva (Seeger, 1955).

Veins:

On the surface in the region of the frontal pole, cerebral veins are almost always to be found either singly or multiply with converging course to Sinus longitudinalis sup., and here they are at risk at their junction in the case of opening of the dura. Contrary to the general view, thoughtless closure of these is not justified even in the anterior region, since Kaplan et al. demonstrated the distribution pattern of these veins which is very extensive in parts. They showed that the connection with the sinus is often situated farther back, whereas anterior portions of the sinus may still be aplastic several centimetres above Foramen caecum.

Therefore, also in the case of big frontal cerebral

---

* Personal op.-demonstration.

veins, attention should be paid to calibre and connections with other veins. In addition, numerous fine veins may lie in Fissura longitudinalis in the vicinity of adhesions attached to the falx. These veins may hinder the approach to Corpus callosum (as in the parietal and occipital lobes).

Superficial veins of Fissura lat. (Sylvii) may pass exactly over the fissure, but also over the first temporal gyrus or over the third frontal gyrus (*A* 4 and *A 5* in Fig. 116, chapter 3). There are hardly an bridging veins in the region of Gyri orbitales. On elevation of Gyri orbitales by spatula, veins of the Sylvian fissure that pass to Ala parva are stretched. They slacken again when the arachnoidal covering of the Sylvian fissure is severed.

Fig. 67 exhibits the basal veins up to the region of the pons; and above A. cerebri post., V. basalis (Rosenthal) can be recognized as the dominating lateral vessel. From the lateral direction it receives veins of Plexus chorioideus and veins of the ventricle wall as well as deep middle cerebral veins. Transverse connections with the opposite side lead over Substantia perforata ant. between Trigonum olfactorium and the terminal stretch of A. carotis int. to Fissura longitudinalis (here connecting with the opposite side). Interpeduncular veins may connect the two Vv. basales (Rosenthal). Above the terminal portion of A. basilaris in the depths of Fossa interpeduncularis, the triangular form of the connection to the median pontine vein can be recognized. In the depths of Fissura longitudinalis there is a paired venous system on the surface of Corpus callosum with drainage to V. cerebri magna (Galeni). Fig. 67 gives a schematic representation taken from injection preparations by the author and from the monograph of Duvernoy (1975), also from Huang and Wolf (1975), as well as from injection preparations according to Stephens and Stilwell (1969).

C. Preoperative Radiology – Some Aspects

For projection of deep-seated processes onto the surface of the skull (Figs. 69 and 73), the position of the lateral roentgenogram must correspond to that of the a-p film (e.g., identical difference in level between Bregma and Lambda). If the cerebral veins are strongly developed (Figs. 69 and 77), the approach must be made so that larger veins are preserved and the projection onto the surface (= trepanation site) is selected accordingly. Before approaches are made over Fissura longitudinalis, attention should be given to the arteries in its vicinity, in particular A. paracentralis (Fig. 69), with a view to their conservation at operation. In comparing a-p and lateral films in the region of the base (Fig. 71), the different heights of Lamina cribrosa/Planum sphenoidale and the orbital roofs should be taken into consideration, as well as the form and position of the anterior clinoid process if it encircles the knee of the carotid siphon before A. carotis interna reaches the intradural space.

The position of the falx edge in the phlebogram follows from the site of Sinus sagittalis inf. (Fig. 71). The position of the free tentorial edge can be determined by connecting Galeni's point to the anterior clinoid process. Planum sphenoidale is variably curved in different individuals, flatly concave in its anterior portion (behind Lamina cribrosa), and variably convex in its posterior portion (Figs. 58 and 72). In the usual a-p projection the highest point of Planum sphenoidale lies in the posterior convex portion. Behind this, Tuberculum sellae drops away and curves somewhat towards the sella lumen.

Diagnosis with contrast media: The localization of Genu corporis callosi follows from the distance of A. pericallosa from the inner surface of the skull (30–40 mm). Regularly only there does A. pericallosa follow closely the surface of Corpus callosum. Cornu anterius lies barely 10 mm behind the knee of A. pericallosa and Genu corporis callosi.

Laterally the roof of Cornu anterius projects beyond the medially inclined Corpus callosum (Fig. 73).

The position of the precentral region is variable; its anterior border is 10 to 30 mm distant from Bregma.

The ventricle width and the distance between the lateral ventricular border and the medial upper region of the insula are 20 mm each. Behind the level of Bregma, in the rostral region of Insula, the distance between Insula and the ventricular system may be reduced to 5 mm (Fig. 58). This corresponds to a width of 5 mm for Corona radiata, and involves the possibility of a lesion of parts of the anterior pyramidal tract (arm paresis) immediately lateral to the ventricular system.

D. Operative Techniques – Some Aspects

Orientation on the midline is important at operations on the convexity (Fig. 75), but its determination is difficult in elderly patients with firmly adherent dura (Fig. 76). If the trepanation is performed laterally to the midline, even tearing of the dura will not involve injury to cerebral veins. The remaining exposure towards the middle can be carried out microsurgically with the drill, while protecting the dura. If at operation on a midline process there is the possibility of a choice of approach from right or left into Fissura longitudinalis (Fig. 77), the side should be chosen where there are no larger connecting veins. The preservation of important vessels should take precedence over the problem of the dominant hemisphere.

Before the extirpation of deep-seated frontal lesions (Fig. 78), the following data should be obtained from radiological examination, also with contrast media: position and distance measurements of the arteries of Fissura longitudinalis, the ventricular system, and the medial portion of Insula with the opercular vessels. The incision of the cerebral cortex should not be made directly at the edge of Fiss. longitud. but rather somewhat laterally to it in the area of overlapping supply between A. cerebri anterior and A. cerebri media. Larger resections of Cortex bring no advantage. The conservation of vesssels and avoidance of oedema are more important than a destructive decompression with resection of large parts of the lobes resulting in secondary malacia of extensive areas of the brain due to elimination of vessels in the vicinity of the resection.

In the frontobasal approach, as in the temporal, Ramus temporalis of N. facialis should be protected. For all incisions the basal incision in the area of the zygomatic arch should be made immediately in front of Tragus (Fig. 74). R. temp. n. facialis lies alongside the anterior branch of A. temp. superfic. in a basal direction. After turning back the skin and galea it is necessary to make a careful exposure of the lateral bony limit of the orbit (Proc. zygomaticus ossis frontalis and Proc. frontalis ossis zygomatici) at its posterior edge (Figs. 80 and 81). From here the temporal muscle with the periosteal sheath can be detached without significant bleeding. If it is intended to open the frontal base and the temporal base, the detachment must be made up to the edge of the zygomatic arch. Instead of the pedunculation of the temporal muscle shown in Figs. 80 and 81, the bone can also be freely removed and the anterior part of the temporal muscle notched (see Chapter 3) in order to reach farther in a temporopolar-basal direction, as in the temporal approach. The zygomatic arch resection performed by the author allows a particularly basal approach (Figs. 80 and 81). Sites at which Tabula externa and interna of the skull are almost parallel should be chosen for the burrholes. Injury to the dura can occur very easily at two places (Fig. 84):

1) With one frontomedian burrhole the dura is injured on both sides before Crista frontalis is bored through as far as the border to Sinus sagittalis sup. It is, therefore, most expedient to make a pair of burrholes, one on each side of the midline.

2) The burrhole at the frontozygomatic point must not be made too far basally, since apart from the dura projecting over Pars orbitalis of the third frontal gyrus, with thinning of the bone, Periorbita in the vicinity of Fossa lacrimalis is also easily damaged.

As in temporobasal trepanation, resection of the small wing of the sphenoid up to the lateral point of Fissura orbitalis sup. allows an approach to be made with only minimal reclination of the frontotemporal basal region of the brain. The distance measurements from the frontozygomatic to the lateral point of Fissura orbitalis sup. (35 mm), and from Fissura orbitalis sup. to Canalis opticus (>20 mm), facilitate orientation (Fig. 85). The distance of Canalis opticus from the frontal pole is more than twice as long.

A frontopolar approach is only justified if a space-occupying lesion reaches in the polar direction, or if the intervention is limited to the polar region. Not only the short distance of the sphenoid region from N. opticus justifies the short temporofrontal approach propagated by Yaşargil, but also the form of the frontal lobe base: medially to the highly arched orbital roofs the rhinencephalon slopes deeply down to the base; it must be reclined before N. opticus can be visualized (Fig. 86 *A*). On the other hand only minimal reclination of the orbital gyrus above the edge of the small wing of the sphenoid is necessary in order to expose N. opticus at shallow depth (Fig. 86 *B*). Dissection of Arachnoidea of Fissura lat. (Sylvii) with a medial incision is suitable in order to expose N. opticus and A. carotis int. over the easily separated Fissura lat. (Sylvii) (Fig. 86 *B*).

For the direct a-p approach the a-p position of the head is customary. For the temporofrontal approach, rotation of the head by 45° is expedient. Fig. 87 illustrates problems of orientation: with slight rotation of the head by 15°–20° the plane of the two Nn. optici (b) is already perceptibly inclined. Orientation can be hampered especially in the presence of deformity at the base – e.g., due to tumours (Fig. 90). Therefore, in Fig. 87 distance measurements have been given. Under normal conditions orientation is easy if an optic nerve is sought and from there the almost always present dural fold connecting the two Nn. optici is exposed. The falx runs vertically to this fold and marks the midline. For the distance of both Aa. carotis intt. a lower-limit value is given in order to avoid surprises at the dissection of suprasellar space-occupying processes which may mask A. carotis int. The reclination of the brain must be kept to a minimum. The site shown in Fig. 88 with extreme reclination is a composite picture of several operative situations. This is also true of the operation sketches in Figs. 89 and 90. It is indeed possible to visualize such an extended operative field all at once, but this is not to be recommended because of the reactions to be expected as a result of compression of the brain. Such large space-occupying processes are the exception, since after their removal the atrophic brain allows a wide view without endangering the vital functions. The thickening of Planum sphenoidale – e.g., in meningeomas, various tumours of the sphenoid-ethmoid region, etc. – can already be seen preoperatively from the roentgenograms (particularly tomograms).

In such cases, after reduction of the tumour, one N. opticus and one A. carotis int. should next be visualized and then the other N. opticus searched for step by step. Here the distance between Canales optici is usually normal; only the position of Nn. optici may be considerably altered by the space-occupying process (Fig. 90). The illustrated displacement of the terminal stretch of A. carotis int. in the case of space-occupying processes is not an indication of an accompanying displacement of N. opticus, since tumours may also push in between N. opticus and A. carotis int., and a basal displacement of N. opticus and A. carotis int. in the same direction, as shown in Fig. 90, is not obligatory (Hänsel and Seeger, 1977). Drilling out the base medially to Canalis opticus is time-consuming. Particular care must be taken in the vicinity of Canalis opticus. The distance measurements given are intended to facilitate rapid work in those areas where N. opticus or A. carotis int. need not be reckoned with.

For suprasellar processes a combined approach before the two Nn. optici, between N. opticus and A. carotis int., and behind A. carotis int. is often convenient (Figs. 91 and 92). Here it is first necessary to open the medial part of Fissura lat. (Sylvii) by resection of Arachnoidea. In this region the basal cisterns, Cisterna ambiens and Cisterna fissurae lat. (Sylvii), meet. The reclination of Uncus and the orbital gyri in one operative procedure allows an alteration of the approach. It is possible to remove space-occupying lesions step by step from all sides, to expose the hypophyseal stalk from various sides, and to proceed along the tentorial edge as far as the prepontine cistern. If there are no arachnoidal adhesions, the approach is simpler. If adhesions are present they may cover over the perforating arteries from A. chorioidea ant. *(C 5)* and from A. communicans post. *(P 5)*. With large tumours the thickening of Arachnoidea may be welcomed and may facilitate the detachment of the tumour from the surrounding tissue (Yaşargil, 1976). If the Arachnoidea is translucent the approach to small processes – e.g., aneurysms or angiomas of the base of the brain – is easier. A view from the front into the suprasellar space as seen in Figs. 91 and 92 *C* is only exceptionally possible, even here only partially with one setting of the microscope.

E. References

Duvernoy, H. M.: The Superficial Veins of the Human Brain. Veins of the Brain Stem and of the Base of the Brain. Berlin–Heidelberg–New York: Springer. 1975.

Hänsel, G., Seeger, W.: Die mikrochirurgische Behandlung der sogenannten Tuberculum-sellae-Meningeome. Acta Neurochir. **37,** 111–123 (1977).

Huang, Y. P., Wolf, B. S.: In: Advances in Cerebral Angiography, Part I, Anatomy: Variations of Basal Cerebral Veins: Embryologic Considerations, p. 82. Berlin–Heidelberg–New York: Springer. 1975.

Kaplan, A.: The lateral perforating branch of the anterior and middle cerebral arteries. Neurosurg. **23,** 305–310 (1965).

Kribs, N., Kleihues, P.: The Recurrent Artery of Heubner. In: Cerebral Circulation and Stroke, editor Zülch, K. J., pp. 40–56. Berlin–Heidelberg–New York: Springer. 1971.

Marino, R., Jr.: The anterior cerebral artery: I. Anatoma-radiological study of its cortical territories. Surg. Neurol. **5,** Feb. 1976.

Mauritz, A.: Das Verteilungsmuster der Rr. perforantes aus A. chorioidea ant. und A. communicans post. Dissertation Freiburg 1978 (in Vorbereitung).

Ostrowski, A. Z., et al.: The proximal anterior cerebral artery: An anatomic study. Arch. Neurol. **3,** 661–664 (1960).

Perlmutter, D., Rhoton, A. L., Jr.: Microsurgical anatomy of the anterior cerebralanterior communicating-recurrent artery complex. J. Neurosurg. **45,** 259–272 (1976).

Renn, H. W., Rhoton, L.: Microsurgical anatomy of the sellar region. J. Neurosurg. **43,** 288–298 (1975).

Seeger, W.: Die opto-chiasmalen Arachnoidalzysten. Dissertation Tübingen 1955.

Sugita, K., Hirota, T., Tsugane, R.: Application of nasopharyngeal mirror for aneurysm operation. Technical note. J. Neurosurg. **43**, 244–246 (1975).

Stephens, R. B., Stilwell, D. L.: Arteries and Veins of the Human Brain. Springfield, Ill.: Ch. C Thomas. 1969.

Yaşargil, M. G., Antic, M. D. J., Laciga, R., Jain, K. K., Hodosh, R. M., Smith, R. D.: Microsurgical pterional approach to aneurysms of the basilar bifurcation. Surgical Neurol. **6**, 83–91 (1976).

Literature for Further Reading

Dunker, R. O., Harris, A. B.: Surgical anatomy of the proximal anterior cerebral artery. J. Neurosurg. **44**, 359–367 (1976).

Koos, W. Th., Böck, F. W. (Editors): Clinical Microneurosurgery. Stuttgart: Thieme. 1976.

Newton, Th., Potts, D. G.: Radiology of the Skull and Brain Angiography. S. Louis: The C. V. Mosby Company. 1974.

Nutik, St., Dilenge, D.: Carotid-anterior cerebral artery anastomosis. J. Neurosurg. **44**, 378–382 (1976).

F. Illustrations

(Figs. 53 to 92)

The illustrations to this and the following chapters contain measurements in millimetres (mm)
We are dealing with approximate measurements. Only where special danger of injury exists are borderline values given; statistical precision is not attempted; the figures are meant to be a useful guide for operative technique.

Fig. 53. Positional relationships between Fissura longitudinalis, Gyrus praecentralis, Insula and Polus frontalis
Watch position of Insula and A. operculofront.
Measurements in millimetres (mm)

FIG. 53

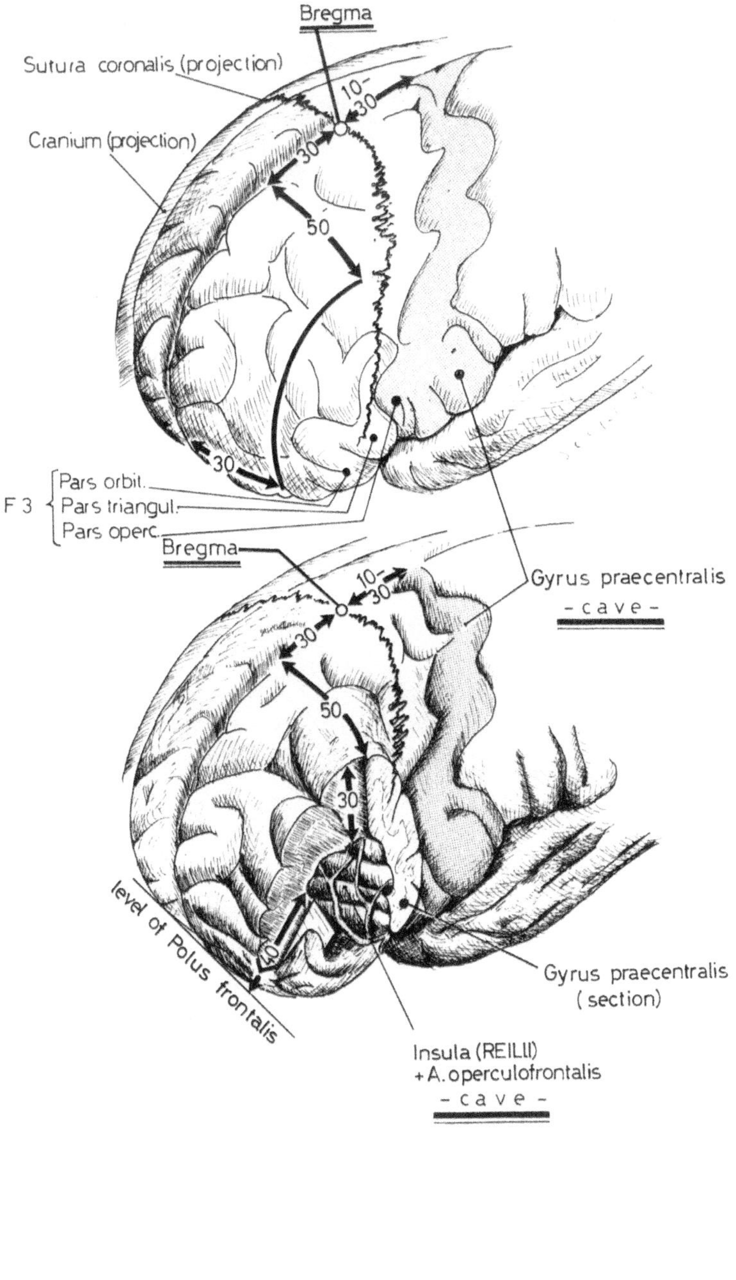
Bregma
Sutura coronalis (projection)
Cranium (projection)
10-30
30
50
30
F 3
Pars orbit.
Pars triangul.
Pars operc.
Bregma
10-30
30
50
30
40
Gyrus praecentralis
- c a v e -
level of Polus frontalis
Gyrus praecentralis
(section)
Insula (REILII)
+ A. operculofrontalis
- c a v e -

Fig. 54. Positional relationships of frontal lobe in Fissura longitudinalis and at the base. Localization of Genu corporis callosi, Lamina terminalis, and projections of the levels of Cornu anterius, Caudatum, Putamen, and Insula. The anterior border of Substantia perforata ant. corresponds to the T-shaped terminal bifurcation of A. carotis int.
?: Variable distances of A. pericallosa from Corpus callosum
Measurements in millimetres (mm)

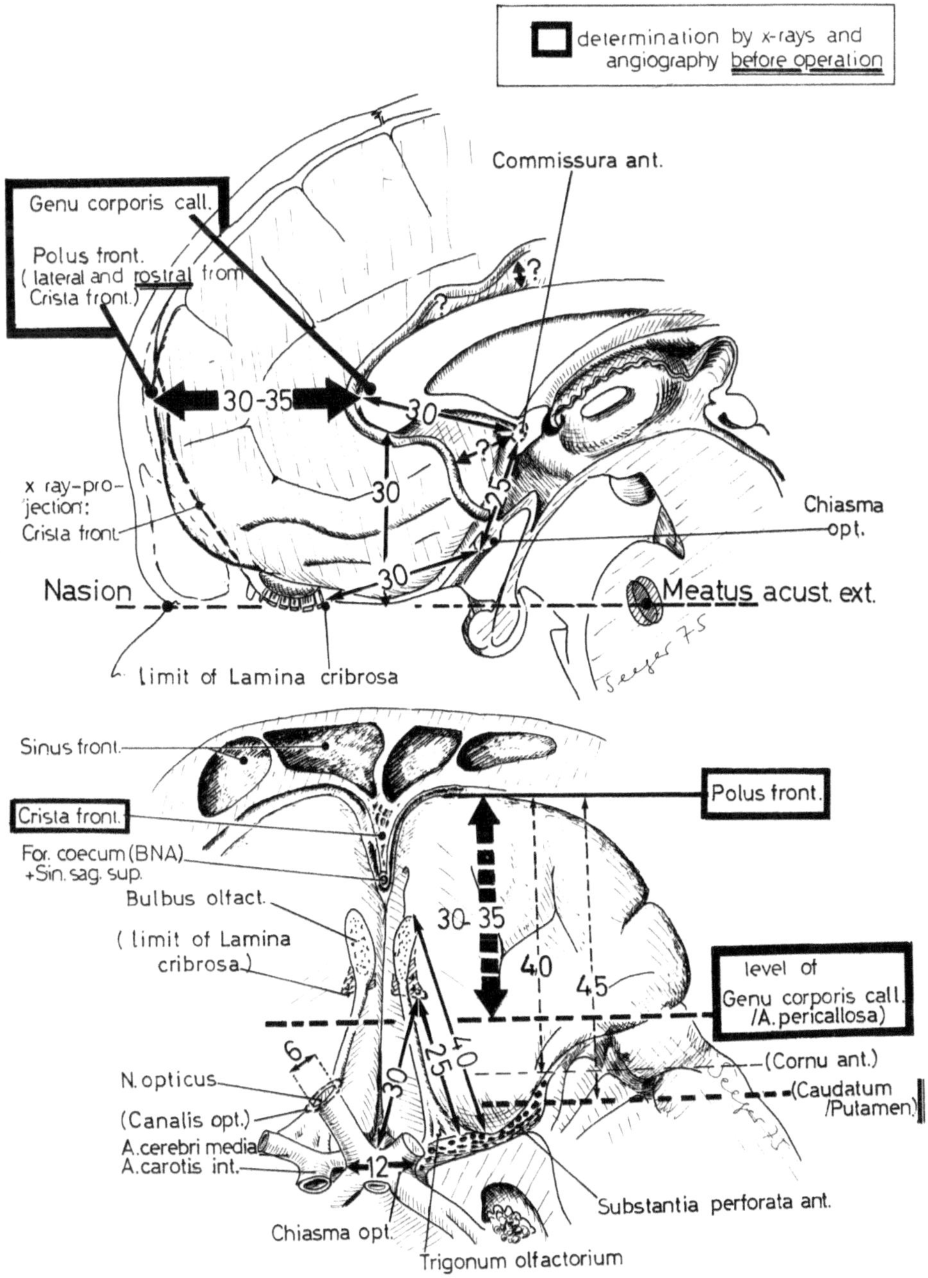
determination by x-rays and angiography before operation
Genu corporis call.
Polus front.
(lateral and rostral from Crista front.)
Commissura ant.
30-35
30
30
30
x ray-projection:
Crista front.
Chiasma opt.
Nasion
Meatus acust. ext.
limit of Lamina cribrosa
Sinus front.
Polus front.
Crista front.
For. coecum (BNA) +Sin. sag. sup.
Bulbus olfact.
(limit of Lamina cribrosa)
30-35
40
45
level of Genu corporis call. /A. pericallosa)
6
40
25
30
N. opticus
(Canalis opt.)
A. cerebri media
A. carotis int.
12
(Cornu ant.)
(Caudatum /Putamen)
Substantia perforata ant.
Chiasma opt.
Trigonum olfactorium

Fig. 55. Frontal section less than 50 mm distant from the frontal lobe pole (section plane *I*).
□: Structures in the vicinity of the section plane
II Section plane of Fig. 56

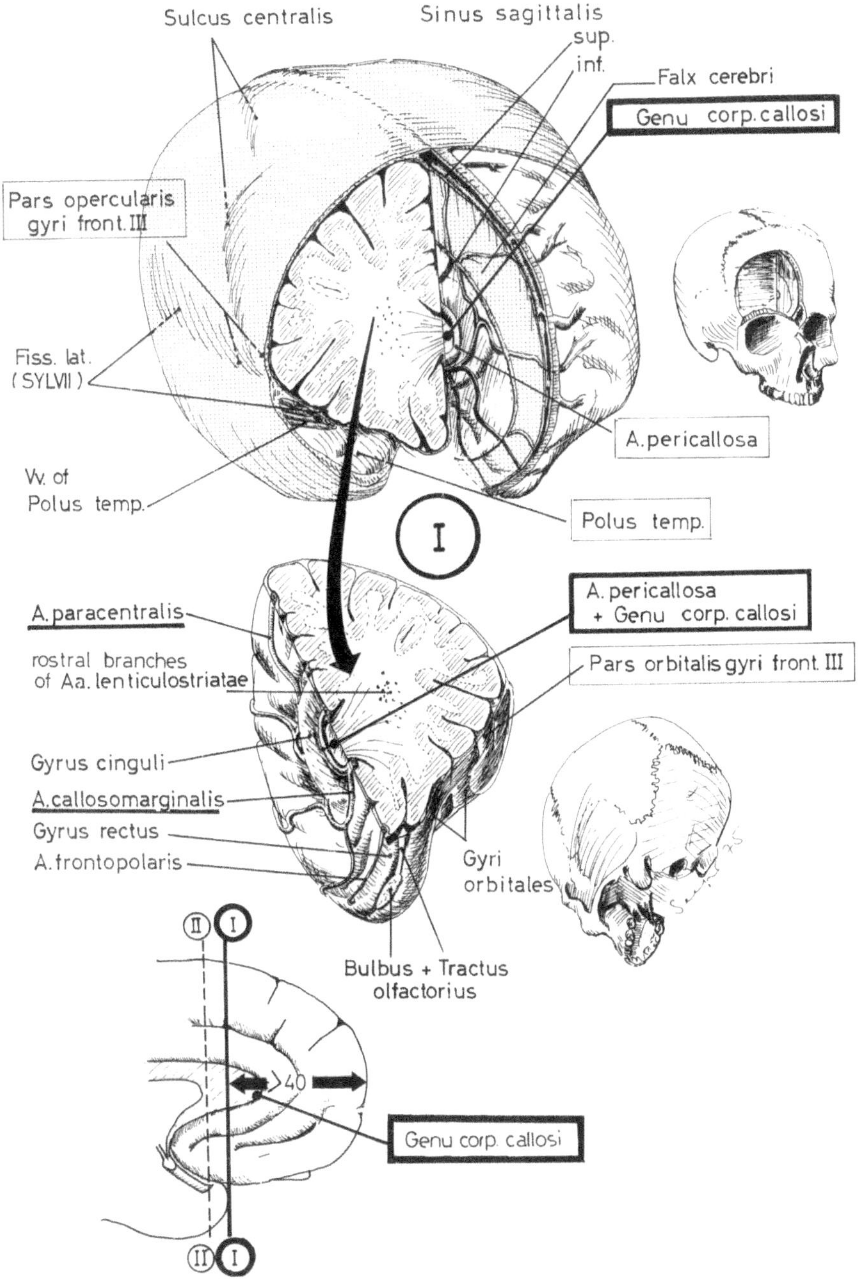
Sulcus centralis
Sinus sagittalis
sup.
inf.
Falx cerebri
Genu corp. callosi
Pars opercularis gyri front. III
Fiss. lat. (SYLVII)
A. pericallosa
Vv. of Polus temp.
Polus temp.
I
A. paracentralis
rostral branches of Aa. lenticulostriatae
A. pericallosa + Genu corp. callosi
Pars orbitalis gyri front. III
Gyrus cinguli
A. callosomarginalis
Gyrus rectus
A. frontopolaris
Gyri orbitales
Bulbus + Tractus olfactorius
II
I
>40
Genu corp. callosi
II
I

Fig. 56. Frontal section 60 mm distant from frontal lobe pole (section plane *II*). For nomenclature see Fig. 55
I Section plane of Fig. 55

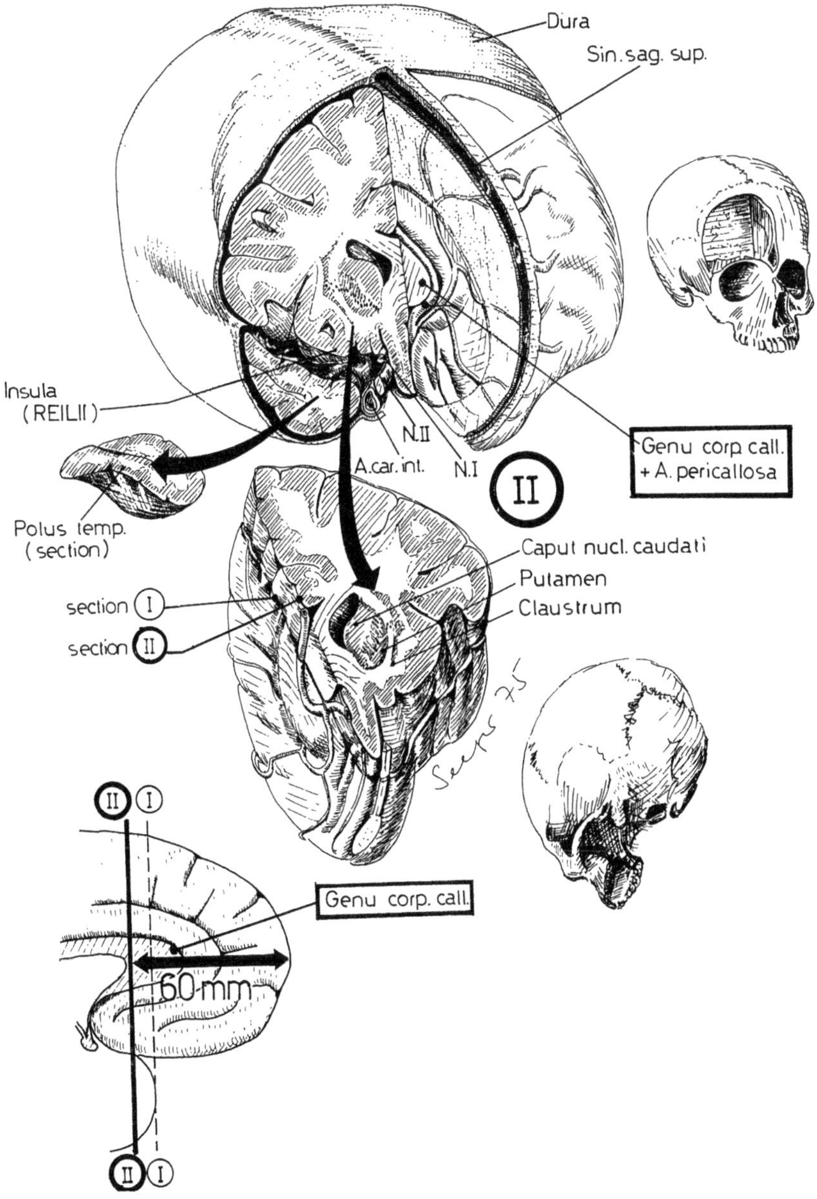
Dura
Sin. sag. sup.
Insula
(REILII)
N.II
A.car.int.
N.I
Genu corp. call.
+ A. pericallosa
II
Polus temp.
(section)
Caput nucl. caudati
Putamen
Claustrum
section I
section II
II I
Genu corp. call.
60 mm
II I

Fig. 57. Projection planes placed tangentially to Genu corp. call., the tip of Cornu ant., and the transition between Caudatum and Putamen. The distances of these structures from the pole of the frontal lobe differ by only up to 15 mm

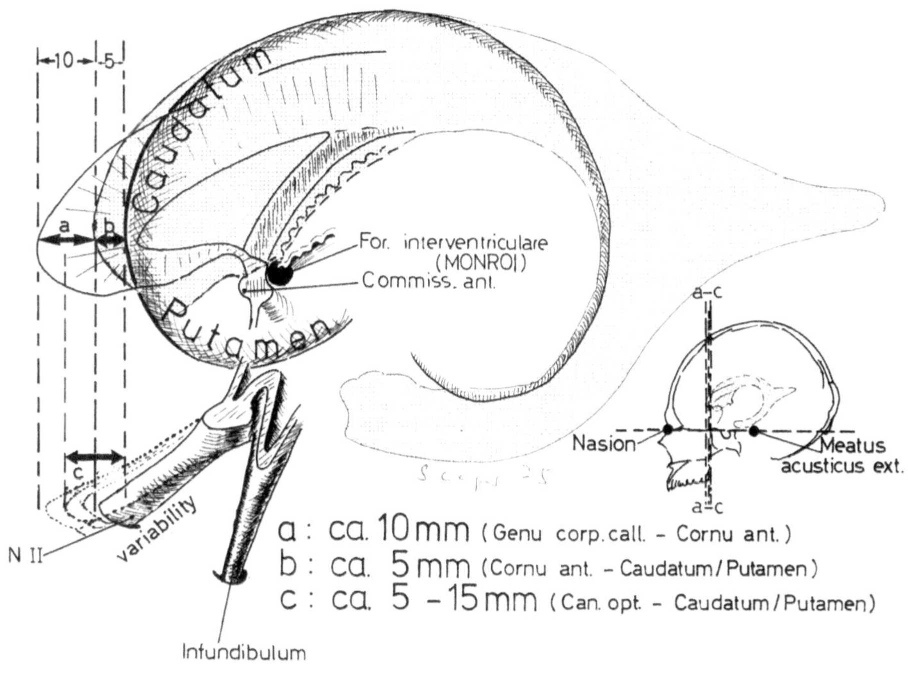
10
5
Caudatum
Putamen
a
b
c
For. interventriculare
(MONROI)
Commiss. ant.
variability
N II
Infundibulum
a–c
Nasion
Meatus
acusticus ext.
a : ca. 10 mm (Genu corp. call. – Cornu ant.)
b : ca. 5 mm (Cornu ant. – Caudatum/Putamen)
c : ca. 5 – 15 mm (Can. opt. – Caudatum/Putamen)

Fig. 58
A Positional relationships of Sulcus cinguli (A. callosomarginalis) to the surface of Fissura longitudinalis cerebri to Insula and to Polus front.
B Positional relationships between tip of Cornu ant., Insula, A. pericallosa, and Genu corporis call. Corona radiata between Insula and tip of Cornu ant. only approx. 5 mm wide in this preparation
C Cornu ant. opened wider than in *B*
Cave injury to A. operculo-frontalis and Insula and underlying basal ganglia! Cave Genu corp. call. + A. pericallosa + callosomarginalis! Measurements in millimetres (mm)

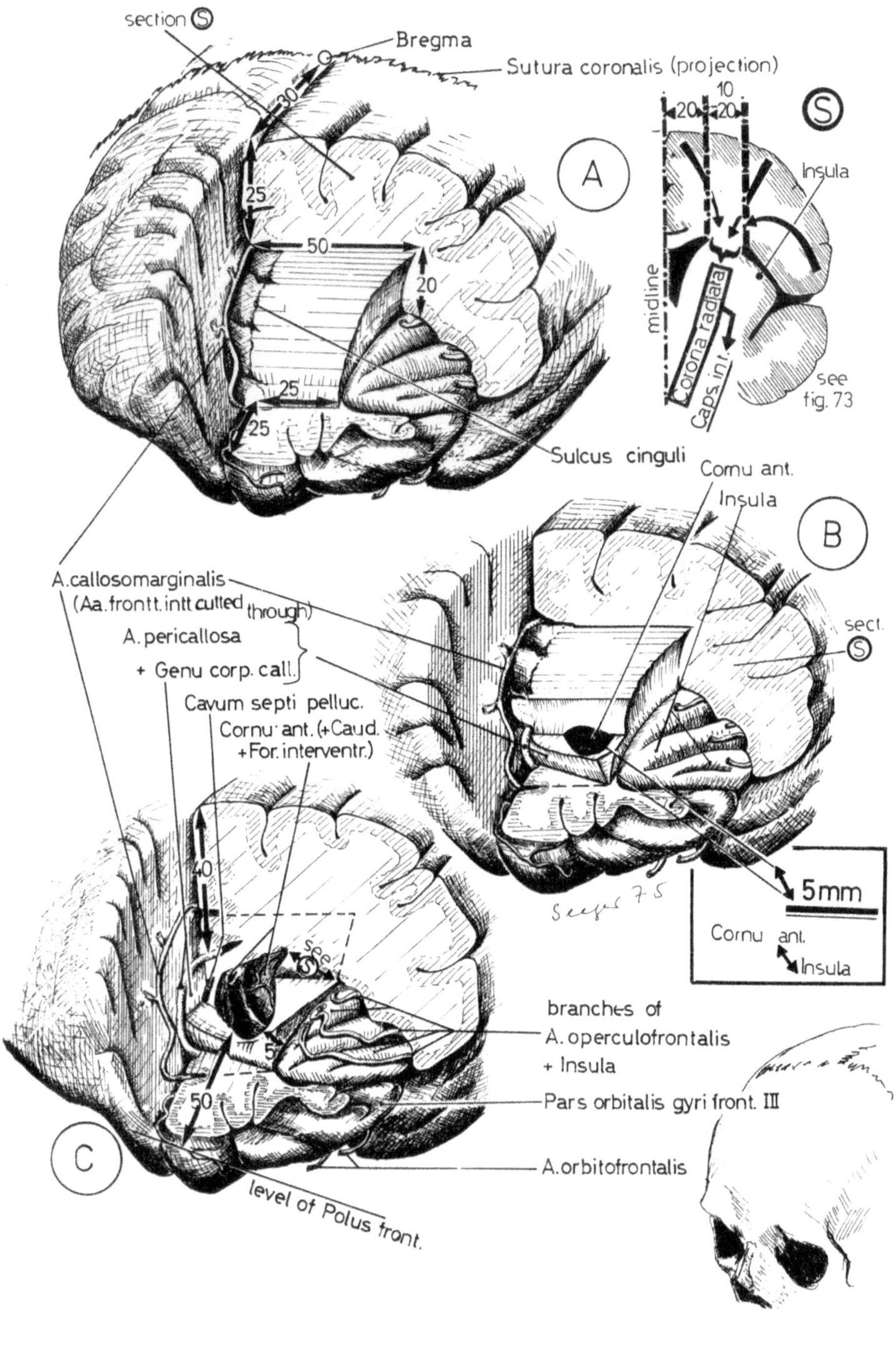
section Ⓢ
Bregma
Sutura coronalis (projection)
30
25
50
20
25
25
A
Ⓢ
10
20
20
Insula
midline
Corona radiata
Caps. int.
see fig. 73
Sulcus cinguli
Cornu ant.
Insula
B
sect. Ⓢ
A. callosomarginalis
(Aa. frontt. intt cutted through)
A. pericallosa
+ Genu corp. call.
Cavum septi pelluc.
Cornu ant. (+Caud. +For. interventr.)
40
see Ⓢ
5
50
C
5mm
Cornu ant.
Insula
branches of
A. operculofrontalis
+ Insula
Pars orbitalis gyri front. III
A. orbitofrontalis
level of Polus front.

Fig. 59
A and *C*
I Section plane of Fig. 55 } Figs. 61 and 62 in
II Section plane of Fig. 56 } similar regions
B Nomenclature of structures illustrated in Figs. 60 and 61

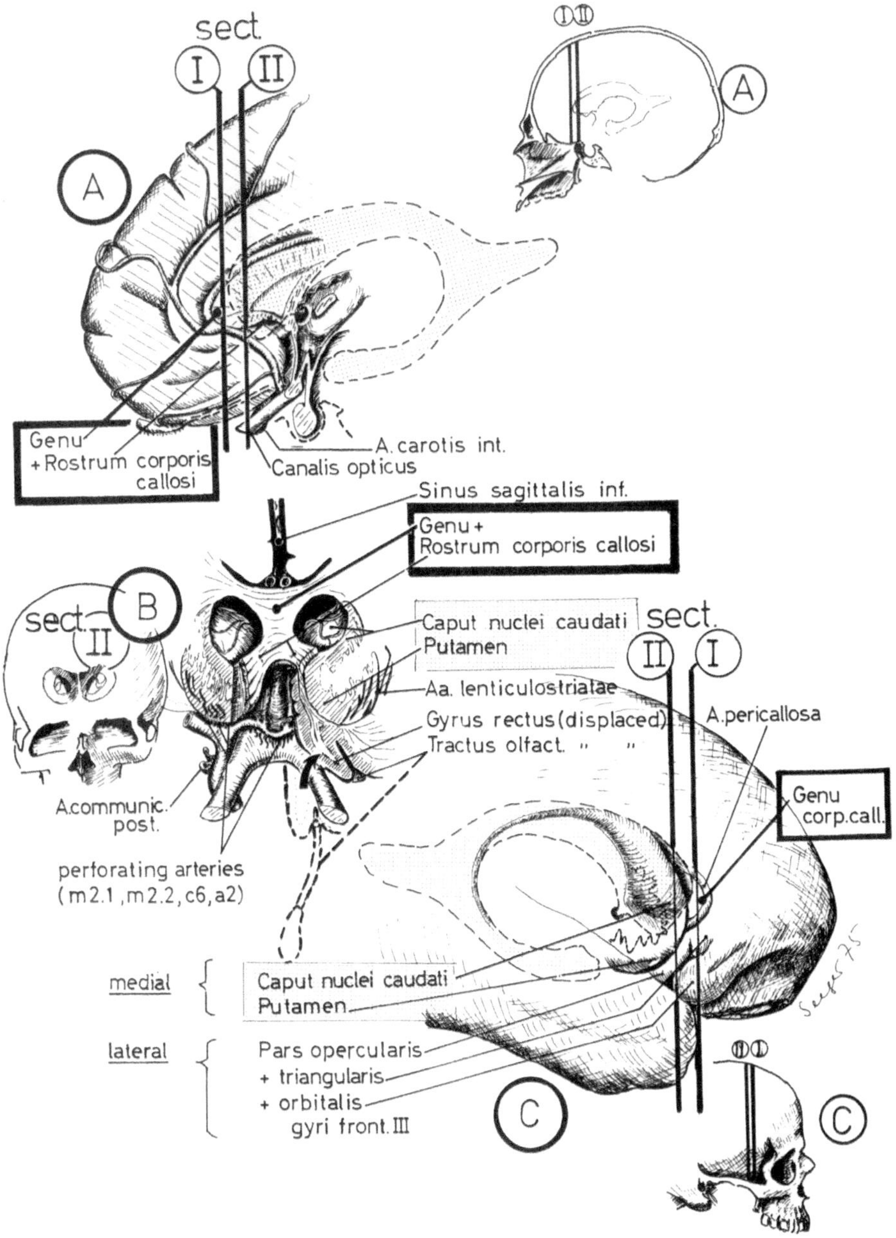
sect.
I
II
A
I II
A
Genu
+ Rostrum corporis callosi
A. carotis int.
Canalis opticus
Sinus sagittalis inf.
Genu +
Rostrum corporis callosi
B
sect. II
Caput nuclei caudati
Putamen
sect.
II
I
Aa. lenticulostriatae
Gyrus rectus (displaced)
Tractus olfact. " "
A. pericallosa
Genu corp. call.
A. communic. post.
perforating arteries
(m2.1, m2.2, c6, a2)
medial
Caput nuclei caudati
Putamen
lateral
Pars opercularis
+ triangularis
+ orbitalis
gyri front. III
C
II I
C

Fig. 60. Fissura longitudinalis ant. in front of the opened Lamina terminalis with Commissura ant.

A In front of Genu corp. call.

B In front of Commissura ant. with bilateral ventricular opening

Note the thin layer of Pallium (Area subcallosa + Rostrum corp., call.) over Putamen, and between Fissura longitudinalis and ventricular system

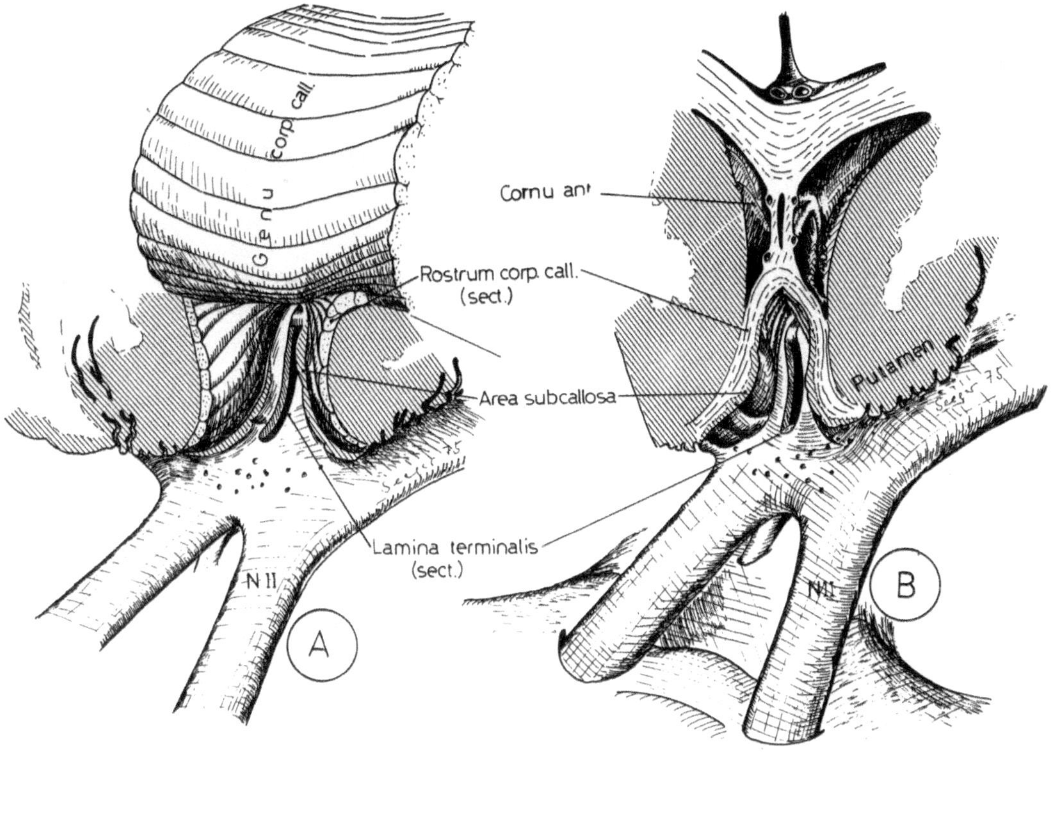
Genu corp. call.
Cornu ant
Rostrum corp. call. (sect.)
Area subcallosa
Putamen
Lamina terminalis (sect.)
N II
A
B

Fig. 61. Positional relationships between terminal branching of A. carotis int., Substantia perforata ant., and its continuation in the basal portion of Lamina terminalis
Note the diverging course of the medial and lateral perforating arteries. Medial groups downwards, lateral groups upwards, corresponding to the bulge of Lamina terminalis and the troughshaped retraction of Substantia perforata ant.

FIG. 61

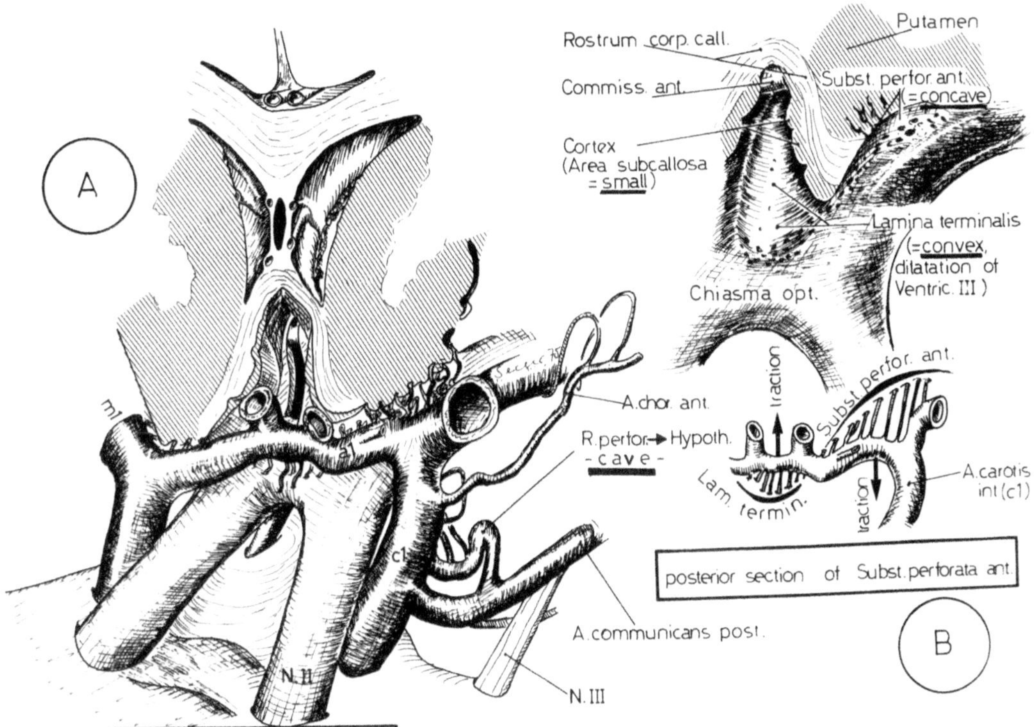
A
m1
c1
A.chor. ant.
R.perfor.→ Hypoth.
- cave -
A.communicans post.
N.II
N.III
anterior section of Subst.perforata ant
Putamen
Rostrum corp. call.
Commiss. ant.
Subst. perfor. ant.
(= concave)
Cortex
(Area subcallosa
= small)
Lamina terminalis
(= convex,
dilatation of
Ventric. III)
Chiasma opt.
Subst. perfor. ant.
traction
traction
Lam. termin.
A.carotis
int (c1)
posterior section of Subst.perforata ant.
B

Fig. 62. Illustration of Lamina terminalis and its neighbouring structures after frontal section of right frontal lobe with longitudinal section of Genu corp. call.

A Without vessels

B With arteries

For nomenclature see Fig. 61

FIG. 62

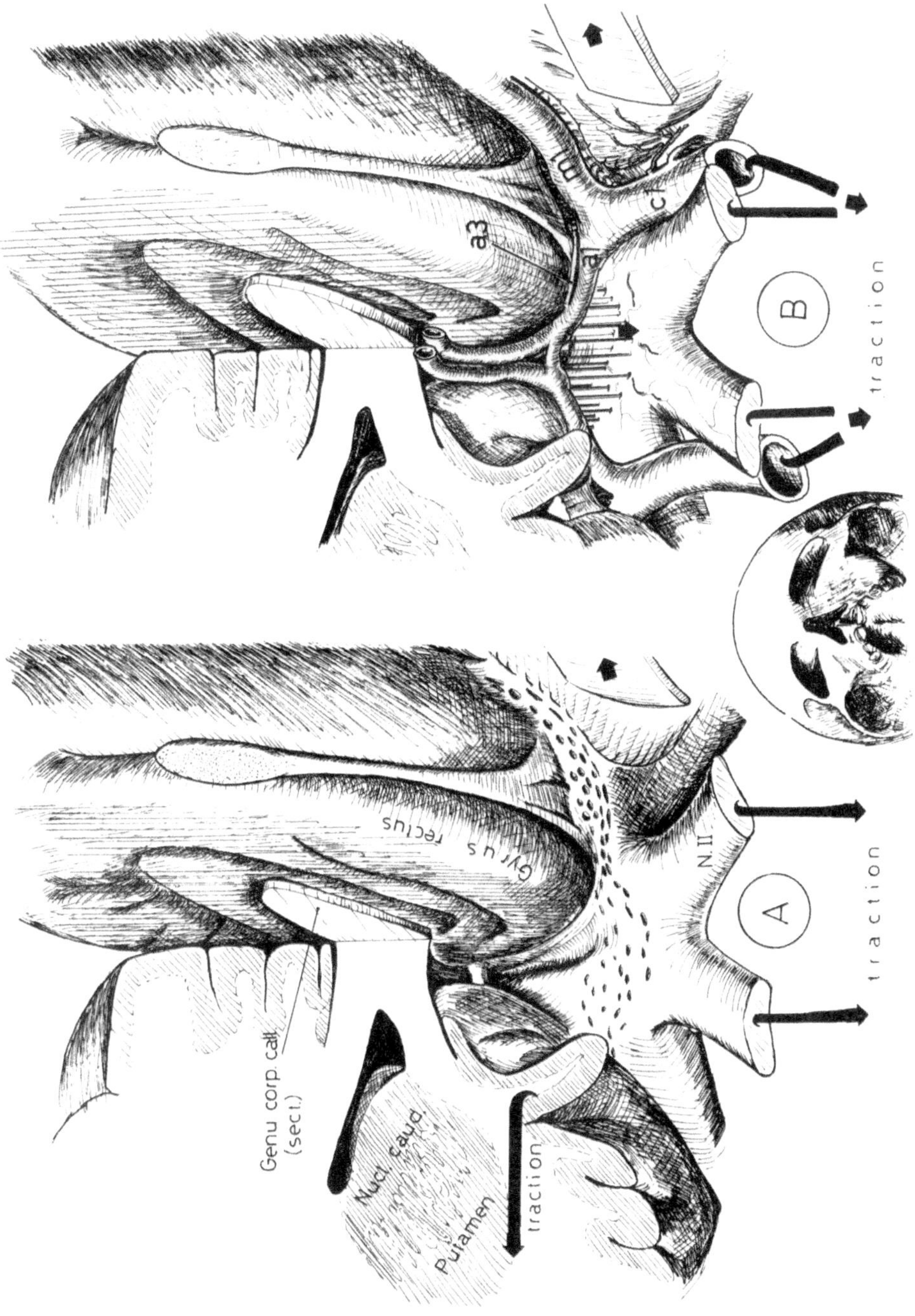
Genu corp. call. (sect.)
Nucl. caud.
Putamen
traction
Gyrus rectus
N.II
A
traction
a3
B
traction

Figs. 63 and 64. Variations in anterior regions of Circulus arteriosus (Willisi) according to Perlmutter and Rhoton (1976, modified). Variable courses of A. recurrens (Heubneri), duplications of proximal anterior segments (*D*), and of A. communicans ant. (*B, C, D, E*). Pronounced meandering of A. cerebri anterior (*A, F*); trifurcation of A. cerebri anterior (*G*)

Fig. 63

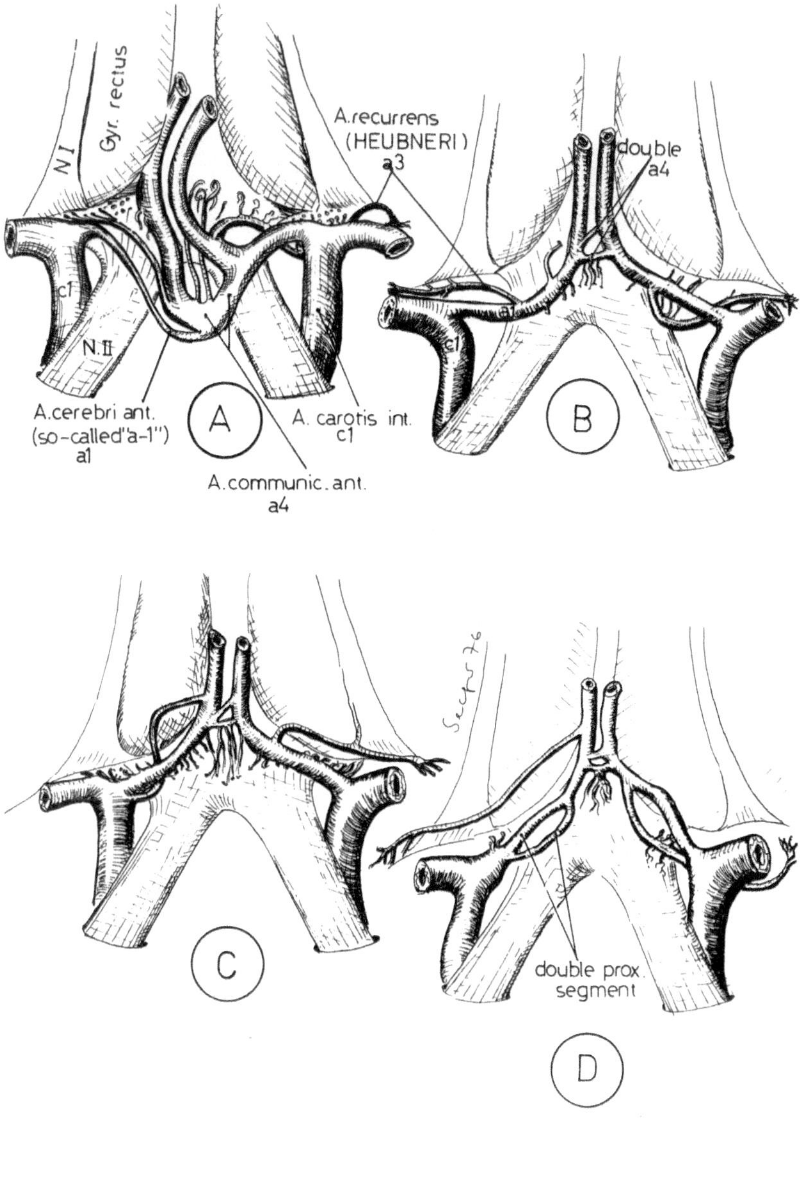
Gyr. rectus
N I
A.recurrens
(HEUBNERI)
a3
c1
N.II
A.cerebri ant.
(so-called "a-1")
a1
A
A. carotis int.
c1
A.communic. ant.
a4
double
a4
a1
c1
B
C
double prox.
segment
D

FIG. 64

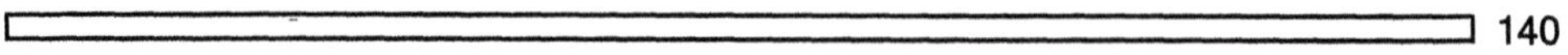

Fig. 64

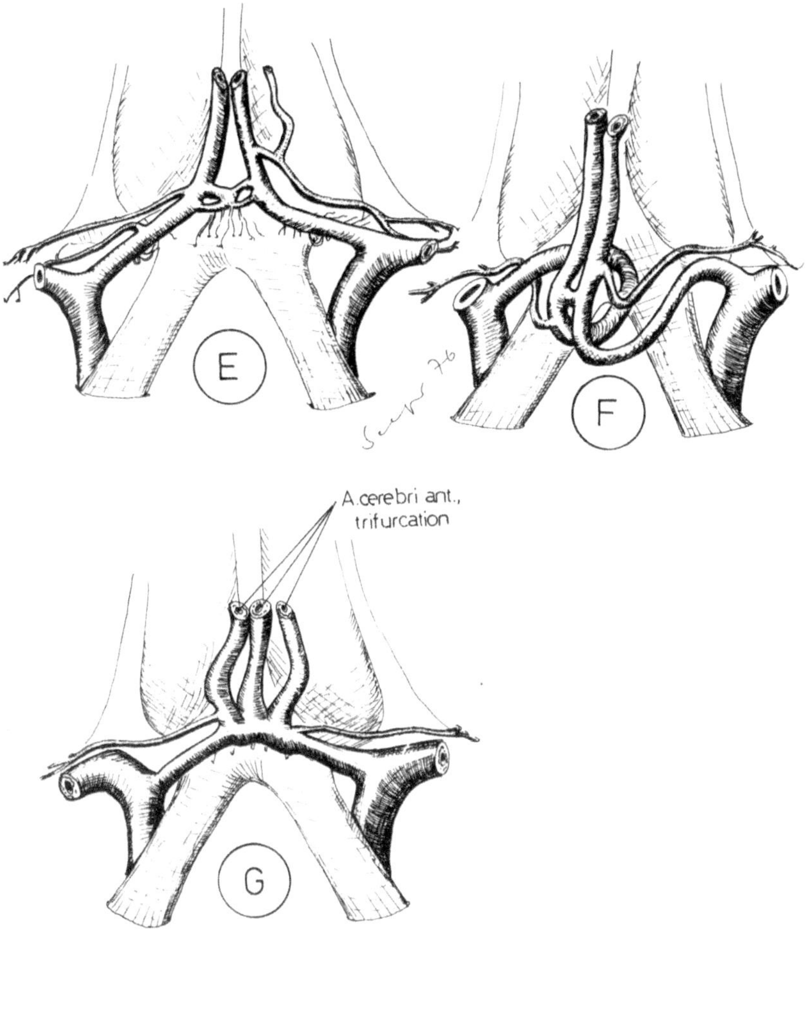
E
F
A.cerebri ant.,
trifurcation
G

Fig. 65. Partial double supply of medial surfaces of both hemispheres from one A. cerebri ant. (Drawing from data given by Marino, 1976)
The case *D* corresponds to Perlmutter's and Rhoton's example *G*

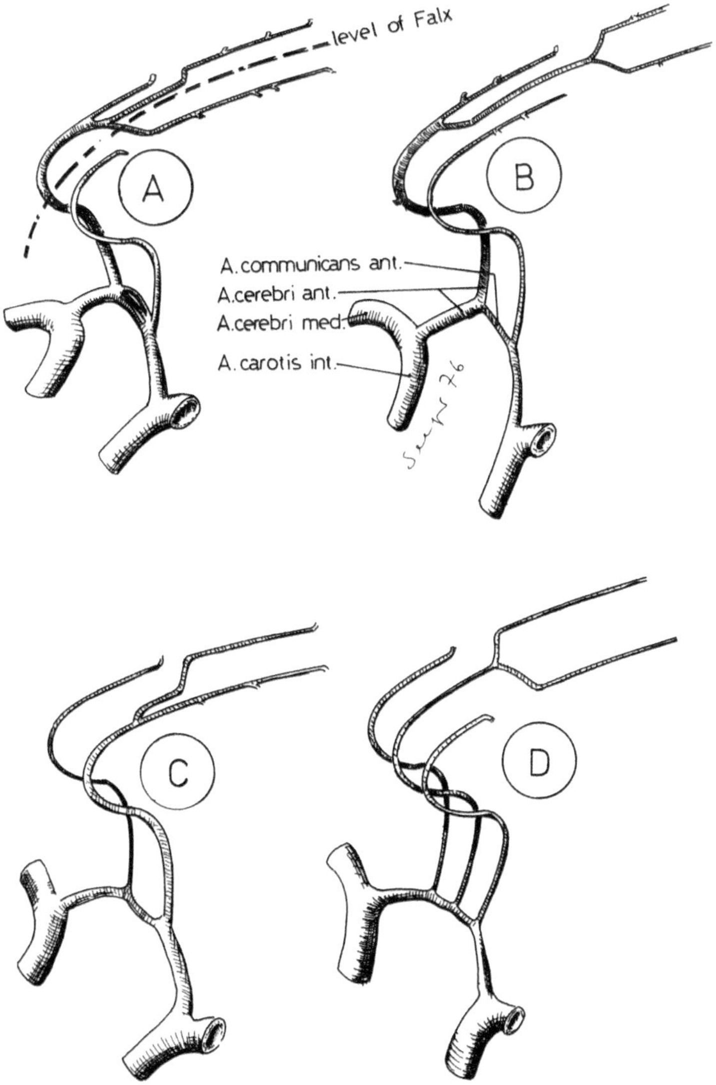
level of Falx
A
B
A.communicans ant.
A.cerebri ant.
A.cerebri med.
A.carotis int.
C
D

Fig. 66
A Perforating arteries in the region of Cisterna chiasmatis and interpeduncularis
B Arachnoid membranes (continuous lines) and arachnoid trabeculae (interrupted heavy lines), which sheath the perforating arteries (see *A*). In the vicinity of Uncus, arachnoid membrane and trabecular system pulled apart (light arrow). Penetration point of N. oculomotorius correspondingly pushed away from Uncus

a Arachnoidea between Uncus and tentorial edge
b Trabecula between A. carotis int. and N. oculomotorius
c Fissura longitudinalis cerebri
d Arachnoid border of Cisterna fissurae lat. (Sylvii)
e Approach to Cisterna chiasmatis from the front
f Approach to Cisterna chiasmatis between N. opticus and A. carotis int.
g Approach to Cisterna chiasmatis and interpeduncularis from the side

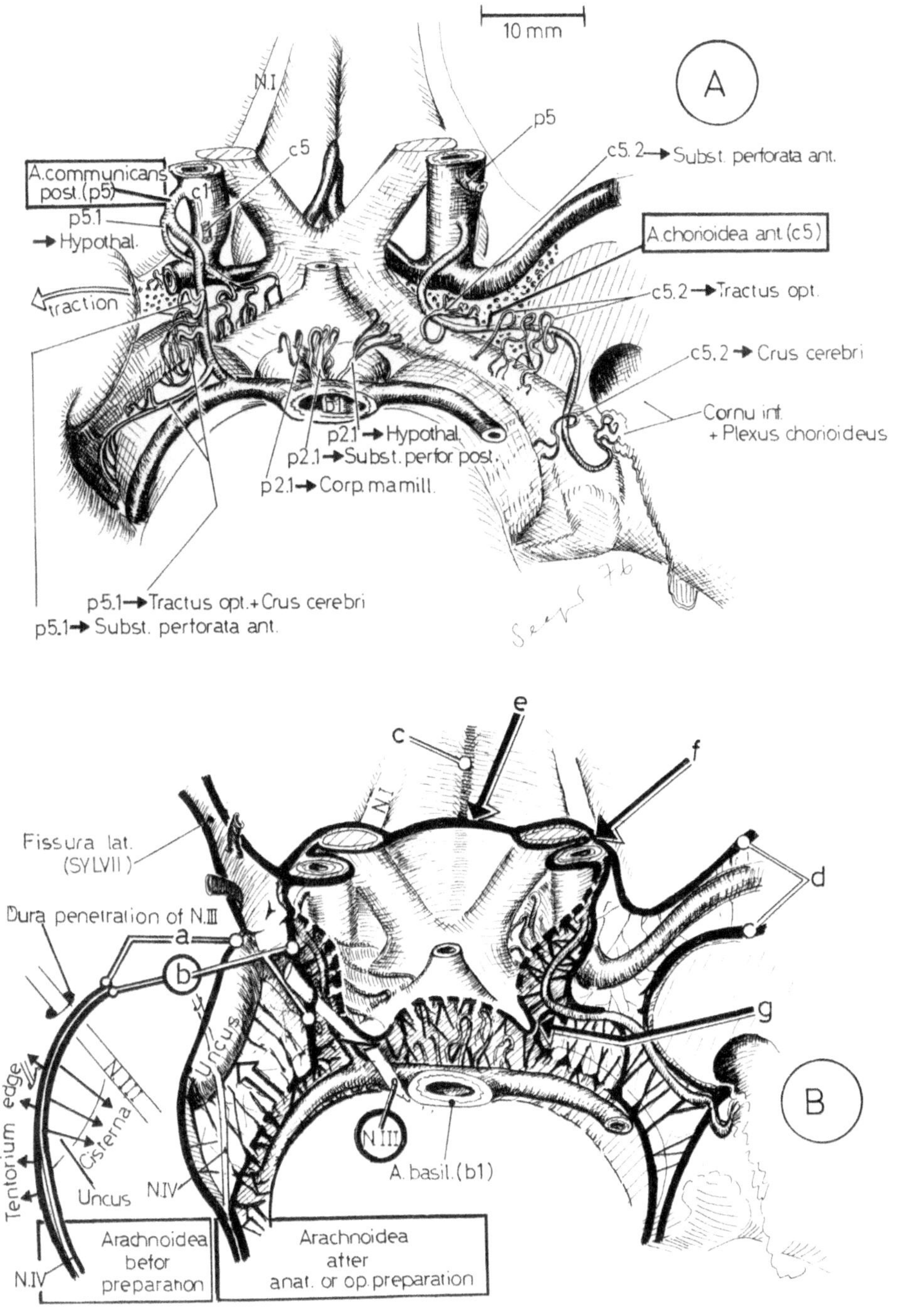
10 mm
A
N.I
p5
c5
A.communicans post.(p5)
c1
p5.1
→ Hypothal.
traction
c5.2 → Subst. perforata ant.
A.chorioidea ant.(c5)
c5.2 → Tractus opt.
c5.2 → Crus cerebri
Cornu int. + Plexus chorioideus
b1
p2.1 → Hypothal.
p2.1 → Subst. perfor. post.
p2.1 → Corp. mamill.
p5.1 → Tractus opt. + Crus cerebri
p5.1 → Subst. perforata ant.
B
e
c
f
N.I
Fissura lat. (SYLVII)
d
Dura penetration of N.III
a
b
g
Uncus
N.III
Cisterna
Tentorium edge
Uncus
N.IV
N.III
A. basil. (b1)
N.IV
Arachnoidea befor preparation
Arachnoidea after anat. or op. preparation

Fig. 67. Venous courses at the anterior cerebral base (according to data of Duvernoy, 1975):

1 Anterior communicating vein
2 Anterior cerebral vein
3 Inferior striate veins
4 Vein of the orbital lobe
5 Interpeduncular vein
6 Posterior communicating vein
7 Premamillary arch
8 Longitudinal tuberal vein
9 Anterior median pontine vein
10 Vein communication to Plexus basilaris of Clivus

FIG. 67

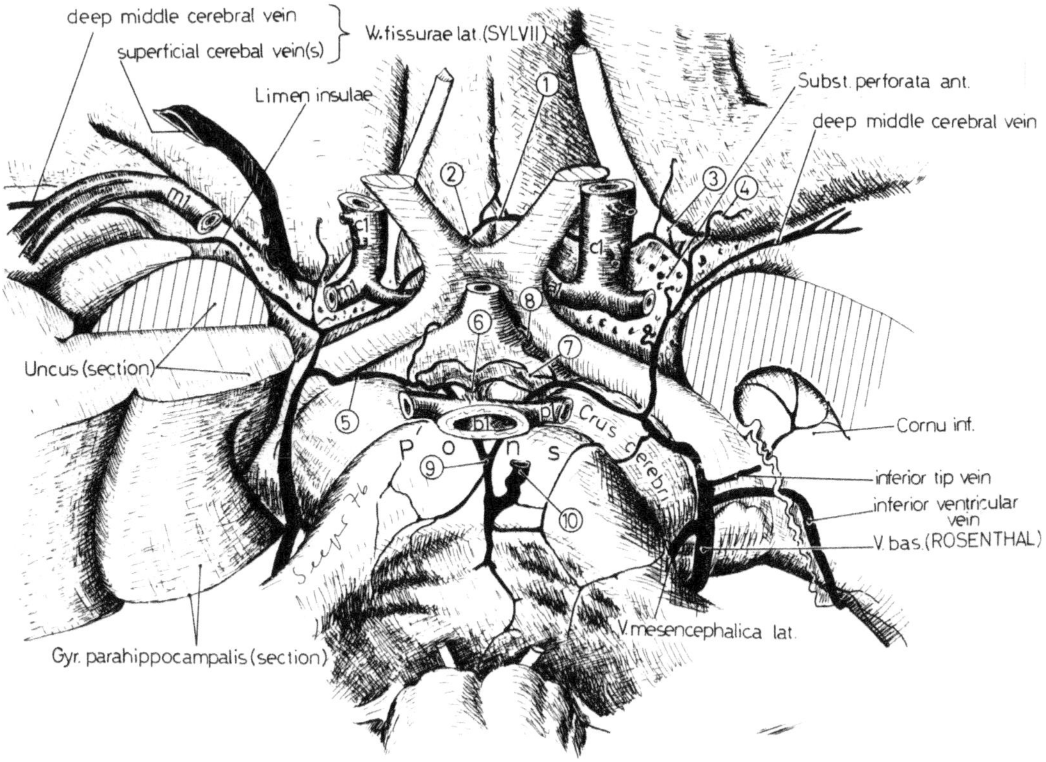
deep middle cerebral vein
superficial cerebal vein(s)
V. fissurae lat. (SYLVII)
Limen insulae
Subst. perforata ant.
deep middle cerebral vein
Uncus (section)
Cornu inf.
inferior tip vein
inferior ventricular vein
V. bas. (ROSENTHAL)
V. mesencephalica lat.
Gyr. parahippocampalis (section)
Pons
Crus cerebri
m1
c1
a1
bk
p1
1
2
3
4
5
6
7
8
9
10

Fig. 68
A View of Cisterna optica from behind (midbrain section). For arterial nomenclature see arterial catalogue
B General view for *A* and *C* (*C* turned by 180°)
C Distribution pattern of perforating arteries after examination of 50 brains (Mauritz, 1977)

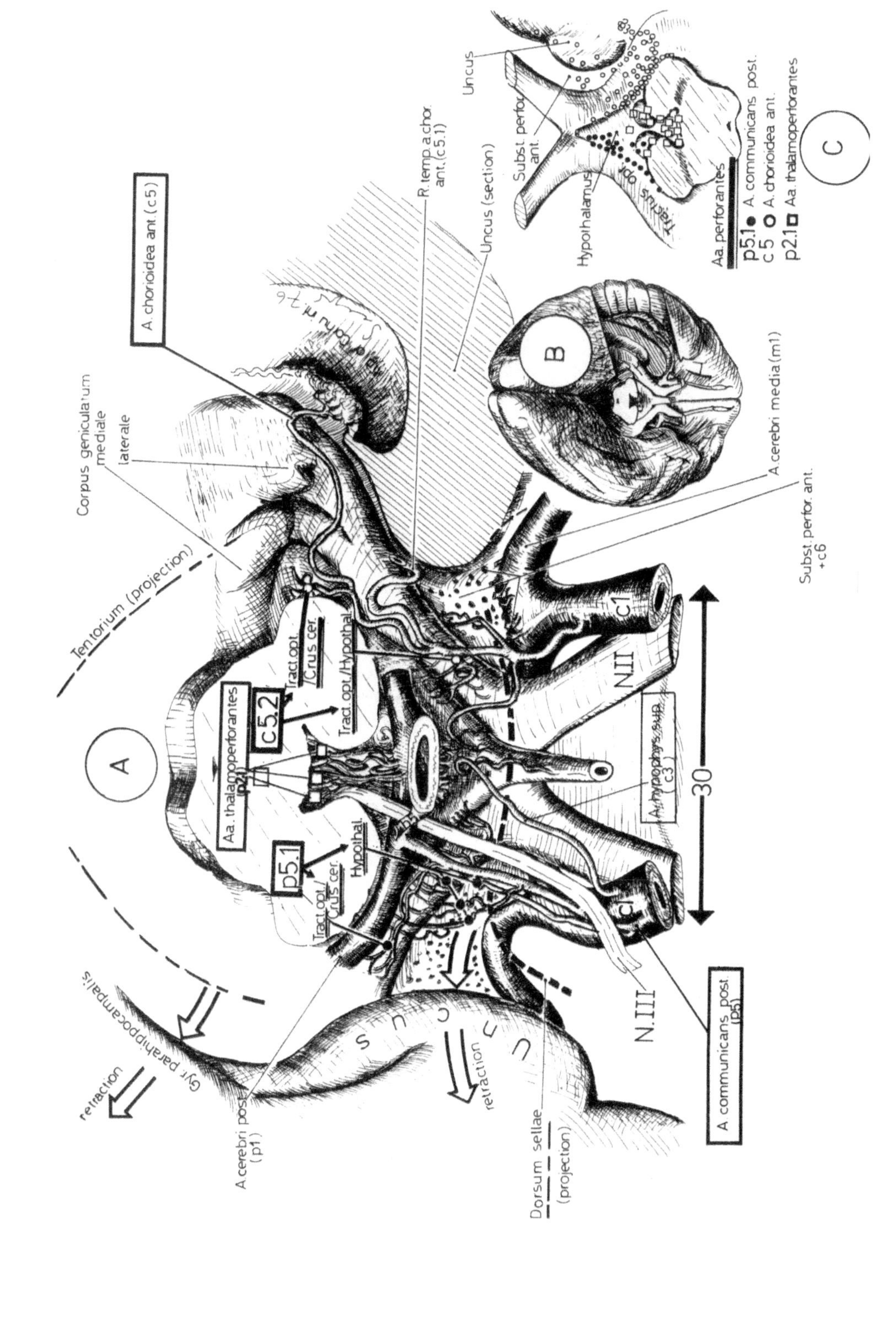
A
B
C
Tentorium (projection)
Corpus geniculatum mediale
laterale
A. chorioidea ant. (c5)
R. temp. a. chor. ant. (c5.1)
Uncus (section)
Uncus
Subst. perfor. ant.
Hypothalamus
Tractus opt.
Aa. perforantes
p5.1 ● A. communicans post.
c5 ○ A. chorioidea ant.
p2.1 □ Aa. thalamoperforantes
A. cerebri media (m1)
Subst. perfor. ant. +c6
Aa. thalamoperforantes (p2.1)
c5.2
Tract. opt.
Crus cer.
Tract. opt./Hypothal.
p5.1
Tract. opt./ crus cer.
Hypothal.
A. hypophys. sup. (c3)
N.II
c1
30
N.III
A communicans post. (p5)
Gyr. parahippocampalis
retraction
A. cerebri post. (p1)
Dorsum sellae (projection)

Figs. 69 and 70. Localization of a right frontal space-occupying intracerebral process. Localization of branches of A. cerebri ant., especially A. paracentralis (*A*), determination of the junction of the communicating veins with the upper Sinus sagittalis sup. by additional angiographic oblique projection (*C*). X-ray projection of the focus onto the surface of the skull before siting the trepanation (*D* and *E*)

Nomenclature:

a–c Junctions of cerebral veins into Sinus sagitt. sup.

d Nasion – lower border of tumour-projection field

e Bregma – upper border of tumour-projection field

f Midline – lateral border of tumour-projection field

g Nasion – roof of Sinus frontalis

Fig. 69

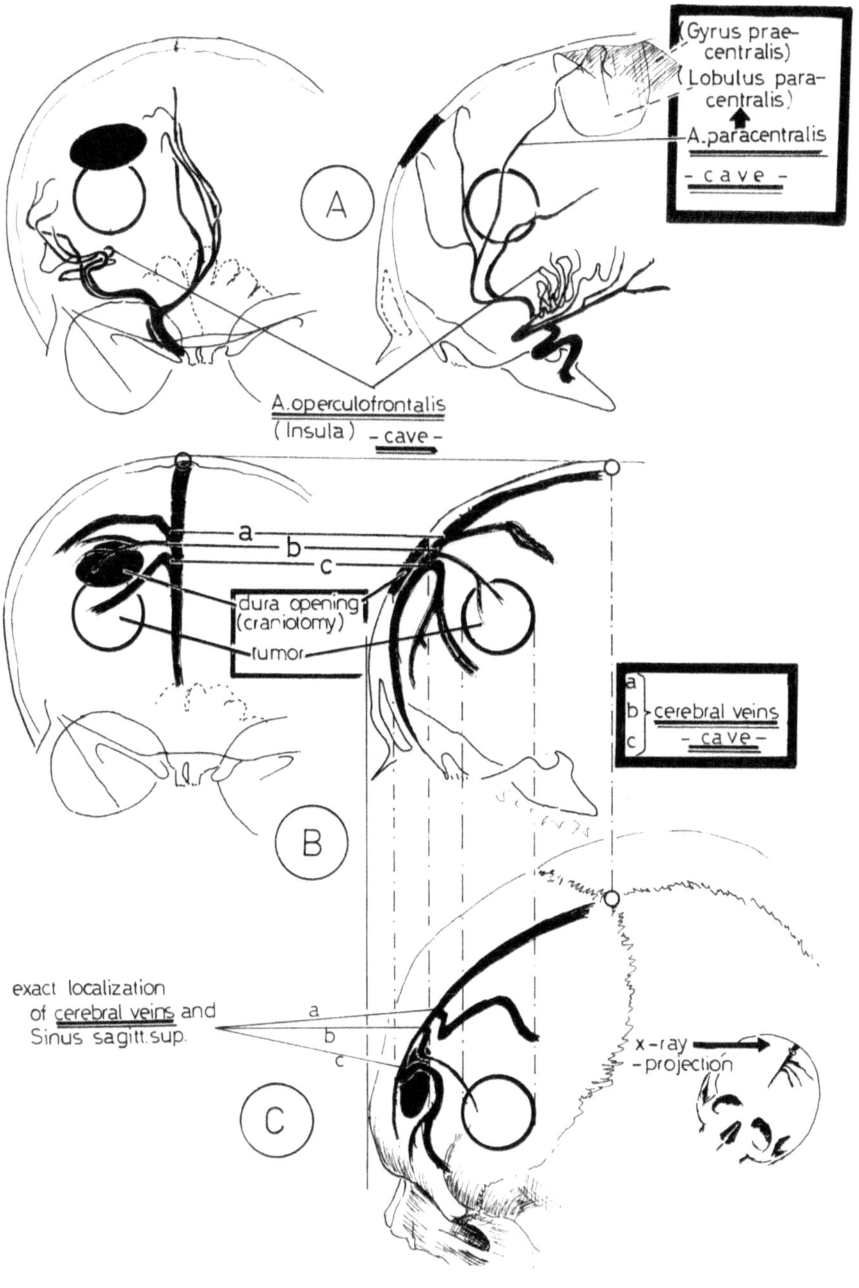
(Gyrus prae-
centralis)
(Lobulus para-
centralis)
A.paracentralis
- cave -
A
A.operculofrontalis
(Insula) - cave -
a
b
c
dura opening
(craniotomy)
tumor
a
b
c
cerebral veins
- cave -
B
exact localization
of cerebral veins and
Sinus sagitt.sup.
a
b
c
x-ray
-projection
C

FIG. 70

152

Fig. 70

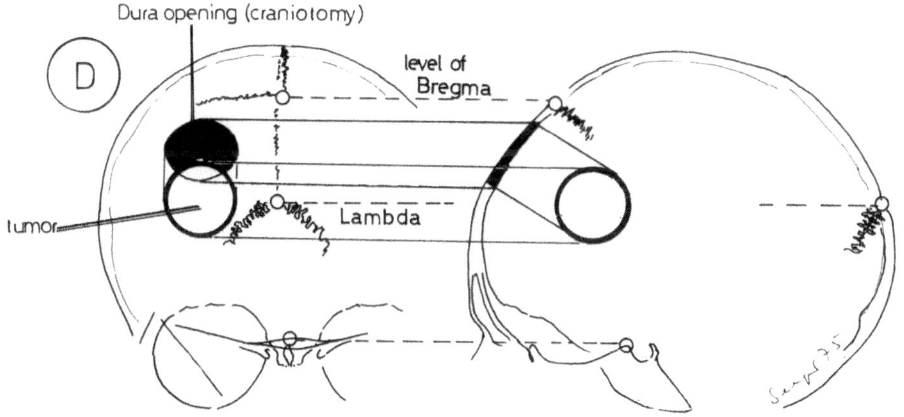
Dura opening (craniotomy)
D
level of
Bregma
Lambda
tumor

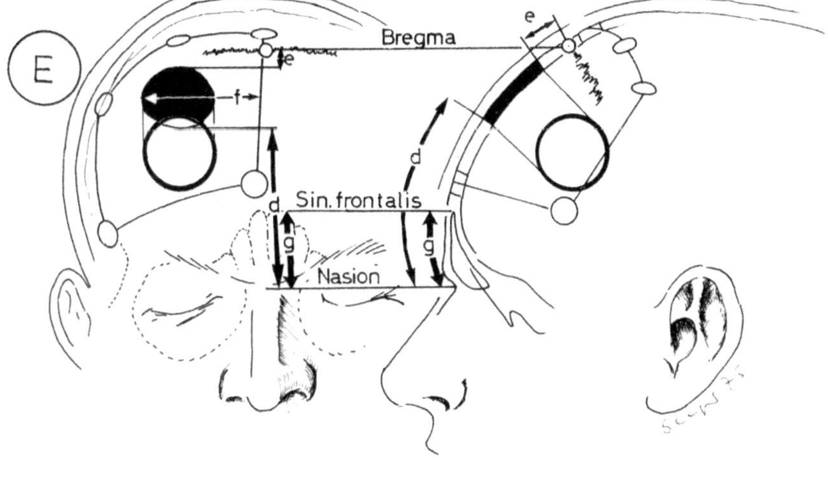
E
Bregma
e
f
d
Sin. frontalis
g
Nasion

Fig. 71. Bony frontal structures (angiogram indicated)

A Skull preparation

B and *C* Roentgenogram

1 a Ala parva, shallow inclination in medial direction to

1 b Planum sphenoidale

1 c Proc. clinoideus ant.

1 d Fiss. orb. sup.

2 a Orbital roof, highly vaulted

2 b Edge of olfactorius furrow between orbital roof and Lamina cribrosa

3 a Crista galli

3 b Foramen caecum (beginning of Sinus sagitt. sup., inconstant)

3 c Lamina cribrosa

3 d Crista frontalis

4 a A. carotis int./For. lacerum

4 b A. carotis int., extradural course

4 c A. carotis int., intradural entry

} see angiogram

5 a Localization of tentorial edge

5 b Edge of Falx/Sinus sagitt. inf.

5 c Falx-tentorial border/Sinus rectus

} see angiogram

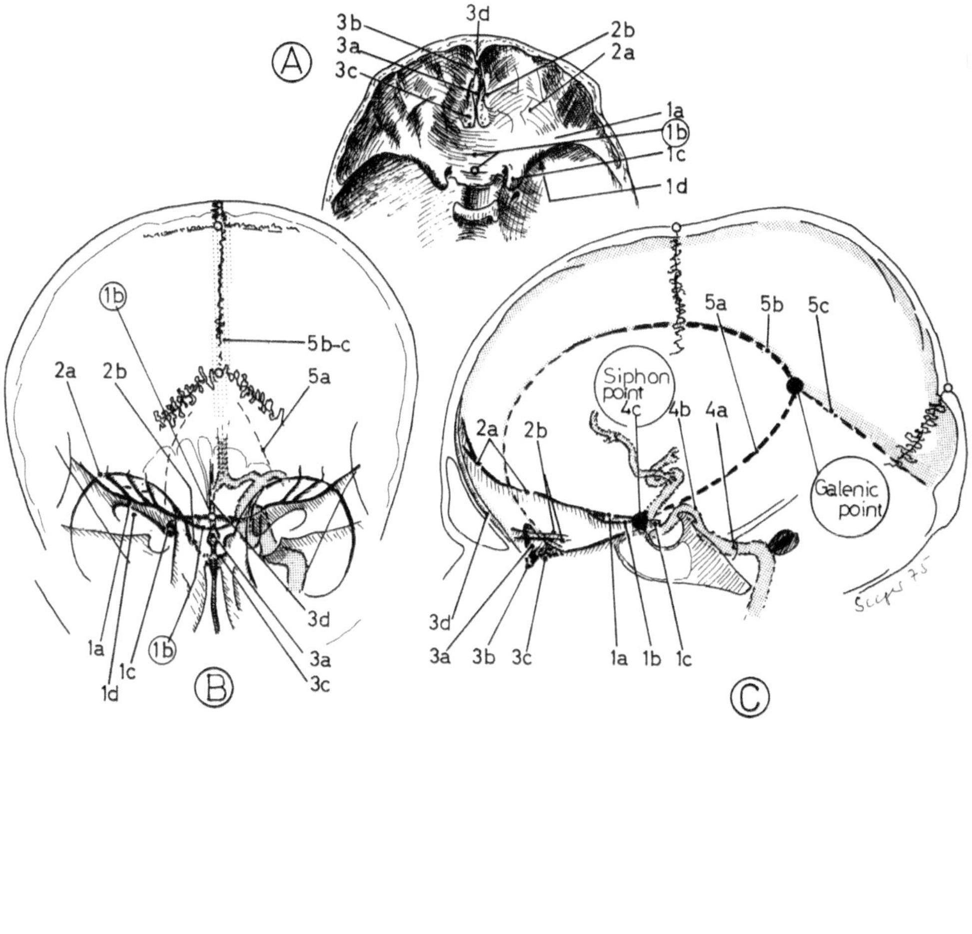
A
3d
3b
3a
3c
2b
2a
1a
1b
1c
1d
B
1b
5b-c
2a
2b
5a
1a
1c
1d
1b
3d
3a
3c
C
5a
5b
5c
Siphon point
4c
4b
4a
Galenic point
2a
2b
3d
3a
3b
3c
1a
1b
1c

Fig. 72. Supplement to Fig. 71: Region of Planum sphenoidale and Ala parva

a Posterior = convex portion of Planum sphenoidale

b Anterior = concave portion, "olfactory groove" anteriorly

c Lateral transition of Planum sphenoidale into Ala parva (flat)

d Transition of Planum sphenoidale laterally forwards into the highly vaulted orbital roof (see also Fig. 86)

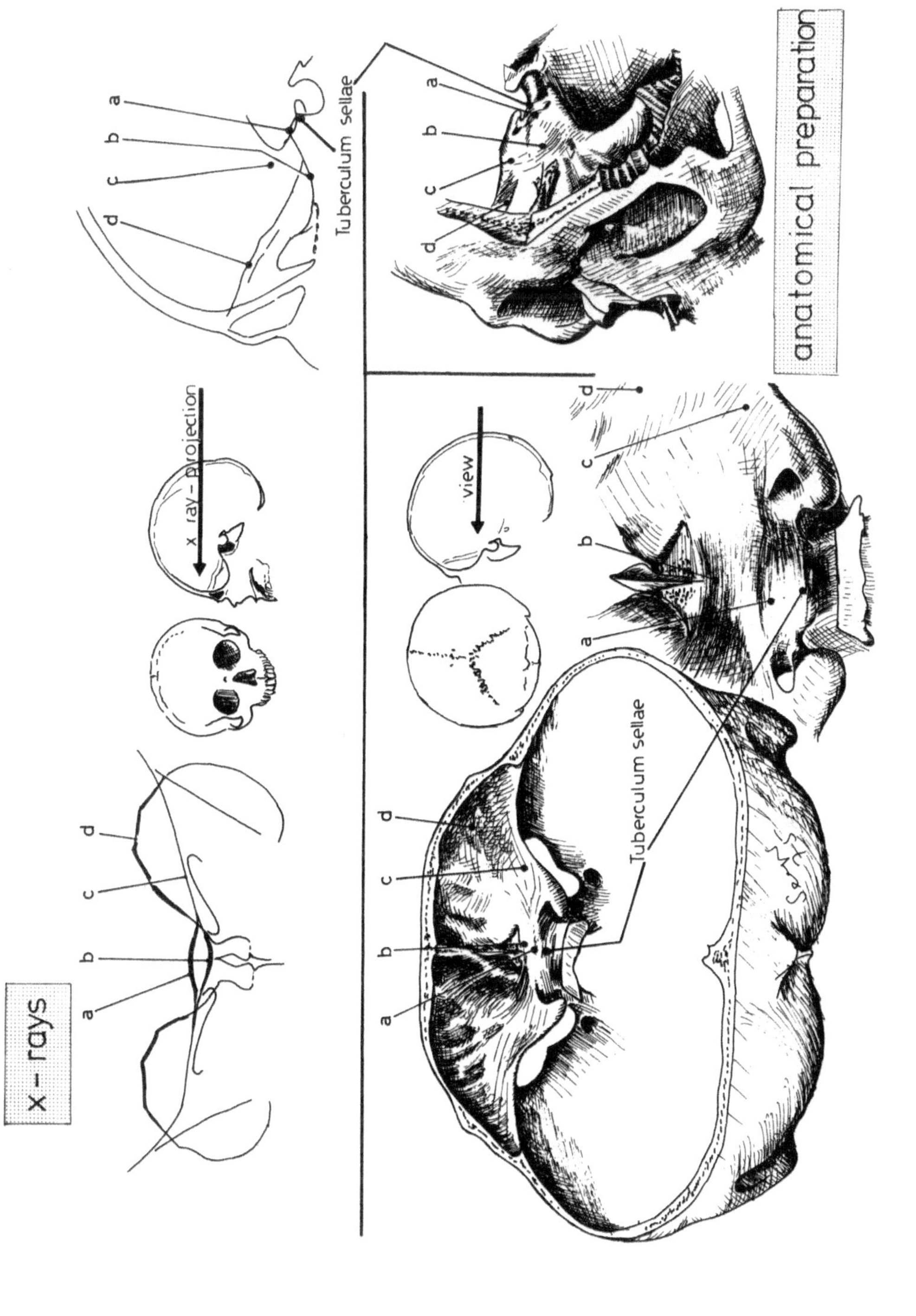
x - rays
a
b
c
d
x ray - projection
a
b
c
d
Tuberculum sellae
view
a
b
c
d
Tuberculum sellae
a
b
c
d
a
b
c
d
anatomical preparation

Fig. 73. Combination of angiogram and air encephalogram (Indian ink copy). Bregma-Lambda distance measured on a-p film (*a*), and lateral film brought into corresponding position (distance Bregma-Lambda plane *a'*). Thus an exact comparison of a-p and lateral films is possible. In the lateral projection A. pericallosa may project into the ventricle; since Fissura longitudinalis with A. pericallosa penetrates deeply above the radiation of Rostrum and Genu corporis callosi (= "forceps"), Cornu ant. vaults over the arteries on both sides (distances *b* and *b'*)
Note the short distance between Cisterna insulae and lateral ventricle. Between them lies Corona radiata with Tractus corticospinalis
Measurements in millimetres (mm)

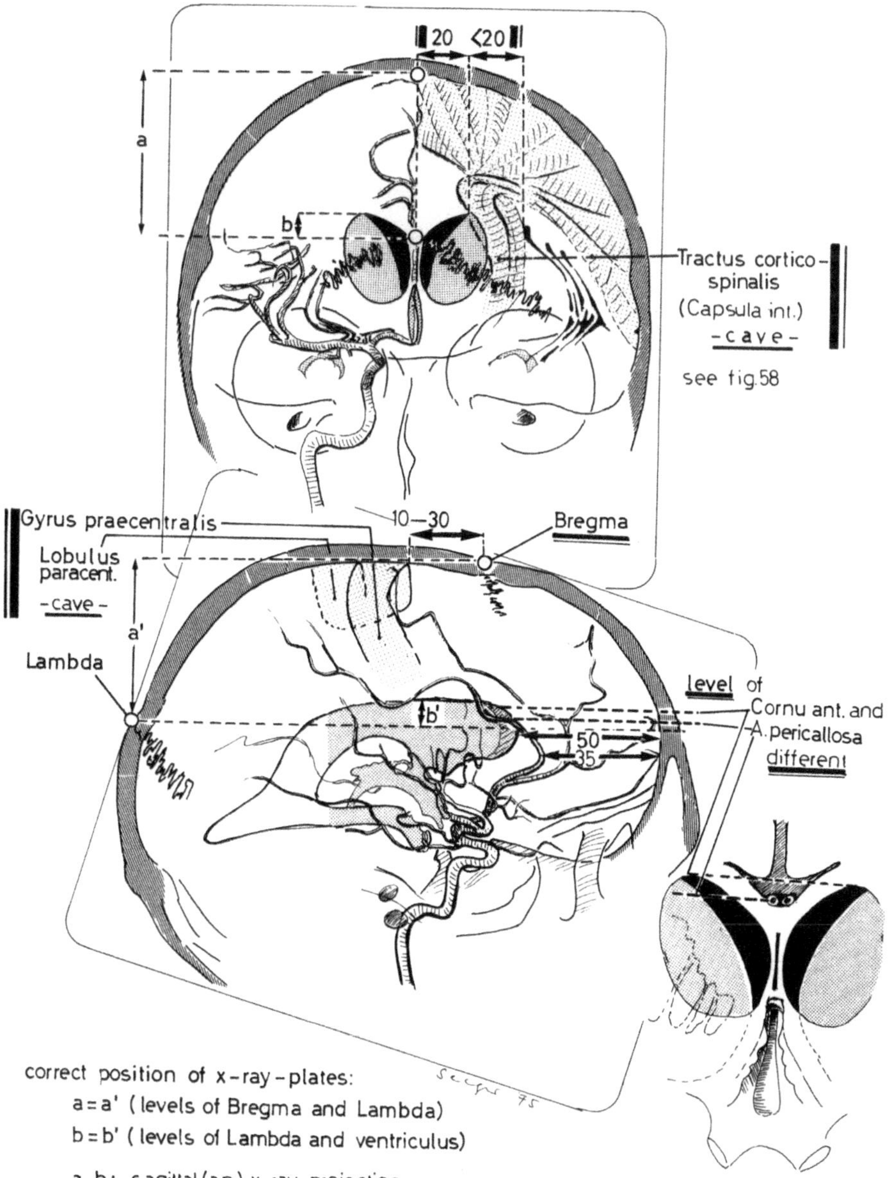

correct position of x-ray-plates:

a = a' (levels of Bregma and Lambda)

b = b' (levels of Lambda and ventriculus)

a, b: sagittal (a.p.) x-ray-projection

a', b': lateral x-ray-projection

Fig. 74. Avoidance of damage to R. temp. N. facialis leading to the frontal muscle (report of Samii and of Yaşargil)*

* Personal communication.

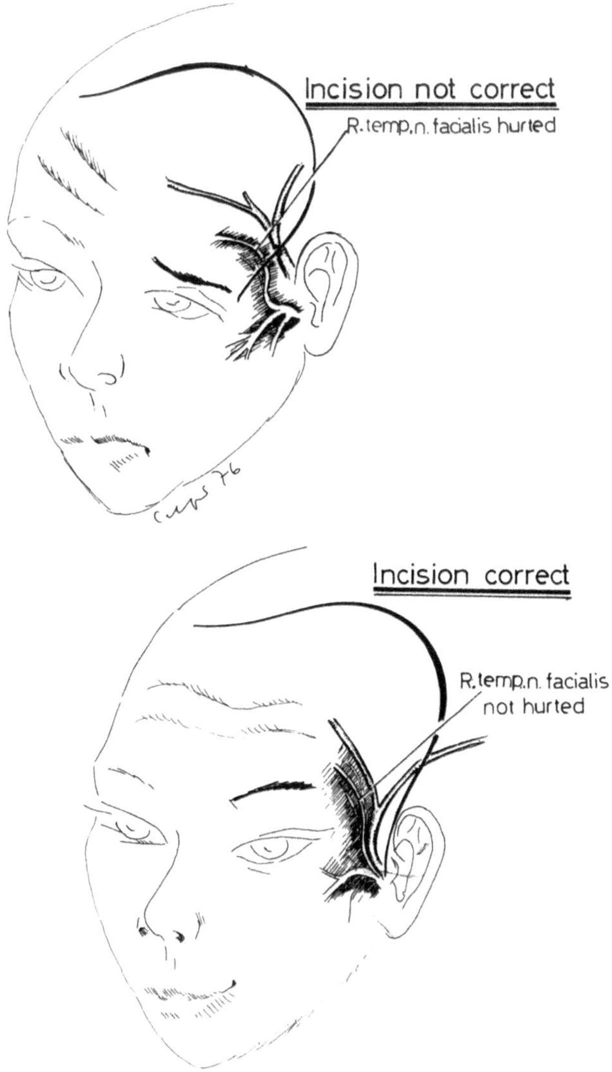
Incision not correct
R.temp.n.facialis hurted
Incision correct
R.temp.n.facialis
not hurted

Fig. 75. Typical frontal trepanation

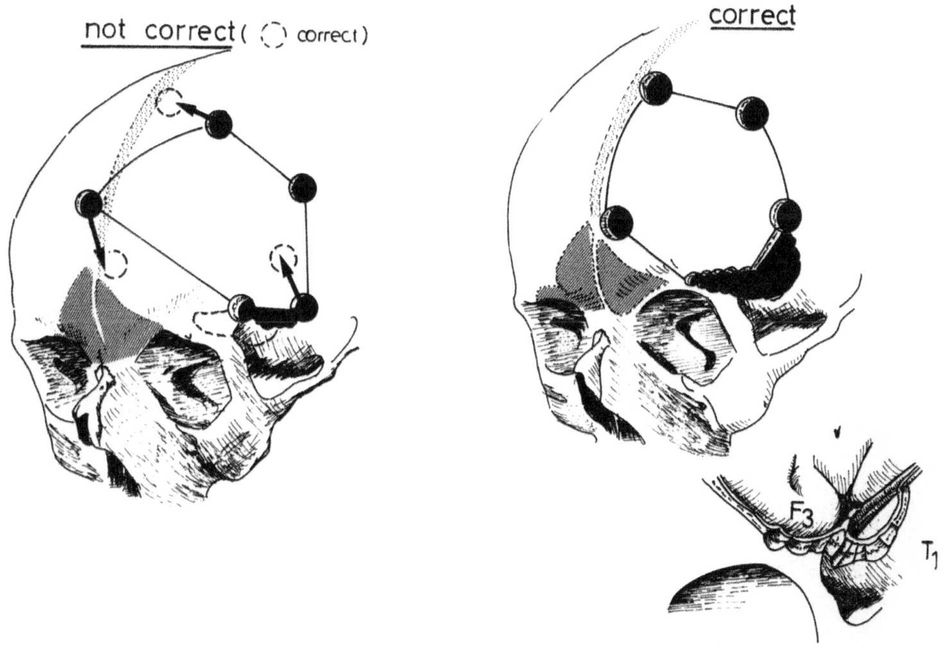
not correct (correct)
correct
F3
T1

Fig. 76. Frontal trepanation avoiding injury to cerebral veins and Sinus in elderly subjects with adherent dura

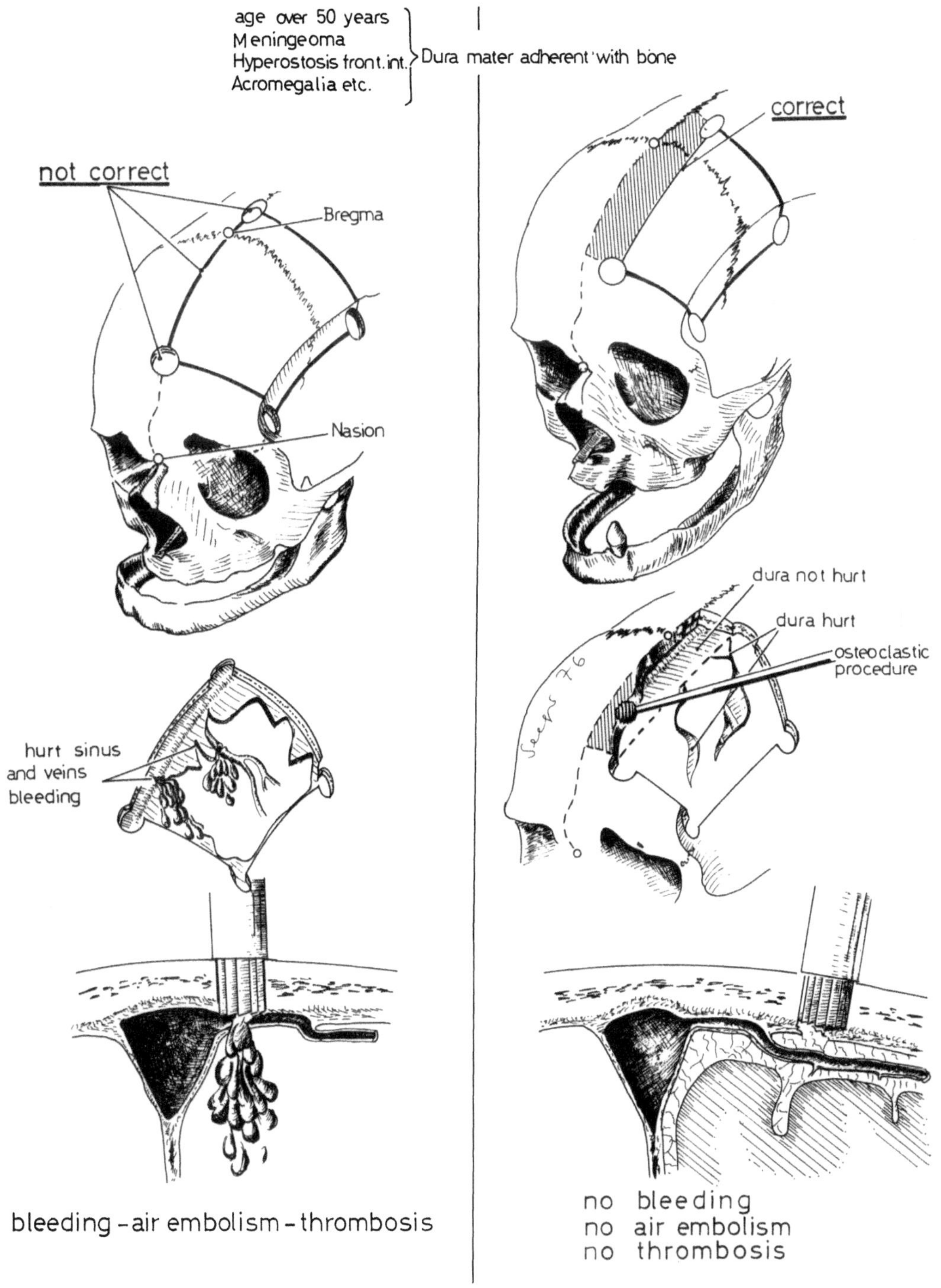
age over 50 years
Meningeoma
Hyperostosis front.int.
Acromegalia etc.
Dura mater adherent with bone
not correct
Bregma
Nasion
hurt sinus
and veins
bleeding
bleeding - air embolism - thrombosis
correct
dura not hurt
dura hurt
osteoclastic
procedure
no bleeding
no air embolism
no thrombosis

Fig. 77. Choice of side for approach to midline processes at Falx not dependent on dominance of hemisphere but on possibility of access (course of cerebral veins to Sinus sagitt. sup. varies on each side)

A Trepanation

B Section from *A* with connection of temporal muscle on the bone flap

C D Lateral localization of cerebral veins (for oblique view see Fig. 69)

E Entry into Fissura longitudinalis on the side of better approach

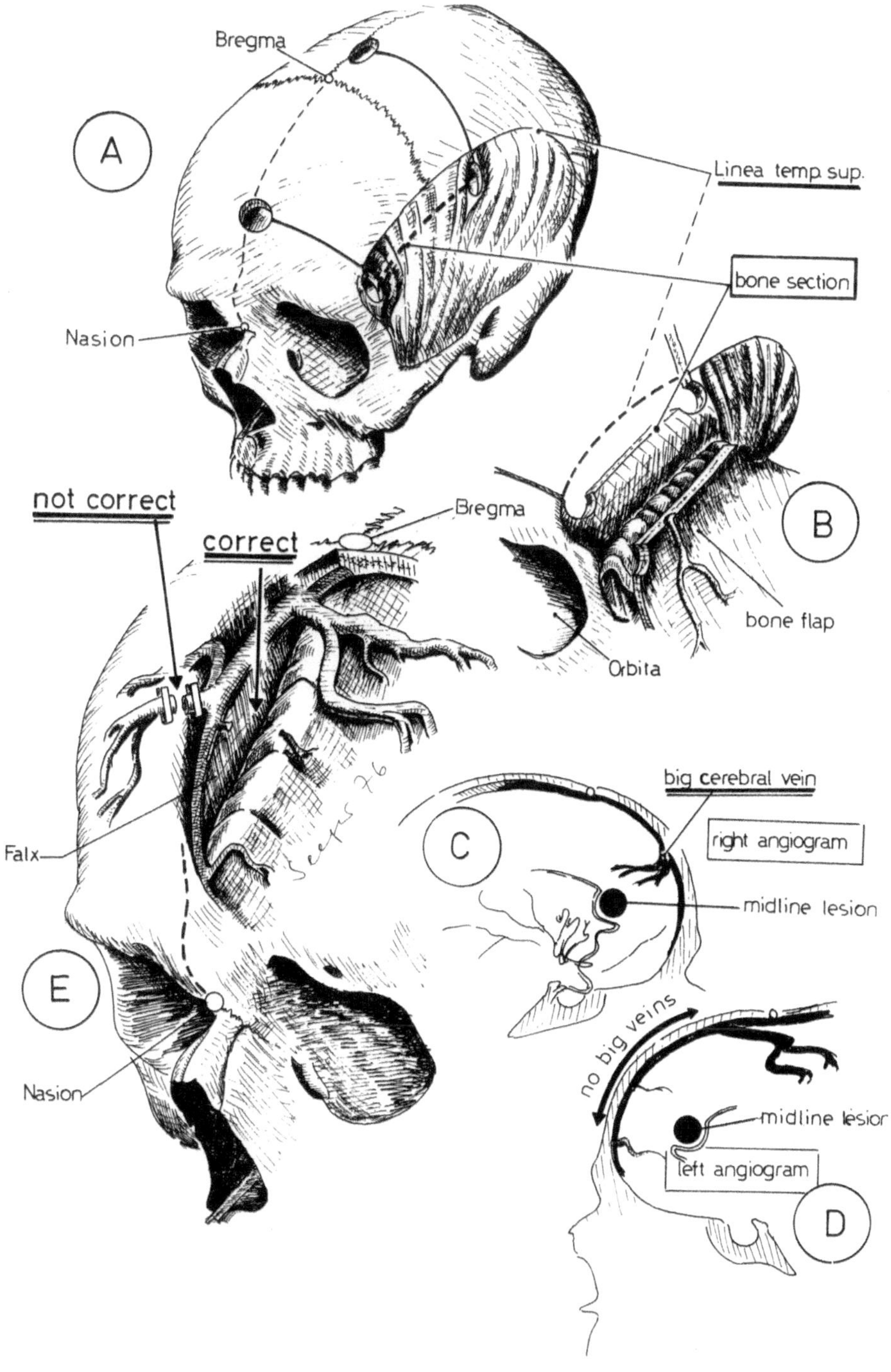
Bregma
A
Linea temp.sup.
bone section
Nasion
B
bone flap
Orbita
not correct
correct
Bregma
Falx
big cerebral vein
C
right angiogram
midline lesion
E
Nasion
no big veins
midline lesion
left angiogram
D

Fig. 78. Typical removal of a frontal process in the white matter with utmost possible conservation of larger arteries and veins. Removal up to unopened roof of ventricle. If border between tumour and white matter is respected, no danger of opening Cisterna insulae or damage of A. operculofront. there

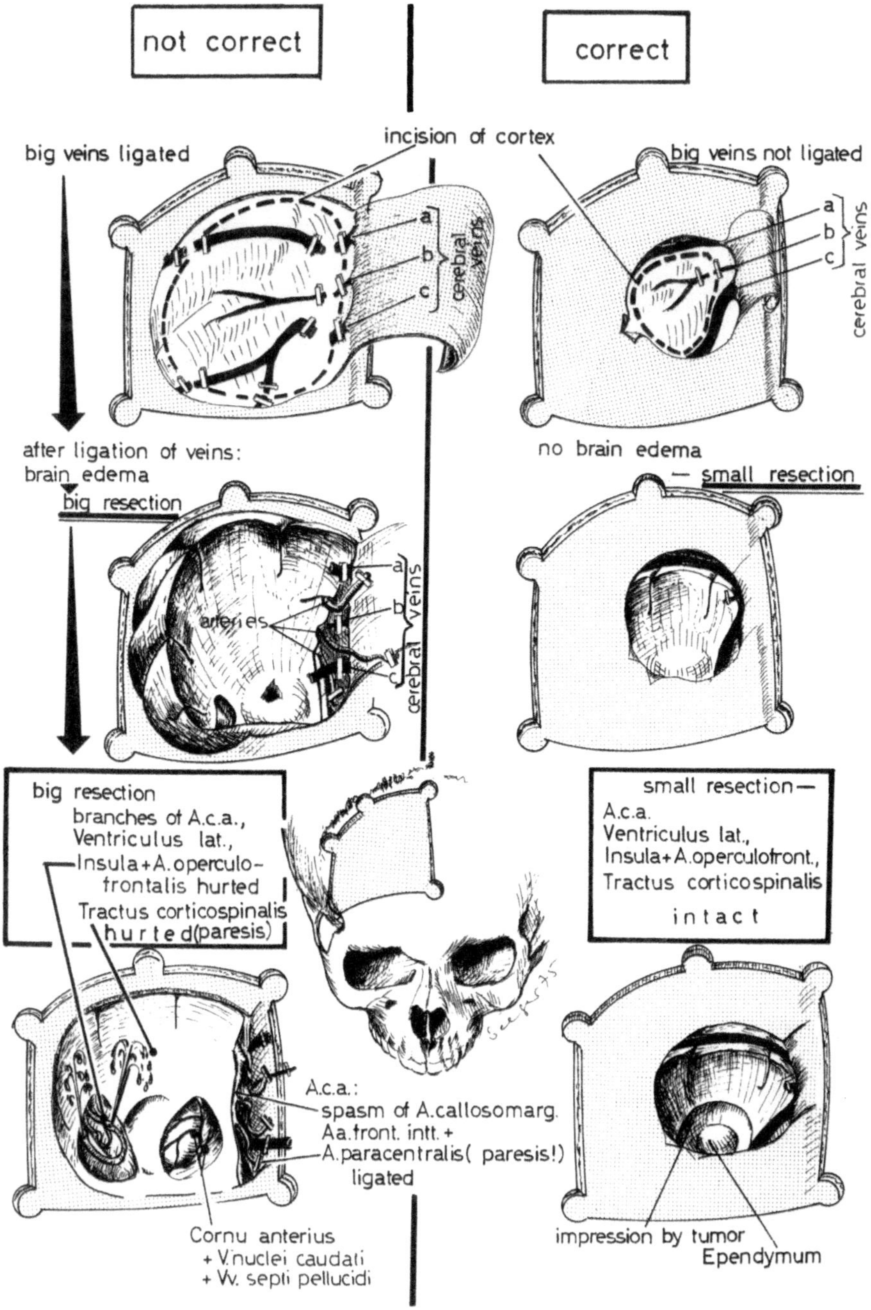
not correct
correct
big veins ligated
incision of cortex
big veins not ligated
a
b
c
cerebral veins
after ligation of veins:
brain edema
big resection
no brain edema
— small resection
arteries
big resection
branches of A.c.a.,
Ventriculus lat.,
Insula+A.operculo-frontalis hurted
Tractus corticospinalis hurted (paresis)
small resection—
A.c.a.
Ventriculus lat.,
Insula+A.operculofront.,
Tractus corticospinalis
intact
A.c.a.:
spasm of A.callosomarg.
Aa.front. intt.+
A.paracentralis(paresis!)
ligated
Cornu anterius
+ V.nuclei caudati
+ Vv. septi pellucidi
impression by tumor
Ependymum

Fig. 79. Basal approach (*A* frontal, *B-D* frontotemp.). Different skin incisions. Embolization – e.g., of meningiomas – carries the risk of skin necrosis. It is prevented by folding the skin flap upwards into parietal direction*

---

* H. Eggert, personal communication.

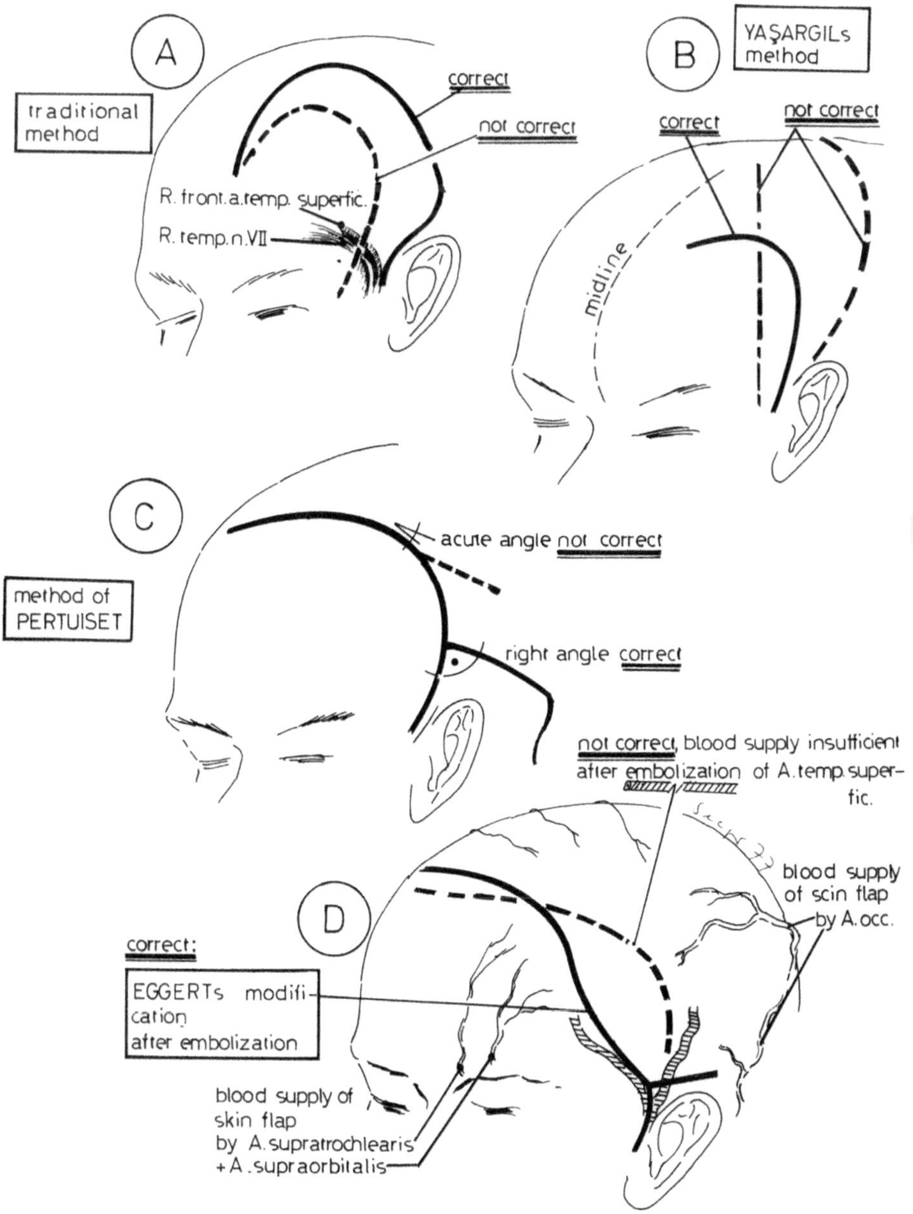
A
traditional method
correct
not correct
R. front. a. temp. superfic.
R. temp. n. VII
B
YAŞARGILs method
correct
not correct
midline
C
method of PERTUISET
acute angle not correct
right angle correct
D
not correct, blood supply insufficient after embolization of A. temp. superfic.
blood supply of scin flap by A. occ.
correct:
EGGERTs modification after embolization
blood supply of skin flap by A. supratrochlearis + A. supraorbitalis

Fig. 80 and 81. Frontotemporal trepanation with subperiosteal removal or temporal muscle at the lateral orbital margin

Fig. 80

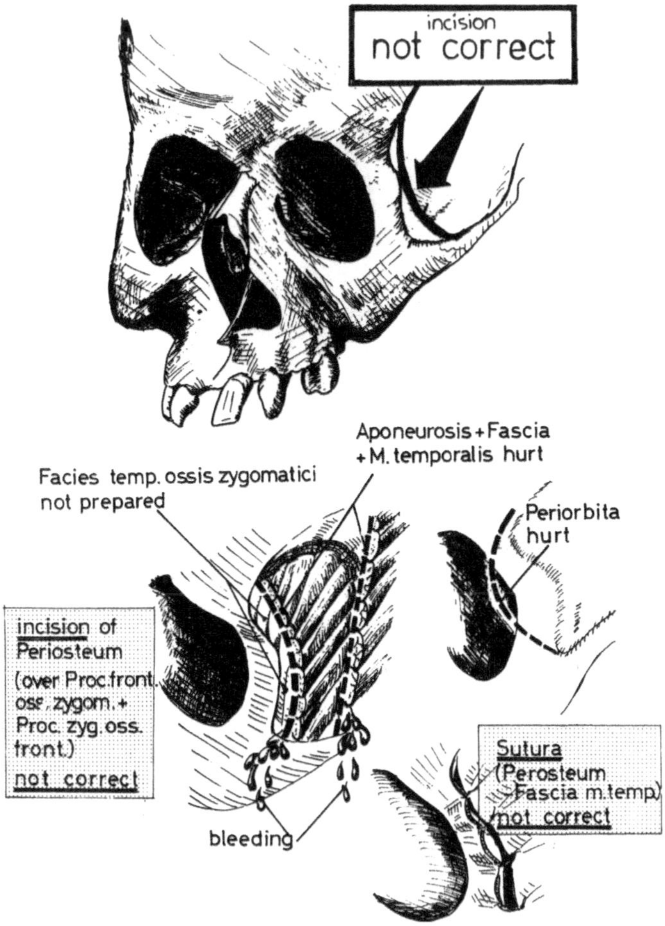
incision
not correct
Aponeurosis + Fascia
+ M. temporalis hurt
Facies temp. ossis zygomatici
not prepared
Periorbita
hurt
incision of
Periosteum
(over Proc. front.
oss. zygom. +
Proc. zyg. oss.
front.)
not correct
Sutura
(Perosteum
Fascia m. temp.)
not correct
bleeding

Fig. 81

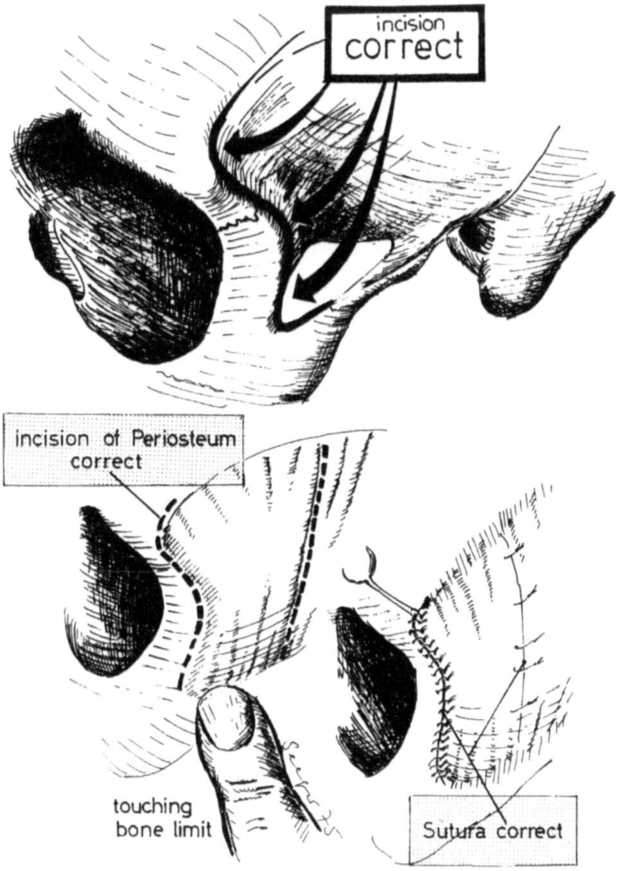
incision
correct
incision of Periosteum
correct
touching
bone limit
Sutura correct

Fig. 82. Frontotemporal trepanation according to Yaşargil, slightly modified

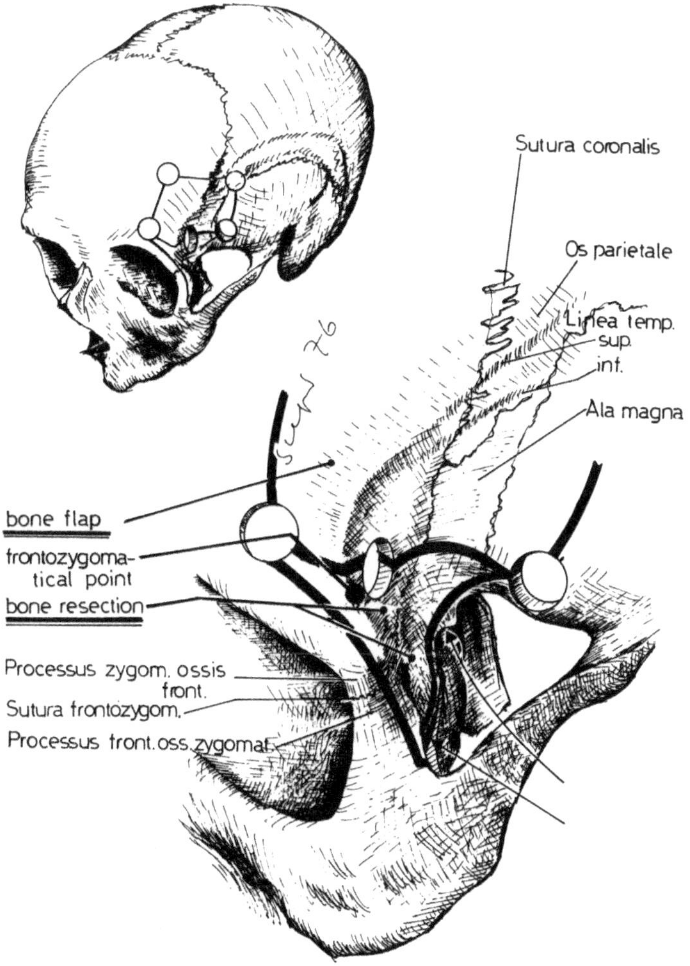
Sutura coronalis
Os parietale
Linea temp.
sup.
inf.
Ala magna
bone flap
frontozygomatical point
bone resection
Processus zygom. ossis front.
Sutura frontozygom.
Processus front. oss. zygomat.

Fig. 83. Yaşargil's muscle dissection at small frontotemporal trepanation

FIG. 83

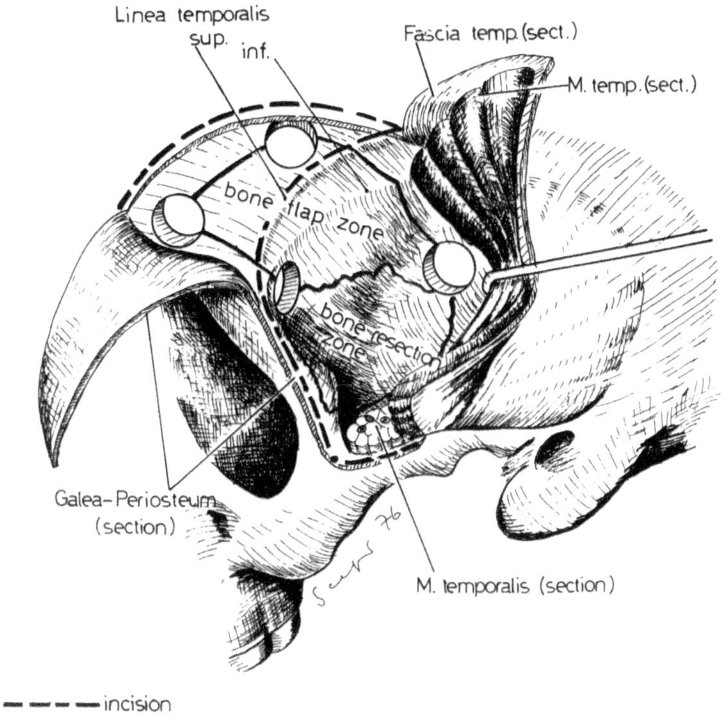
Linea temporalis
sup.
inf.
Fascia temp.(sect.)
M. temp.(sect.)
bone flap zone
bone resection zone
Galea-Periosteum (section)
M. temporalis (section)
incision

Fig. 84. Trepanation if possible in areas with plane parallel skull thickness in order to avoid damage to Dura and Periorbita

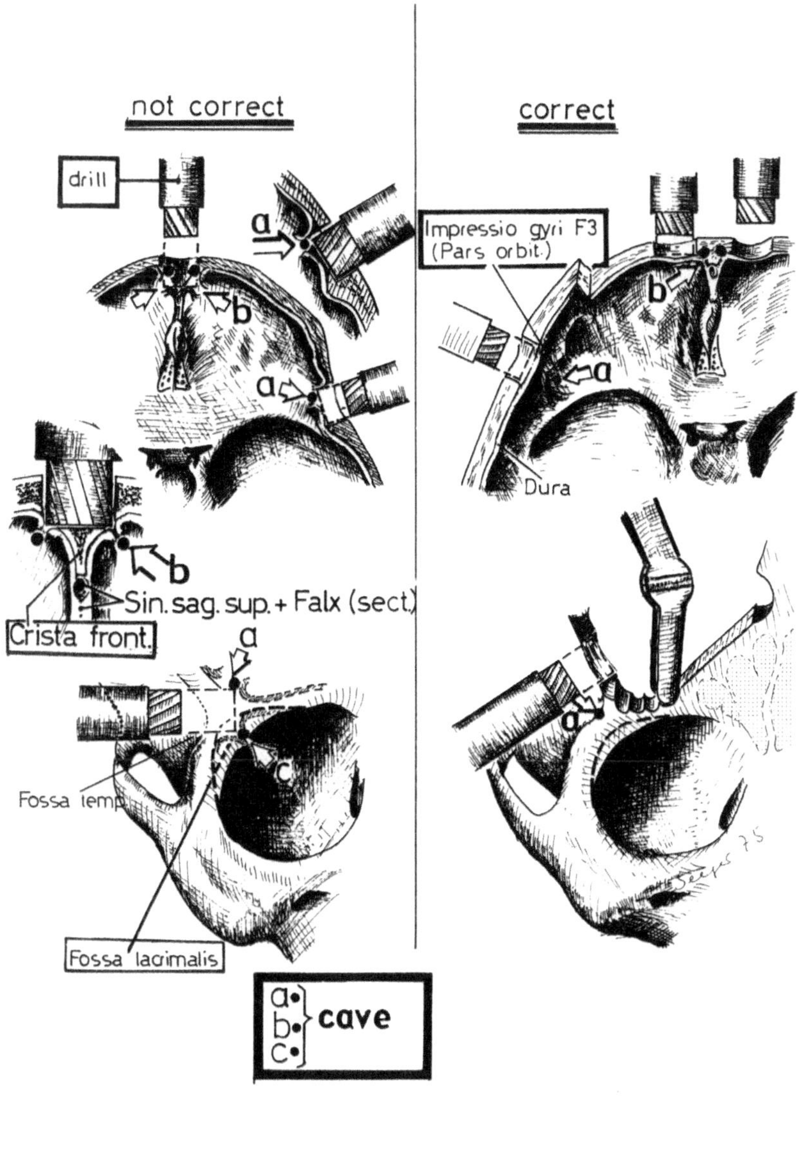
not correct
correct
drill
a
b
a
Impressio gyri F3
(Pars orbit.)
b
a
Dura
b
Sin. sag. sup. + Falx (sect.)
Crista front.
a
c
Fossa temp
Fossa lacrimalis
a
a•
b•
c•
cave

Fig. 85. Positional relationships between Canalis opticus and pole of frontal lobe, Fissura orbit. sup., and lateral orbital margin
Measurements in millimetres (mm)

A 1 Schematic drawing of base from above

B 1 Example of a frontoorbital approach with distance of lateral orbital margin from lateral point of Fissura orbit. sup.

A 2 Frontotemporal transition from behind

B 2 Bony resection from the front

In the frontolateral approach the orbital arch is preserved. Resection of small wing of sphenoid in a medial direction up to lateral point of Fissura orb. sup. without opening Fissura orb. sup.: Distance of medial trepanation border from Canalis opticus only 20 mm, from frontal pole 50 mm

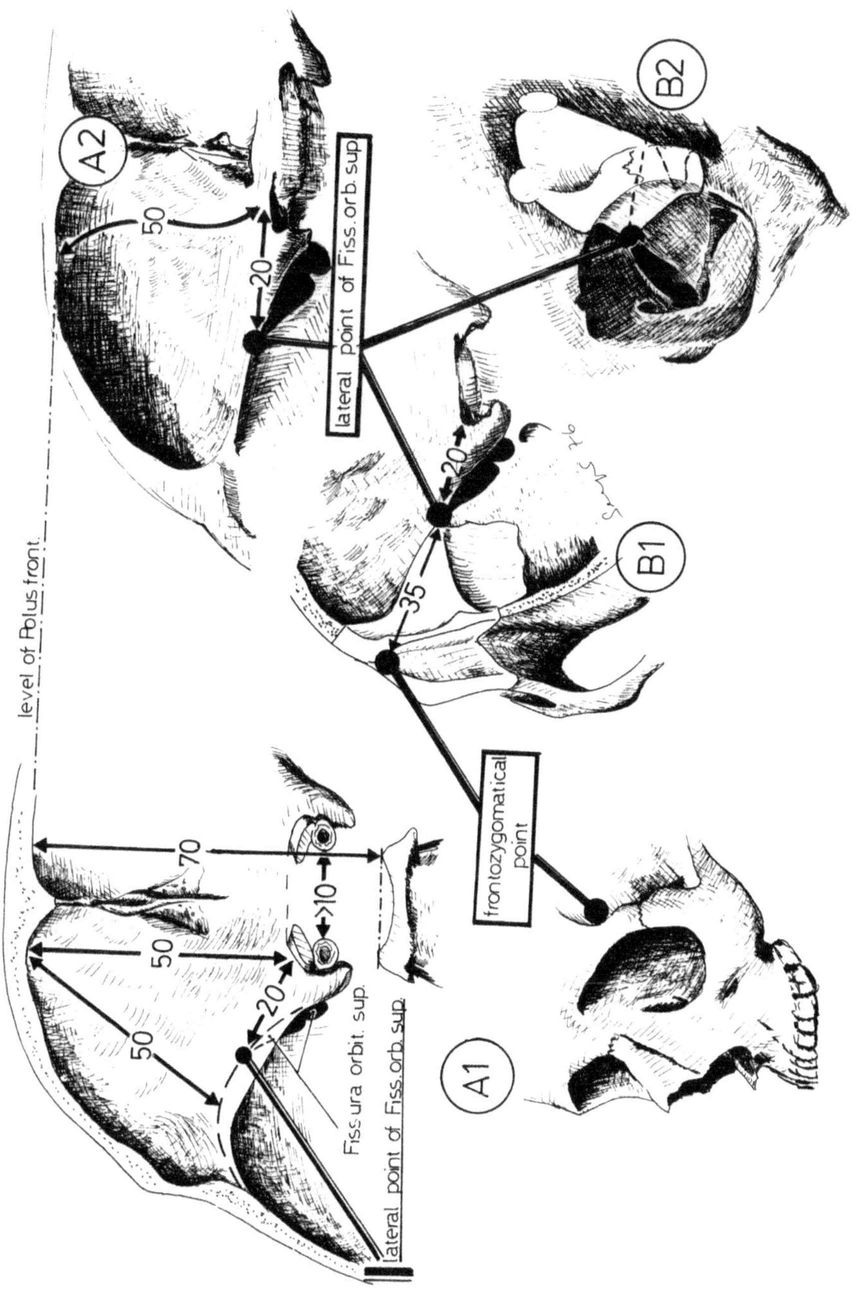
A1
A2
B1
B2
level of Polus front.
lateral point of Fiss.orb.sup
lateral point of Fiss.orb.sup
Fissura orbit. sup.
frontozygomatical point
70
50
50
50
20
20
20
>10
35

Fig. 86. Traumatization of frontal lobe at approach to N. opt. from the front by compression of Gyrus rectus with spatula (*A*). Minimal reclination of frontal and temporal brain at approach over the opened Fissura lat. (Sylvii) (*B*). See also Fig. 85

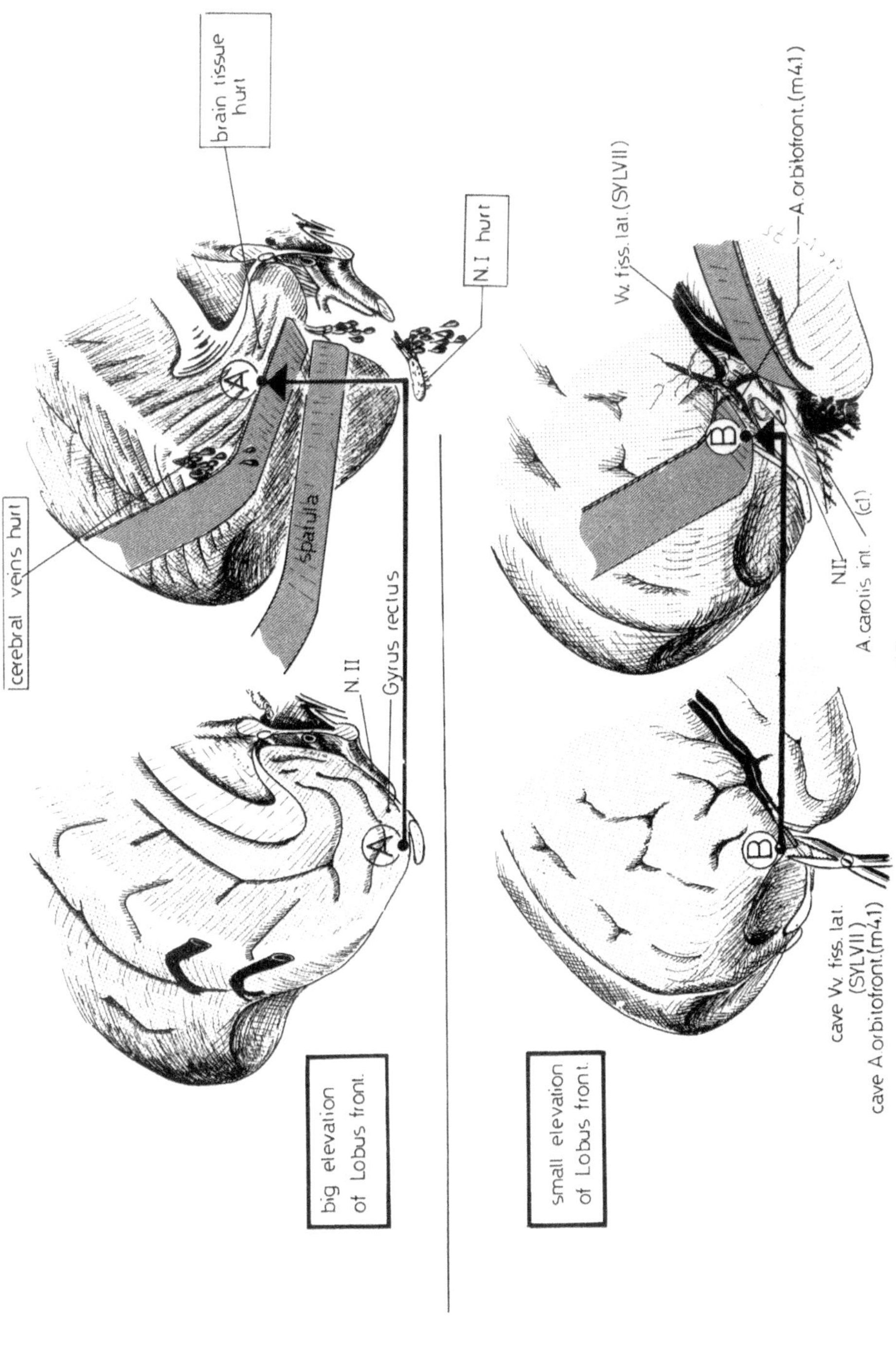

big elevation of Lobus front.
cerebral veins hurt
brain tissue hurt
N.I hurt
Spatula
N.II
Gyrus rectus
A
small elevation of Lobus front.
Vv. fiss. lat. (SYLVII)
A. orbitofront. (m4.1)
NII
A. carotis int.
(c1)
B
cave Vv. fiss. lat. (SYLVII)
cave A orbitofront. (m4.1)

Fig. 87. Head rotation of 20° already hampers orientation in vicinity of both Nn. optici, if a median Falx (not shifted by tumour) is unavailable as reference structure. Distance measurements for intraoperative determination of Nn. optici and Aa. carotis intt. – e.g., for extracerebral tumours with destruction or shift of Falx and deformation of base

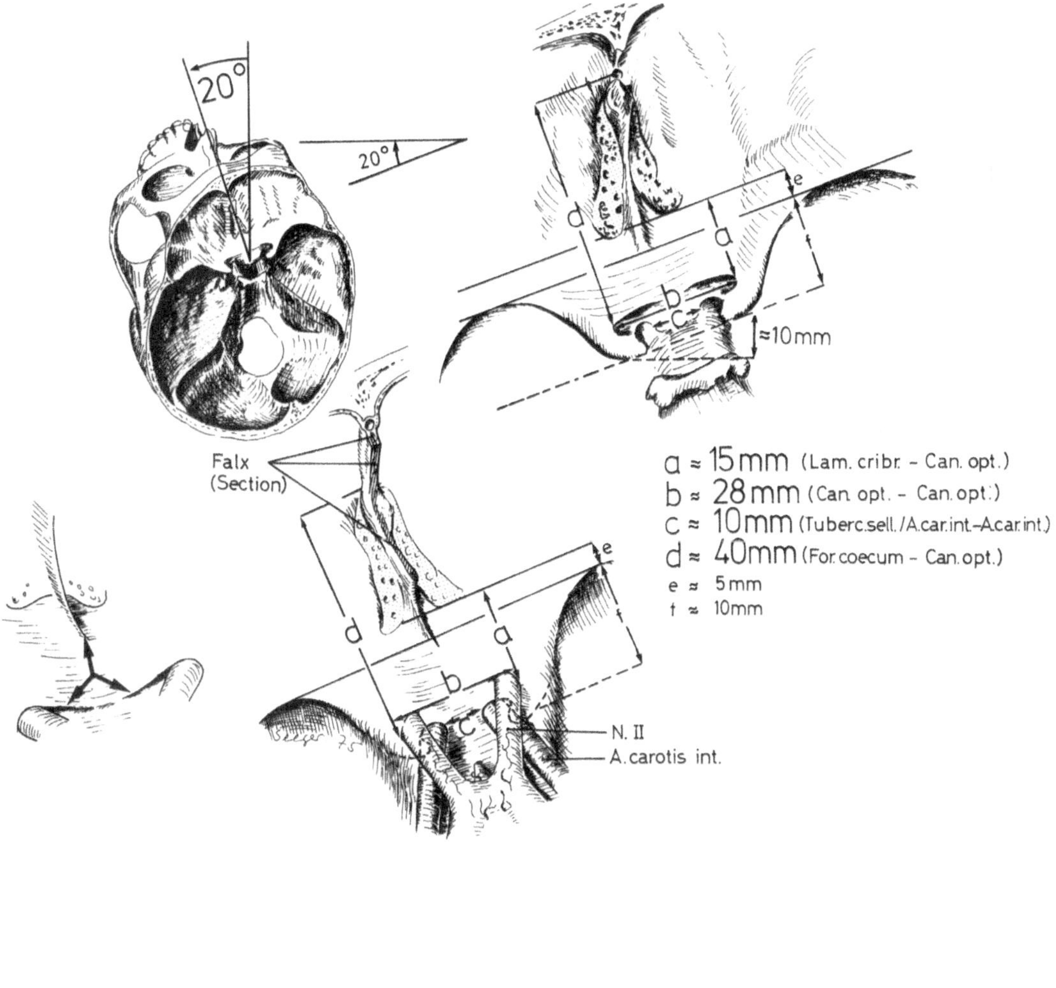
20°
20°
Falx
(Section)
d
a
b
c
e
f
≈10mm
N. II
A. carotis int.
a ≈ 15mm (Lam. cribr. - Can. opt.)
b ≈ 28mm (Can. opt. - Can. opt.)
c ≈ 10mm (Tuberc. sell. / A. car. int.-A. car. int.)
d ≈ 40mm (For. coecum - Can. opt.)
e ≈ 5mm
f ≈ 10mm

Fig. 88
A Search for N. olfact. which is followed in posterior direction as far as crossing of Canalis opticus
B Focussing of N. opt. after opening Fissura lat. (Sylvii) and preparation of veins at Ala parva
C and *D* Preparation of Chiasma region
Designation of Fig. 71:
1 a Ala parva
1 b Planum sphenoidale
2 a Orbital roof
2 b Medial area of orbital roof
3 a Projection of Crista galli
3 b Projection of Foramen caecum
3 c Lamina cribrosa
5 b Border of Falx
a 1 A. cerebri ant.
a 2 Perforating arteries to Chiasma, covering Lamina terminalis
a 3 A. recurrens (Heubneri)
a 4 A. comm. ant.
c 1 A. carotis int.
m 1 A. cerebri media
(See catalogue of arteries)

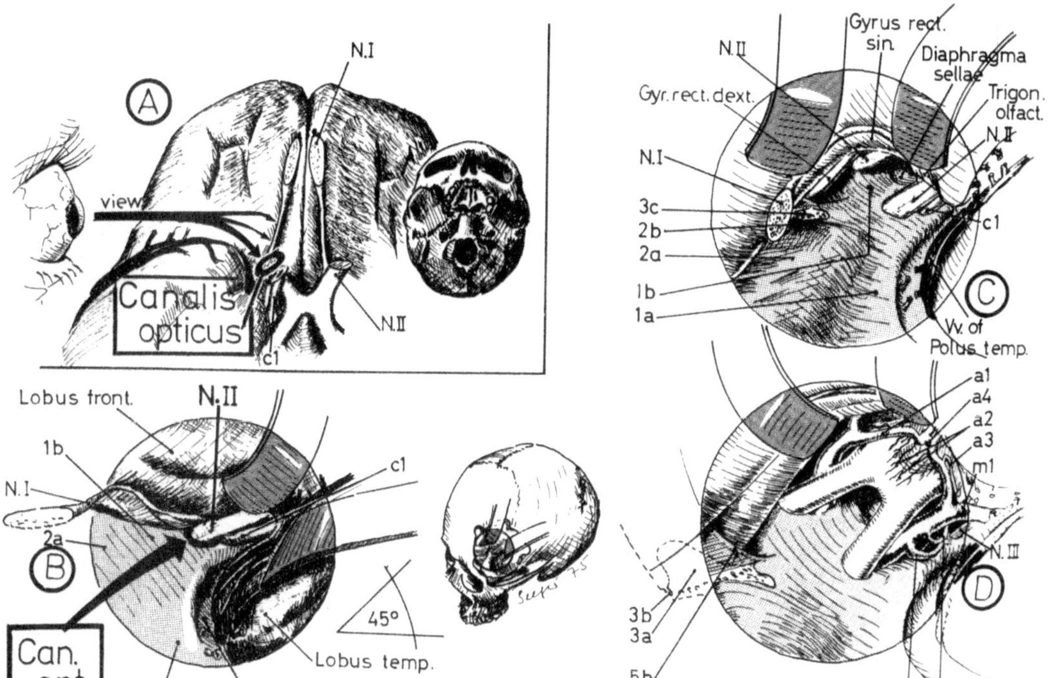
A
N.I
view
Canalis opticus
c1
N.II
Gyrus rect. sin.
N.II
Diaphragma sellae
Gyr. rect. dext.
Trigon. olfact.
N.II
N.I
3c
2b
2a
1b
1a
c1
C
Vv. of Polus temp.
Lobus front.
N.II
1b
N.I
c1
2a
B
Can. opt.
45°
Lobus temp.
1a
Fossa cranii media
a1
a4
a2
a3
m1
N.III
3b
3a
5b
D
p6
c5

Fig. 89 (see also Figs. 63 to 65). Variants in course of A. carotis int. and A. cerebri ant. Arrows: Displacement as against normal findings

A Course of A. cerebri ant. above perforating arteries to Chiasma (70%)*

B Deep course of A. cerebri ant. at margin of Chiasma (30%)

C Variant of penetration of A. carotis int. through the dura (arrow) and of A. communicans post. (P 5)

For vessels nomenclature see catalogue of arteries (pages 3–4)

---

* After Perlmutter and Rhoton (1976).

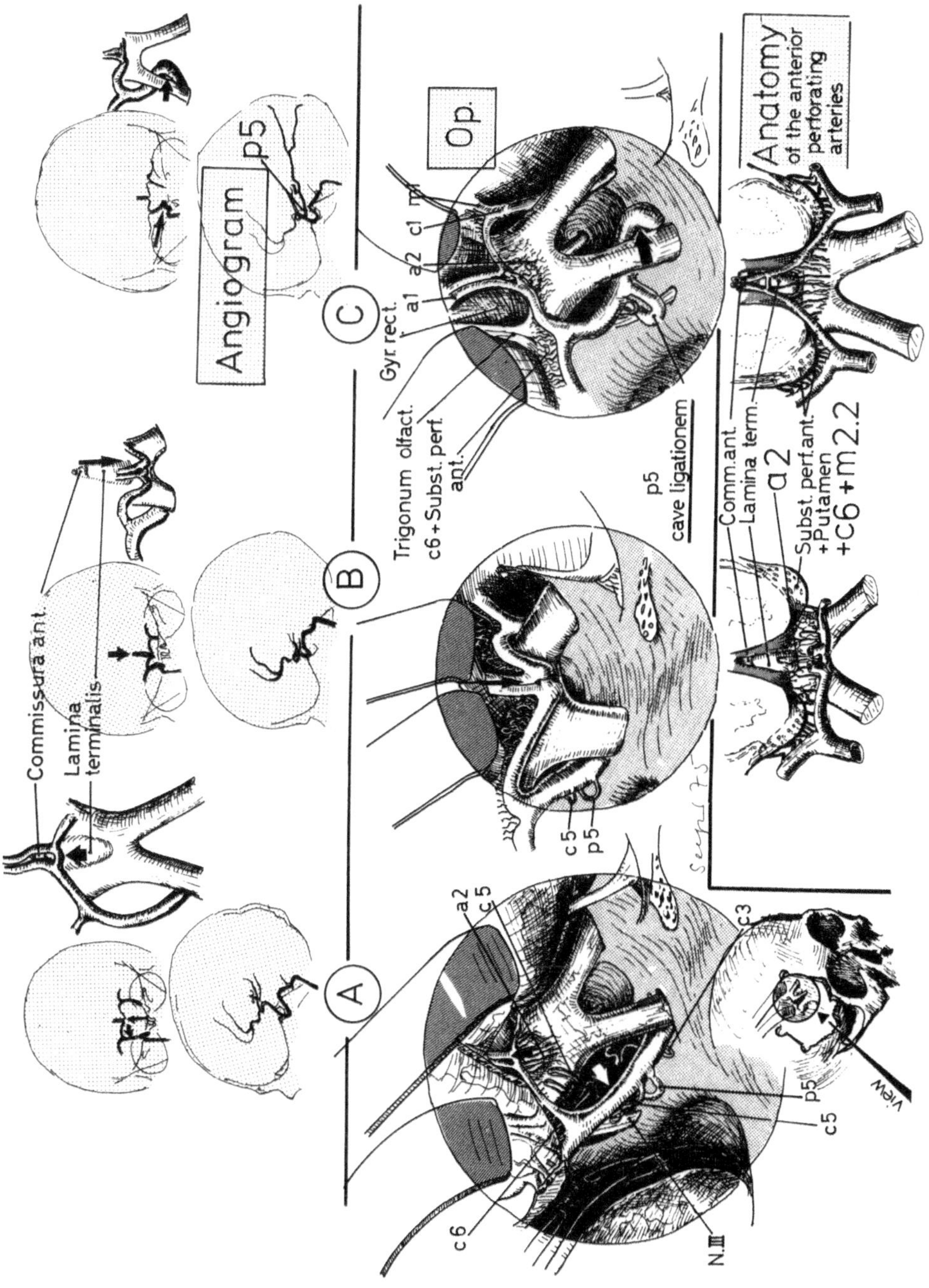
A
B
C
Commissura ant.
Lamina terminalis
Angiogram
p5
Op.
Gyr. rect.
a1
a2
c1
m1
Trigonum olfact.
c6+Subst. perf. ant.
p5
cave ligationem
Comm. ant.
Lamina term.
a2
Subst. perf. ant.
+Putamen
+c6+m2.2
Anatomy
of the anterior
perforating
arteries
a2
c5
c5
p5
c3
p5
c5
c6
N.III
view

Fig. 90. Drilling out of Planum sphenoidale with bony deformation due to tumour. For positional relationships and distance measurements see Fig. 87. For nomenclature of vessels see catalogue of arteries (pages 3–4)

FIG. 90

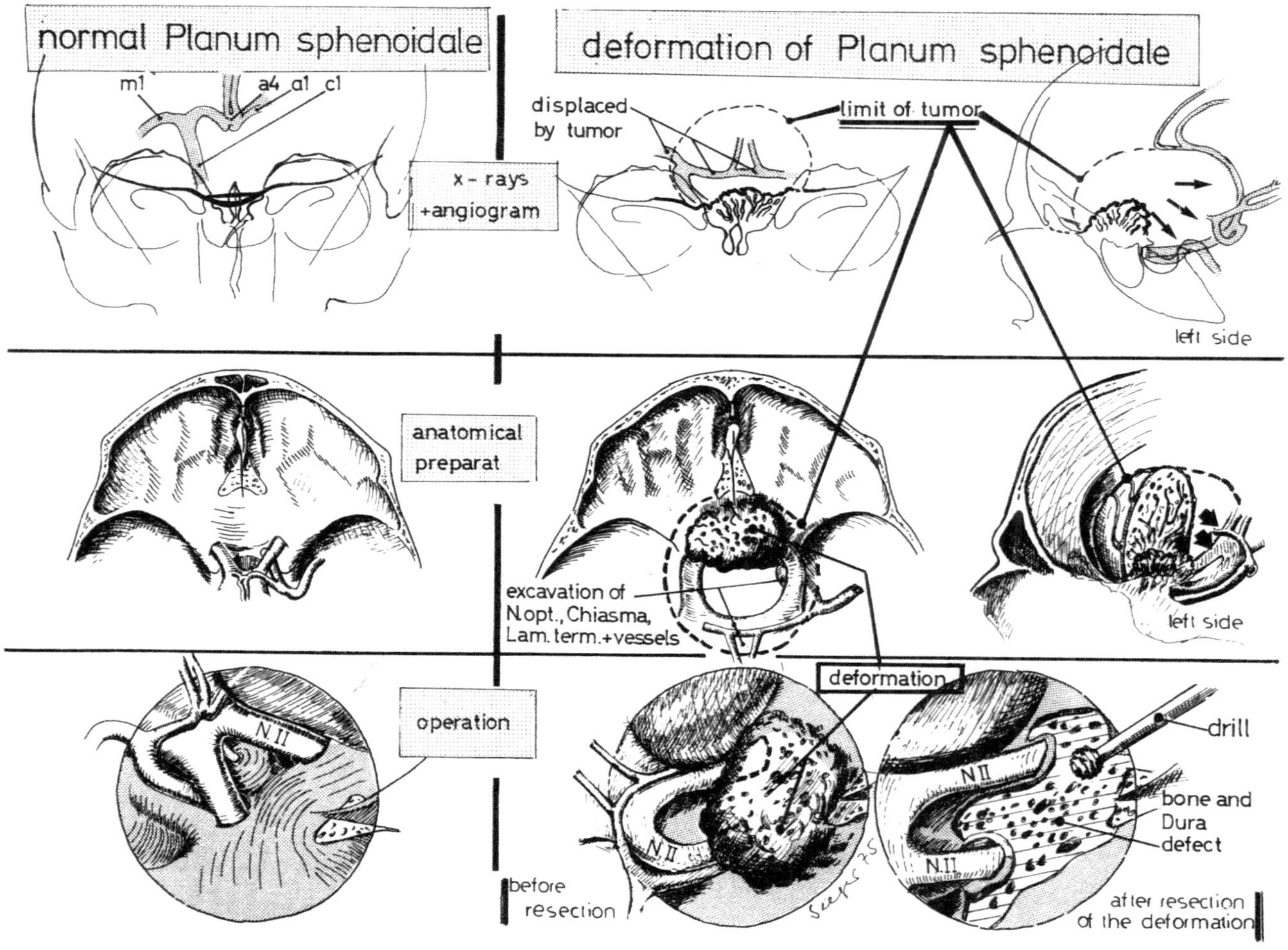
normal Planum sphenoidale
deformation of Planum sphenoidale
m1
a4 a1 c1
x - rays
+angiogram
displaced
by tumor
limit of tumor
left side
anatomical
preparat
excavation of
N.opt., Chiasma,
Lam. term.+vessels
left side
operation
N.II
deformation
drill
bone and
Dura
defect
before
resection
after resection
of the deformation

Figs. 91 and 92. Neighbourhood relationships between Cisterna fissurae lat (Sylvii), Cisternae basales, and Cisterna ambiens at site of operation
A A topographical diagram
B Lateral view into Cisterna chiasmatis after opening of Arachnoidea at the tentorial border and of the trabecular system that touches medially and sheathes the perforating arteries
C View into Cisterna chiasmatis after opening of Arachnoidea from the front at extremely basal approach (e.g., after frontobasal removal of tumour with reclinable frontal lobe)

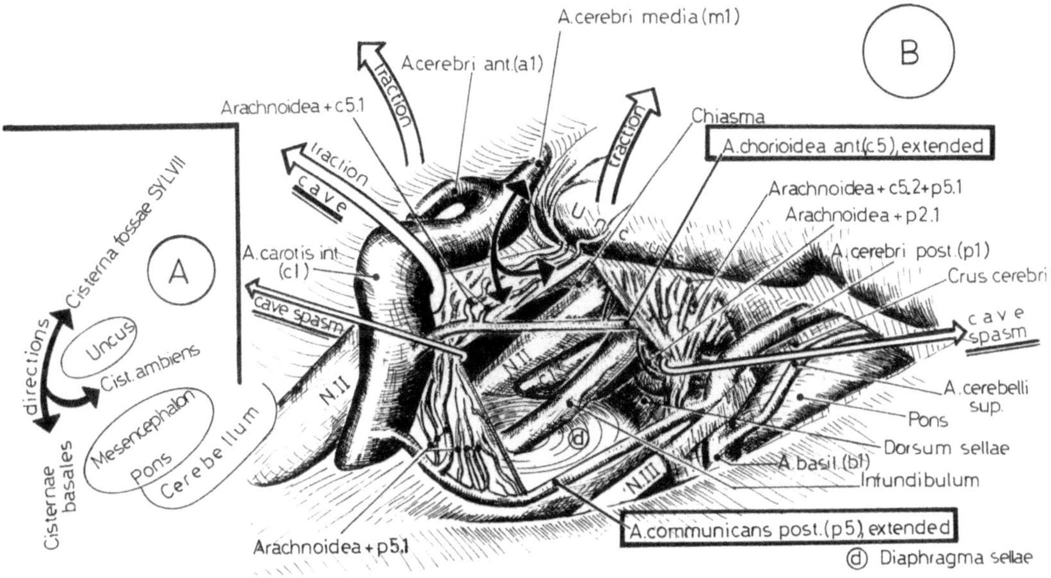
B
A
A.cerebri media (m1)
A.cerebri ant.(a1)
traction
Arachnoidea + c5.1
traction
Chiasma
A.chorioidea ant.(c5), extended
traction
cave
Arachnoidea + c5.2 + p5.1
Arachnoidea + p2.1
A.cerebri post.(p1)
Crus cerebri
Cisterna fossae SYLVII
A.carotis int. (c1)
cave spasm
cave spasm
Uncus
Cist. ambiens
directions
N.II
A.cerebelli sup.
Pons
Dorsum sellae
A.basil.(b1)
Infundibulum
Mesencephalon
Pons
Cerebellum
Cisternae basales
N.III
A.communicans post.(p5), extended
Arachnoidea + p5.1
d Diaphragma sellae

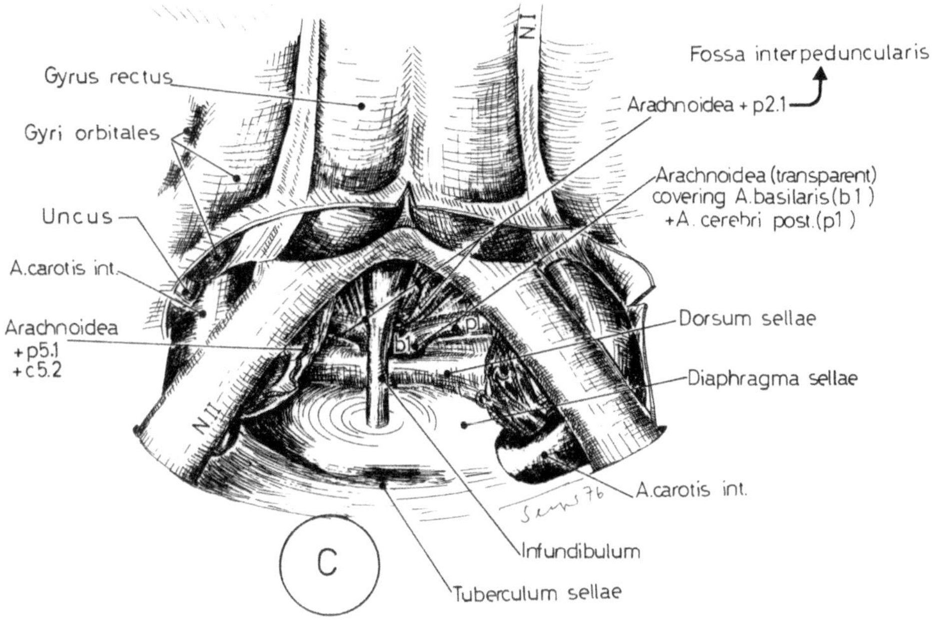
N.I
Fossa interpeduncularis
Gyrus rectus
Arachnoidea + p2.1
Gyri orbitales
Arachnoidea (transparent) covering A.basilaris (b1) + A. cerebri post.(p1)
Uncus
A.carotis int.
Dorsum sellae
Arachnoidea + p5.1 + c5.2
Diaphragma sellae
N.II
A.carotis int.
Infundibulum
Tuberculum sellae
C

Chapter 3
Temporal Lobe and Upper Brainstem

A. Outer Surface (Fig. 93)

At the pole, the outer surface of the temporal lobe is almost flat and inclined mediobasally. Posteriorly it rises and becomes laterally increasingly rounded. With the third temporal gyrus it curves round towards the base. The area of the pole is convexly arched forwards into the middle cranial fossa. Over Impressio petrosa the under surface becomes concave, and the curve towards the edge of Tentorium becomes flatter. Impressio petrosa of the temporal lobe base reaches forward medially from the lateral point of Margo superior partis petrosae as far as the mid-uncus area at the level of the anterior border of the pons. Not until it reaches the occipital lobe crossing over Tentorium does the temporal lobe again rise increasingly steeply in a medial direction. The highest point is at the upper border of the petrous bone (lateral point of Margo superior partis petrosae), 75 mm behind the temporal pole over the entrance of Sinus petrosus superior into Sinus transversus. The surfaces of Uncus, Gyrus parahippocampalis, and of flattened Gyrus occipitotemporalis lateralis are not very variable.

Surface Arteries (Fig. 94)

One big A. temporalis post. (*m8*) is almost always present, whereas A. temporalis media (*m5*), usually arising from the distal trunk, and the group of smaller Aa. temp. antt. (*m2.1*), originating from the proximal trunk of A. cerebri media, vary considerably in number and calibre. Only the last-named of these (apart from branches of A. orbitofrontalis) cross over Fissura lateralis (Sylvii) in order to reach the convexity by way of the superior margin of the first temporal gyrus. Here they can impede dissection in Fissura lateralis (Sylvii).

Surface Veins (Figs. 93 and 116)

The group of Sylvian veins, which is not constantly present, ends mediobasally at Ala parva ossis sphenoidalis (Sinus alae parvae). If of large calibre these bridging venous branches can only be ligated if sufficiently strong anastomoses of the Sylvian group of veins to V. Labbé or over the convexity to the upper bridging veins are present (Fig. 93). Due to the effects of superimposition, angiograms do not show the anastomoses reliably, and the posterior Sylvian region must, therefore, be directly inspected in cases with large Sylvian veins. This procedure is usually unnecessary, as the basal connections are mostly of thin calibre and unimportant (Fig. 93, above). The position of the Sylvian veins does not coincide exactly with the course of Fissura lat. (Sylvii) (Fig. 116, A 4 and A 5).

B. Deep Brain Structures

The narrow field during operation only allows the observation of a few important structures – e.g., N. opticus and A. carotis int. It is particularly important to be aware of the localization of structures lying in the immediate neighbourhood which cannot be demonstrated operatively. In no other supratentorial region of the brain are the conditions so complicated as in the temporomedial area.

As an aid to better understanding, a preparation has been chosen (Figs. 105 to 108) which shows a frontoparallel section (Fig. 105) of the middle temporal lobe. Plexus chorioideus of Cornu inf. has been removed, so that Fissura chorioidea gapes wide open (arrows). The base of Uncus, which is the anterior connection of the temporal lobe to the area of the basal ganglia – Uncus base – is horizontally cut.

The connection of the temporal lobe to the rest of the brain is particularly broad anteriorly between Substantia perforata ant. and the tip of Cornu inf., but between the wall of Cornu inf. and Insula it is only approximately 10 mm wide (see Fig. 109) and it broadens out only at the end of the Sylvian fissure where the temporal lobe merges without demarcation into the occipital lobe. Taenia chorioidea lies hardly recognizable at the lateral border of

Tractus opticus and Corpus geniculatum lat., but may also run medially over Pulvinar thalami or laterally directly over Corpus geniculatum lat. Even under the microscope Corpus geniculatum lat. – usually multilobular – cannot always be clearly recognized, whereas the rounded Corpus geniculatum med. is always very prominent.
At the border between Cisterna ambiens and Cisterna fissurae lat. (Sylvii) lies Substantia perforata ant., bounded anteriorly by Trigonum olfactorium and posteriorly by Uncus insertion (at the transition to Putamen). Substantia perforata ant. passes medially without a sharply defined borderline into Lamina terminalis, and laterally into Limen insulae. The most anterior part of the insertion of Uncus behind Limen insulae is almost free from perforating arteries. The transition to the orbital gyri may be shallow. The borders of Trigonum olfactorium are hardly recognizable from an oblique, lateral viewpoint.

Fissura lateralis (Sylvii) (Figs. 94, 95, and 99 A)

Difficulties of orientation in the surface relief in a restricted operative field are not seldom due to bridging formations between the first temporal gyrus and the parietal lobe (a factor rarely taken into account in the anatomical literature). Here the opercular gyri may merge directly into the temporal lobe (Fig. 94, below left). In these cases the Sylvian arteries emerge from the fissure and may again disappear into the depths beyond the bridging gyrus. After pulling apart the frontal, partietal, and temporal lobes, two-thirds of the floor of Fissura lateralis (Sylvii) is formed by Insula. The lateral part of Insula (normally 5–10 mm deep) may reach the surface of the brain. The anterior, upper part lies under the opercular gyrus (gyri) of the frontal lobe (distance from the frontal pole 40–50 mm). The sharply ending posterior parts is deepest, 25 mm under the surface of the parietal lobe. (In this region the parietal gyri may run parallel in columnar formation in a medial direction and roll up to cover the upper half of Insula).

Arteries of Fissura lateralis (Sylvii) (Figs. 95, 100 B, 110 A) (Ring, 1969, Potts et al., 1974)

Perforating arteries arise from the proximal stem of A. cerebri media similarly as from the carotid bifurcation, and pass to Substantia perforata ant. usually increasing in calibre laterally (2–3 Aa. lenticulostriatiae to Putamen). They arise against the direction of arterial flow from the proximal trunk of A. cerebri media, or may develop marked looping and hang down into Cisterna fissurae lat. (Sylvii) (Fig. 95). After about 20 mm, on the far side of Limen insulae, A. cerebri media separates at the so-called 'trifurcation' into its terminal branches. There are, however, seldom three, usually two or more than three, branches (Fig. 101). A. cerebri media lies approximately on the lateral margin of Insula and A. operculofrontalis lies with its branches on the upper half of Insula covered by Pars opercularis. The branches of A. operculofrontalis usually curve back before the highest point of Insula (transition between Insula and opercular gyri), extend caudally but usually not as far as the lower margin of the opercular gyri, and thus do not reach the Sylvian fissure itself. This course gives the branches of A. operculofrontalis a downward convex arch* (Fig. 100 *B*). The farther back the arteries lie in the fissure (A. sulci centralis, A. parietalis post., A. angularis), the more horizontally they run**, parallel to the parietal gyri which extend above the bottom of Fissura lat. (Sylvii) like columns (Fig. 100 *A*). These arteries tend to arise directly from the fissure, and not from neighbouring sulci, to the brain surface (Fig. 100 *A*).

Deep Veins of Fissura lateralis (Sylvii) (Figs. 113 and 114)

At the bottom of Fissura lat. (Sylvii) – at a deeper level than the arteries – there is sometimes a small vein (V. cerebri media) which crosses through the perforating arteries to Substantia perforata ant. and may make contact with V. basalis (Rosenthal), V. interpeduncularis, and also to veins of Plexus chorioideus of Cornu inf. (Fig. 114, below). In the area between Crus cerebri, Uncus, and Trigonum olfactorium very variable venous connections supply V. basalis (Rosenthal) with blood from the basal ganglia, Insula, the basal thalamus, and hypothalamus. They have been described in detail by Huang and Wolf (1975) and by Duvernoy (1975). See also Newton and Potts et al. (1974).

C. Region of Cisternae basales (Figs. 102, 103 and 109)

Figs. 102 and 103 show the relationship of the bony and duracovered medial base to the neighbouring

* "U-type".
** "L-type".

intracranial structures. Uncus always projects about 10 mm beyond the medial edge of Tentorium. Its anterior border may adhere to A. carotis int. and may cover the exit of A. communicans ant. and A. chorioidea ant., as well as the lateral part of N. oculomotorius.

The posterior edge of Uncus is demarcated by an indentation from Gyrus parahippocampalis, which lies just behind the frontal plane of the anterior margin of Crus cerebri. This location can be identified at neurosurgical preparation. Both Crura cerebri converge caudally and run at a steep angle forwards towards the base, in contrast to the pons, which shows a backward bend in relation to the axis of Crus cerebri (Fig. 109).

Temporomedial structures in lateral projections (see Fig. 104):

Particularly in coagulations of the temporomedial dura it must be considered which structures are threatened by the effects of deeply penetrating heat. Almost the whole of the medially rising dural surface passes over N. trigeminus region, and, medially from this, N. abducens and A. carotis int., whereas the remaining cranial nerves initially run along the edge of the tentorium and soon disappear under Proc. clinoideus ant.

Distance measurements: Although Tuberculum sellae with its posterior margin is more clearly recognizable on the bony base, the connection between the anterior margins of Nn. optici was chosen as the line of reference, because here despite smoothly delineated bones there is regularly a fold of dura connecting both Nn. optici.

The distance measurements should, in addition to facilitating intradural orientation, also be used as an indication of the position of extradural bony structures, in order, for example, to enable the course of N. trigeminus to be projected onto the dura according to the position of N. opticus and A. carotis int. (Figs. 102 and 103).

Distance Measurements:

Figs. 102–104

	mm
Canalis opticus – Apex partis petrosae	30
Canalis opticus – Proc. clinoid. post.	20
Proc. clinoid. post. – Apex partis petrosae	>10
Foramen ovale – Foramen rotundum	>10
Foramen lacerum – Foramen ovale	< 5
Apex partis petrosae – Meatus acusticus int., lateral limit	25
Foramen spinosum – Hiatus canalis facialis (N. petrosus superficialis major)	15
For. spinosum – Canalis caroticus (For. lacerum)*	5
Level of Canales optici – Infundibulum (perforating Diaphragma sellae)	15
Canalis opticus – Foramen ovale	<30
Anterior limit of Canalis opticus – N. trochlearis (penetrating dura)	30
Anterior limit of Canalis opticus – anterior limit of N. trigeminus (penetrating dura)	30
Canalis opticus – Canalis opticus (lateral limits)	25
Canales optici – edge Tentorium – Falx (Vena cerebri magna – "Galenic point")	65
Midline – Tentorium edge	20
Anterior – posterior crossing of Tentorium edge by Uncus	20
Posterior Tentorium crossing of Uncus – level of Corpora quadrigemina (posterior mesencephalic border)	30
Crus cerebri anterior medial – posterior lateral	20
Sagittal depth of mesencephalic tegmentum	15
Length of N. oculomotorius between anterior border of Crus cerebri and dural exit (N. III)	15
Anterior border of Chiasma – Infundibulum penetration point on Diaphragma sellae very variable**	
Penetration point of Infundibulum on Diaphragma sellae – A. cerebri post. (= ant. border of Pons cerebri)	20
N. opt. – lateral point of Fissura orbit. sup.	>20
N. opt. – anterior edge of preganglionic trigeminus root at dural penetration	30
N. opt. – N. oculomotorius penetration	20
N. opt. Canalis rotundus (measured along the dura)	25
N. opt. – temporal base at the level of Foramen ovale (measured over the dural curvature)	25
Difference in height: Canalis opticus – Foramen ovale	20
Dural penetration of N. III – anterior margin of dural penetration of N. V	10
Dural penetration of N. III – N. IV	5
Dural penetration of Nh IV – N. V	5
Foramen rotundum – Foramen ovale	10–15
Length of Foramen ovale	approx. 10

Reference Figures of Distances Between Cerebral Structures in the Region of Cisterna Ambiens and its Neighbourhood (Fig. 109)

	mm
Length of temporal lobe insertion between beginning of Fissura lat. (Sylvii) and posterior end of Fiss. lat. (Sylvii)	55
Temporal lobe insertion anteriorly between beginning of Fiss. lat. (Sylvii) and tip of temporal horn (= main trunks of A. cerebri media and tip of temporal horn)	15-20
Width between Insula and roof of temporal horn (Cornu inf.)	10
Exit of Crus cerebri at level of Corpus geniculatum laterale – Taenia chorioidea	5
Posterior margin of Crus cerebri – Lamina quadrigemina rostral	10

* The obsolete anatomical designation 'Foramen lacerum' is used here, although Canalis caroticus lies in its medial anterior segment only, and its lateral part is covered by Synchondrosis sphenopetrosa. Here, too, since there is a possibility of carotid damage at sharp dissection, the variable foramen must be taken into account (Fig. 104).

** Variability of this region – see Renn and Rhoton (1975).

	mm
Posterior margin of Crus cerebri – Lamina quadrigemina caudal	15
Length and height of Crus cerebri	15
Shortest distance between Infundibulum and anterior surface of Pons (penetration point of Infundibulum – Pons see Fig. 102)	10
Margin of Pons at intersection point with Trigonum lemnisci and posterior margin of Crus cerebri – superior margin of N. trigeminus exit from Pons	10
Length of basal margin of Pons between Crus cerebri and Medulla oblongata	25
Recessus lateralis – inferior margin of N. trigeminus	15
Ventral surface of Medulla oblongata – Recessus lat. ventriculi quarti (in lateral projection)	10
Shortest distance between Infundibulum and ant. margin of Crus cerebri	15

The lateral measurements in the lower brainstem region are given in consideration of interventions by the temporal access, in which the approach is made into the posterior cranial fossa from the prepontine and pontolateral direction.

Arteries of Cisternae basales (Figs. 107–114)

Substantia perforata anterior is covered anteriorly to an extent of approximately two-thirds by the bifurcation of A. carotis int. The base of Trigonum olfactorium and the anterior margin of the T-shaped carotid bifurcation nearly coincide. The perforating arteries lie dorsally, and with a basal or lateral approach are only visible if they form substantial coils which hang down and are not covered by the arachnoid membranes. The lateral Aa. perforantes are the strongest (Aa. lenticulostriatae, *m2.3*); they run from their origin (A. cerebri media) in the brain substance to the lateral parts of Putamen (Figs. 107 and 108, *m2.3*). In the presence of Uncus processes they must be reckoned with extending into the region of the basal ganglia (Nucl. amygdalae and Putamen), especially if Uncus is aspirated subpially and one inadvertently reaches medially up into Putamen. This can be avoided when there is tumorous enlargement of space in this area, if at the same time the region of Cisternae and Cornu inf. has been sufficiently visualized.

A. communicans post. sends mainly anterior perforating arteries to Hypothalamus, whereas the hypothalamic perforating arteries penetrating farther back between Tractus opticus and Hypothalamus originate from A. chorioidea ant. (*p5.1* and *c5.2*, Figs. 107 and 108). In the chapter "Frontal Lobe" it was shown that the perforating arteries from A. communicans post. and A. chorioidea ant. can mutually replace each other in their area of overlap on the medial margin of Tractus and that they are especially variable. They can only be demonstrated if the temporal branches of A. chorioidea ant. (*c5.1*) are previously cut. At the tip of Cornu inf. the terminal courses of A. chorioidea ant. and the anterior parts of A. chorioidea-posterior group converge (Figs. 107 and 108, *c5* and *p6.1*). The largest part of A. chorioidea-posterior group *(p6.7)* runs forwards and upwards in the middle region of Crus cerebri (Figs. 110 and 111). This vessel is also stretched when the temporal lobe is everted, and therefore in Figs. 107 and 108 the typical knee at Corpus geniculatum laterale is missing. A. thalamogeniculata *(p8)* is particularly variable, and in contrast to the specimen shown in Figs. 107 and 108 it has often a network of connections of Trigonum lemnisci (Fig. 114, above).

In Figs. 109-114 the temporal lobe has been removed, thereby opening the ventricular trigonum (cut surface of posterior portion of Hippocampus – o in Fig. 109). Anteriorly the peduncle of the temporal lobe is encircled by A. cerebri media. The axis of Crus cerebri (*Cc* in Fig. 109) nearly corresponds to the vertical axis of the body in the erect position. The pontine vein runs in accordance with the known flexion of the brainstem at an angle of approximately 60°.

Under the microscope it can be seen that perforations for the entrance of arteries lie not only at sites of predilection – Substantia perforata ant. and post. and anterior surface of the pons and Medulla oblongata in the median region – but also especially in the area of Trigonum lemnisci, the quadrigeminal region, the border between Crus cerebri and the margin of the pons, as well as farther caudally at the border between Brachium pontis and Lobulus quadrangularis and the cerebellopontine angle. The distance between Infundibulum and the ventral surface of the pons is one-third shorter than that between Infundibulum and Crus cerebri caudally at the entrance to the pons. Corpora mamillaria in the depths of Fossa interpeduncularis are hardly recognizable from an oblique lateral viewpoint, as they are covered by A. basilaris and its branches. Here orientation is easier from the base (Figs. 107 and 108).

With oblique visualization and reclination of the temporal lobe the arterial region can be demonstrated above the edge of Tentorium up to the region of Cornu inf. (in the stiffer formolfixed preparations only by means of resection of the temporal lobe). Whereas in Figs. 110-114 (above) typical vascular courses are shown, Fig. 114 (below) shows a rare variant which would hardly have been identifiable in the conventional angiogram. Here A. calcarina (*p13*) arises directly out of A. chorioidea ant.; the hitherto existing angiographic technique is not adequate to determine such variants preoperatively. Enlargement and tomoangiography will make the analysis easier in the future.

The strongly coiled Aa. perforantes pose a problem in the approach to the arteries of Cisterna ambiens, particularly at the border between Crus cerebri and the pons, since they can in principle arise from all of the arteries (*p1, p3, p4, b5*) encircling Crus cerebri. Trigonum lemnisci and Lamina quadrigemina can be supplied from all these arteries, and not only from A. quadrigemina (*p4*) and A. thalamogeniculata (*p8*). The smaller accompanying arteries of the proximal A. cerebri posterior (*p6.1* and *p4*) usually run above N. oculomotorius; under it lies N. trochlearis, which crosses laterally over A. cerebelli sup. (*b5*) which is closer to the pons. In the region of Trigonum lemnisci the N. trochlearis (*N. IV*) may be crossed laterally and medially by perforating arteries. Distally the perforating vessels lie medially of *N. IV* and show, in distinction to other perforating arteries, a network of mutual connections, which for this reason and because of their deeper position allow isolation of N. trochlearis by operative and anatomically preparative isolation up to the quadrigeminal region. In Fig. 112 A. cerebri post. (*p1*), with its smaller parallel-running accompanying vessels [A. chorioidea post. med. (*p6.1*), A. quadrigemina (*p4*)], has been drawn rostrally to the side out of its typical position on the superior margin of the pons. This technique, which is possible at operation as well as in dissection, leads to severe tension on the loops of perforating arteries at Crus cerebri. It may be seen that all the vessel trunks surrounding Crus cerebri cover a large number of perforating arteries, which can hardly be seen from the lateral direction. In a number of cases, as in Fig. 112, the density of the vessels in the region of Trigonum lemnisci is particularly great. Apart from the arterial network already mentioned, this region is also interspersed with veins (Tamaki et al., 1976). In contrast to the region of Crus cerebri, an interruption of arteries is possible here if network connections are secured. In the injection preparation this can be demonstrated with the magnifying glass, as in vivo with the surgical microscope.

Veins of Cisternae basales (Figs. 113 and 114)

The large venous trunks are, like nearly all veins of the brain, inconstant. V. basalis (Rosenthal) with its numerous variants was described in great detail in 1975 by Y. T. Huang and B. S. Wolf. Fig. 113 (centre) shows the typical course with particularly frequent variants according to the author's own observations. Particularly important are the strong venous connections, which may emerge at different points of Plexus chorioideus and take blood not only from Plexus chorioideus but also, farther rostrally, from various parts of the basal ganglia (atrial veins, see Chapter 6).

Resections of Plexus chorioideus in these variants lead one to expect damage of the brainstem, since in the parenchyma itself there are not more anastomoses. Typical for these veins is their tendency to hug the surface structure closely, whereas the overlying arteries, also smaller branches, show numerous coil formations lying freely in the cisternal space. Only in the basal region of Cisterna ambiens may small initial branches of V. basalis (Rosenthal) be woven through with the perforating arteries. One of the variants in Fig. 113 (lower right) shows a strong connection of V. basalis (Rosenthal) laterobasally with the point of entry of the group of Sylvian veins in the temporobasal dura or at the edge of Ala parva of the sphenoid bone. The interruption of connecting veins between Fissura lat. (Sylvii) and basal dura at the wing of the sphenoid is only without danger for the venous drainage of the brainstem if the typical strong connection of V. basalis (Rosenthal) to V. magna (Galeni) has been reliably confirmed by angiography. If V. mesencephalica lat. is of a large calibre its interruption could impair drainage from the midbrain, pons, and the region of Lobulus quadrangularis. In the variant illustrated in the upper part of Fig. 114 the venous drainage of the lateral midbrain region follows mainly a common course with the upper cerebellar drainage to V. petrosa sup., which can in other cases be ligated without risk.

D. Preoperative Radiology – Some Aspects (Figs. 115, 116, 118–121)

The floor of the middle cranial fossa lies deeper than the student imagines (Fig. 115), since the fine double contour of the polar regions of the middle cranial fossa projecting over one another is masked by the body of the sphenoid with its air-filled spaces, and the fact is overlooked that the foremost frontal plane of the temporal pole projects about 20 mm* forward of that of Proc. clinoideus ant. The more heavily drawn lateral insertions of Alae parvae into Alae magnae already correspond to Fissura lat. (Sylvii).

The position of the temporal horn is very variable. There is, therefore, no exact method for its localization on the basis of bony structures. Thus Fig. 115 is merely intended as a rough guide in a lateral x-ray projection: temporal pole, deepest point of the middle cranial fossa, and tip of the inferior (temporal) horn form an almost equilateral triangle with length of sides 40 mm, whereby the tip of the inferior horn lies approximately at the level of Dorsum sellae and is at the same time a measure of the medially steeply rising basal part of the temporal lobe. Its pole region leans anteriorly against the floor of the middle cranial fossa and flattens out in an anterior direction, whereas the principal direction of this cerebral lobe coincides approximately with the course of A. cerebri media. Since at the surface relief of the brain Fissura lat. (Sylvii) and the inferior margin of the temporal lobe run nearly parallel, their direction is almost identical with the connecting line between the deepest point of the middle cranial fossa and the anterior point of Sulcus and Sinus transv. behind the lateral point of Margo superior partis petrosae on the convexity of the skull.

Medially the temporal lobe extends upward to the tentorial edge. Above this lies the medial border of the inferior horn, separated from the tentorial edge by the narrow-edged Uncus and Gyrus parahippocampalis, which rolls inwards towards the hippocampus into the inferior horn. The tentorial edge and the medial border of the inferior horn lie equidistant from the midline: 20 mm. This corresponds to half the width of the tentorial space. Fig. 115 is the tracing of a ventriculogram.

Fig. 116 shows the simplified copy of an angiogram. The sketched – in inferior horn tip projects just underneath the Sylvian arteries and, corresponding to the thickness of the temporal lobe peduncle, approximately 1 cm medially of them. The distance between the inferior horn tip and carotid bifurcation is only 10 mm (corresponding to the distance Subst. perf. ant. to inferior horn tip). The superficial Sylvian veins run higher than the Sylvian arteries, corresponding to the slope of Fissura lat. (Sylvii) from laterally in a mediobasal direction. Nevertheless in the example shown the venous variants *A4* and *A5* of Fig. 116 are to be reckoned with Fissura lat. (Sylvii) and veins of the fissure do not always dovetail.

In operations on the terminal section of A. carotis int., particularly for aneurysms of A. communicans post. or carotid ligatures at the penetration point through the dura, an exact previous angiographic localization of the exit of A. communicans post. (and A. choriodea ant.) is necessary in order to avoid inadvertent ligature of these two branches and/or their perforating arteries. The first of the up to 50 perforating branches leaving A. communicans post. is often the biggest and may leave A. communicans post. immediately after the carotid exit of the vessel. The projection of A. chorioidea post. at the exit from the carotid onto the anterior clinoid process allows conclusions to be drawn as to whether this vessel leaves A. carotis int. immediately above the dura or somewhat farther away in the area of the basal cisternae (Fig. 116, *A2* and *A3*). The superimposition of the arterial branchings may, especially if there is much looping, be so extreme that even posterior parietal branches with a more horizontal course and operculofrontal ramifications taking a basal convex course cannot always be clearly differentiated. Of the perforating arteries especially Aa. lenticulostriatae are almost always recognizable. Between them and the proximal branches of A. cerebri media, marking the surface of Insula, lie Capsula extrema, Claustrum, Capsula externa, and the lateral margin of Putamen (Fig. 116, *B1*).

An illustration of the smaller perforating arteries has not been included, despite the current angiographic enlargement techniques, since these arteries have been more clearly demonstrated several times in anatomical preparations.

Collaterals between the Sylvian group of veins and other superficial veins [connections to Sinus sagitt. sup. and V. Labbé (Fig. 116, *A1*)] cannot always reliably be assessed by angiography. Their absence in the presence of strongly developed Sylvian veins should be a warning to exercise reserve in lifting and interrupting these veins at Ala parva. The same

* Measurement taken from skull preparations (often lateral roentgenograms without exact projection).

applies to V. Labbé, which occasionally hinders the approach to the middle cranial fossa.
In the angiographic demonstration of A. basilaris and its branches the direction of projection in the a-p roentgenogram is of particular importance. In old people the reclination of the head, and thus the correct x-ray position, is difficult to achieve. The angiogram of a young person (Figs. 118 and 119) has, therefore, been contrasted with that of an older patient (Figs. 120 and 121). The inclination of the head can be seen for example from the position of Bregma and Lambda as well as from the level of the petrous bone in relation to Orbita. The preceding sketch in Fig. 117 shows the different direction of projection of an imaginary midbrain cross-section. Lateral roentgenograms that are not quite exactly adjusted or asymmetries in the course of vessels (Fig. 119) allow an evaluation of the vessels on both sides.
The inferior horn tip can be located at the division point of A. chorioidea ant. (Fig. 119, *c5*). In the case of cerebral atrophy or hydrocephalus in Figs. 120 and 121 the anterior horn extension is larger, also rostrally and basally, than in the ventricular system of normal width. Although the perforating arteries and choroidal post. group are frequently recognizable, single branches are difficult to differentiate due to superposition, so that only gross displacement is recognizable. Only in children is a more exact analysis possible. Here too the enlargement technique is an important prerequisite of adequate preparation for microsurgical intervention.

E. Operative Techniques – Some Aspects
(Fig. 122)

For the incision of skin and underlying tissue the same techniques should be used as in the frontal exposure, to protect Ramus temporalis n. facialis. After turning back the skin and galea, the temporal muscle together with the periosteum should be carefully separated from the bone. Whether the temporal muscle should be partly left on the bone or completely detached, in the method of Yaşargil, will not be further discussed here. It is important that the approach should be made far towards the base, and through a narrow access the anterior part of the temporal muscle transversely notched somewhat above the zygomatic arch (Fig. 122, *1*). The muscle should be separated at Linea temporalis sup. and not in its parenchyma (Fig. 122, *3*). In this way its function will be at least partly preserved, and the tendency to haemorrhage from the heavily branched A. temporalis prof., which runs mainly in its anterior part, reduced. The anterior burrhole should not be placed too low in order to avoid penetration of the orbit (Fossa lacrimalis, Fig. 122, *2*). The basal burrholes should also not be made too low because of the danger of opening the "knee" of Sinus transversus or Tegmen tympani (Fig. 122, *4*). It is better to remove the last part of the bone osteoclastically towards the base (Fig. 122, *5*, *6*). The higher the burrholes lie, the easier it is to lead the dura protector round the insertion of Ala parva et magna (Fig. 123). In Yaşargil's method with the temporal muscle isolated, the bone flap can be made a little farther towards the base. Both for frontolateral and for anterotemporal processes Yaşargil's modification so-called "pterional" (sphenoidal) approach offers the possibility of reaching mediobasal structures in the neighbourhood of N. opticus, A. carotis int., Infundibulum, and Pons without extreme reclination of the temporal brain, overcrossing N. III. The bony resection in a medial direction is limited by the lateral fold of Fissura orbitalis sup. (Figs. 124 and 125). The transition of the dura into Periorbita is here characterized by a sharp-edged fold that could be mistaken for a harmless vein and coagulated. This could result in thrombosis of V. ophthalmica sup. (Fig. 124 *B*), the farthest laterally lying structure of the fissure, which is surrounded by this fold, and would explain the postoperatively observed symptoms of thrombosis of Sinus cavernosus.
R. frontalis of A. meningea media regularly passes over the lateral dural fold at the fissure from the middle cranial fossa through an opening in the sharp-edged Ala parva into the anterior cranial fossa. During interruption of A. meningica media (R. front.) it is likewise necessary to protect the dural fold and its contents. Fissura orbitalis inf. with Vv. ophthalmicae inferiores is also endangered if the temporal muscle is not pulled back from the fissure on coagulation of the branches of A. temporalis profunda. The localization can be seen in Fig. 124 *A* and *B*, and in Fig. 125. In drilling off the insertion of Ala parva and Ala magna it should be noted that the lateral orbital wall behind Pars orbitalis of Os zygomaticum is thinwalled over Fissura orbitalis inf. so that the lateral orbital region is easily opened, in contrast to the strong bony block of the medial parts of Ala magna lying immediately

behind the thinwalled part of Proc. orbitalis of Os zygomaticum and above Fiss. orbitalis inf. (Fig. 125, below). The distance between the lateral end of Fissura orbitalis sup. and Canalis opticus measures only 20 mm, whereas the distance of N. opticus from the frontal pole is about 60 mm. If the reclination of the brain should be insufficient, the zygomatic arch can be resected subperiosteally, and M. temporalis luxated. Dural tack-up sutures at the base are usually attached to the temporal muscle, and these hinder chewing. For the past year the author has used with success the procedure of pinning the dura along the bony base (developed by his predecessor Prof. Dr. T. Riechert).

The varying slope and curvature of the temporal lobe already described (Fig. 93, below) should be borne in mind during placing and adjusting of the self-retaining spatulae. Fig. 126 demonstrates how the brain is traumatized by a too sharply bent and wrongly applied spatula, without the field of vision being particularly extensive.

The view of the area between N. olfactorius and N. trochlearis shown in Fig. 126 requires careful preparation, especially of the arachnoid membranes. This is, for example, after subarachnoid haemorrhages, very time-consuming because of the adhesions. In Fig. 127 the dangers are shown: in preparing Cisterna chiasmatis, the perforating arteries and branches of A. cerebri ant. lying in front of N. opticus and Chiasma (R. orbitalis of A. frontopolaris) (Fig. 127, *a6.1*, Fig. 127, *a2*) must be protected. For most operations in this region it is necessary initially to push back Gyrus rectus on a wide front from the surface of N. opticus. At the posterior margin of N. opticus the opening of Cisterna fissurae lat. (Sylvii) and the arachnoid membrane between N. opticus and A. carotis int. allows an approach to Diaphragma sellae, which is normally very narrow but can become occasionally very wide by preparation, pushing apart A. carotis int. and N. opticus (Fig. 127, above). In these cases the main danger is injury to perforating vessels originating from A. communicans post., A. chorioidea ant., and the posterior surface of A. carotis int. (superior hypohyseal artery). After removal of space-occupying lesions, A. carotis int., N. opticus, N. oculomotorius, and Tentorium fold of the opposite side, as well as Infundibulum, can be seen through this crevice under the microscope (Fig. 127 left above, after extirpation of a craniopharyngeoma).

The brain surface adjacent to A. carotis int. corresponds to the anterior part of Uncus, injury to which involves a greater risk of epilepsy. Premature pulling back of Uncus can cause a medially lying aneurysm to be torn off and/or N. oculomotorius to be stretched if it is adherent to Uncus. In addition, the presence of A. communicans post., its perforating branches, and, somewhat higher, A. chorioidea ant. (also with perforating branches) must be expected. The anterior margin of Uncus is poorly differentiated from the gyri in the polar region of the temporal lobe. Its posterior margin is almost always clearly notched. Only farther dorsally are Rr. temporales (Fig. 127, *p11.1, p11.2*) to be expected. The anterior level of Crus cerebri is thus already passed. Further lifting of the temporal lobe causes tension of the temporobasal branches of A. cerebri post. (*p11.1, p11.2*) and the vessels to the midbrain. Loose loopformations facilitate the reclination of the brain, but cannot be recognized initially. After further opening of Arachnoidea between the medial inferior margin of the temporal lobe (Gyrus parahippocampalis) and the tentorial edge, N. trochlearis is to be expected. It is fixed between two arachnoid layers and runs just above or below the tentorial edge. Bevor Tentorium is split, N. trochlearis must be freed with good visualization (Fig. 127).

Tentorium is always incised behind the level of Sinus petrosus sup. in order to avoid damage to N. trigeminus, A. carotis int., and other cranial nerves. Since Sinus petrosus is hardly transparent, the surgeon must palpate with the dissector whether the hard bony middle cranial fossa and surface of the petrous bone or the elastic tentorium has been reached laterally. Occasionally bridging veins running from the surface of the temporal lobe to the tentorium are a hindrance on the way. It is better to push some elastic material (muscle, gelfoam, or something similar) into the venous opening rather than to carry out a thorough coagulation of the tentorium, which would only lead to shrinkage of the tentorium and widening of the opening. The tentorium is diffusely interspersed by lacunar treelike branches which are connected with Sinus rectus. If the tentorium is incised, the old method of clipping is still the safest way to prevent extensive thromboses that can propagate as far the sinus region. After turning back the split tentorial edge, the view is opened onto Lobulus quadrangularis, A. cerebelli sup. (*b5*), A. basilaris, (*b1*) and, with further reclination of Uncus, also onto A. cerebri post. with its perforating branches (Fig. 126). N. trigeminus is only visible if the tentorium is turned far back or if it is pushed upwards, together with N. trochlearis which crosses over it, by an underlying tumour (Friedrich and Seeger, 1976). The whole ascending dural region between the tip of the petrous bone and Sinus petrosus sup. on the one hand and Proc. clinoideus ant. and N. opticus on the other, is filled by the formations of dural duplicatures lying here laterally to Sella. This region is demonstrated in Fig. 127, and for the sake of clarity N. oculomot. and N. ophthalmicus have been resected. Nothing can be seen of Sinus cavernosus. As Parkinson et al. have proved, Sinus cavernosus lies mainly medially between A. carotis int. and the periosteal lining of Sella. Our own dissections carried out on fresh cadavers confirm these findings*.

The largest part of the temporomedial dural surface is underlaid by Ganglion semilunare (Gasseri) and the three branches of N. trigeminus. This must be taken into account during coagulations in this region – e.g., for meningiomas – as well as particularly the neighbourhood of the very variable extradural pathway of A. carotis int., and the remaining cranial nerves (*N. III, N. IV, N. VI*) running between A. carotis int. and N. trigeminus obliquely from above and behind towards the front and below laterally. In addition, the reader is referred to the distance measurements given at the beginning, which allow a projection of these structures onto the surface of the dura. Martins and Umbach reported in 1975 on a simple localizing method of Foramen ovale.

F. Appendix

Parasellar and Sella Region (Figs. 128 and 130)

The tentorial edge continues as a small fold up to the point of passage of N. oculomotorius. Widened out into a plate, it covers the anterior clinoid process and is perforated by N. opticus and A. carotis int. (Fig. 128, above). In contrast to the sharp edges of Tentorium· and Ala parva of the sphenoid, the elevation of the dura in the opticus-carotid – region is blunt, whereby difficulties of orientation may arise. A. carotis int. may at its point of penetration cross under the medial margin of N. opticus. In the case of tumours, A. carotis int. may pass far laterally of N. opticus through the dura of the base. This, however, cannot always be recognized with certainty on previous angio – and tomographic examination. A. hypophyseos sup. may arise out of the medial carotid wall (Fig. 128, above). Diaphragma sellae normally makes a moderately concave bend in a basal direction between the extended tentorial folds. About 5 mm behind the dural point of exit of N. oculomotorius that of N. trochlearis is to be expected. The point of dura entry of N. trigeminus is arched over to an even greater extent by the tentorial edge than that of N. trochlearis. The trigeminal trunk itself may be visible from a temporal approach if basal tumours raise and stretch it rostrally or if Tentorium is split. Then N. trochlearis lies stretched across the trigeminal root, which it would normally cross over without close contact (Fig. 128, lower picture).

Acess to N. abducens is difficult from the supratentorial direction; its point of dural perforation lies 20 mm behind Dorsum sellae, and, after a diverging extradural course of approximately 10 mm, passes through under the dura-covered strap of bone (or Gruber's ligament*) at the tip of the petrous bone (Apex ossis petrosi) in front of N. trigeminus, to follow medially Ganglion semilunare (Gasseri) and N. ophthalmicus before it reaches the lateral carotid wall as the deepest and most basal nerve of the tentorial fold (Fig. 128, below).

N. trochlearis and N. trigeminus run most superficially between two layers of the dura (Fig. 128, below). Only N. nasociliaris as one of the three branches of N. ophthalmicus dips before it reaches Fissura orbitalis sup. into a deeper, fibrous layer before N. trochlearis runs alongside N. ophthalmicus (Fig. 128, below). N. oculomotorius also runs in this deeper layer, and 5 mm after perforating the dura reaches the lateral edge of Processus clinoideus ant., where it likewise passes under the inner layer of the double-layered dura. This laminated structure is demonstrated in Fig. 129: between the two layers of the dura outside Anulus tendineus (Zinnii) Nn. trochlearis, frontalis, and lacrimalis pass into the superior and lateral part of Fissura orbitalis sup. and laterally of those run one or more Vv. ophthalmicae superiores. The deeper-lying Nn. nasociliaris, oculomotorius, and abducens are enclosed by Anulus tendineus (Zinnii). Between these nerves and A. carotis int. is a loose space which i

* Thanks are due to Prof. Sandritter, Director of the Departmental Group, Pathological Institute, University of Freiburg, for providing the material.

* Quoted after Parkinson (1965).

filled by numerous trabeculae, formerly wrongly believed to be Sinus cavernosus. In particular, the investigations of Parkinson (1965) and of Bedford (1966) have shown that Sinus cavernosus is confined essentially to the fissure between the medial carotid wall, the periosteal lining of Sulcus caroticus, and the lateral border of the sella. If both the outer dural layers are removed as well as all nerves except N. abducens, which lies close alongside A. carotis int., Sinus cavernosus will be visible medially and the meningohypophyseal artery laterally (arising from the carotid wall).

Fig. 130 gives information on the structure of these medial parts of the dura including the vessels supplying the sella and hypophysis. Between the periosteal lining of Clivus and the overlying tough dural layer lie venous lacunae, which form a spongy mass permeating the whole region up to the occipital foramen (so-called Plexus basilaris). They are connected with Sinus cavernosus, Sinus petrosus sup. and inf., and Sinus marginalis. Practically the whole basal dura is permeated by such lacunae. Probably for the sake of simplicity the current anatomical atlases show only the larger branches. Particularly dense vascular areas lie all around the hypophysis, penetrating different layers of the dura; they cannot be separated from Sinus cavernosus and Plexus basilaris. In opening the capsule of a hypophyseal tumour, the increased venous vascularization in the region of Tuberculum sellae is also noticeable. In coagulating, care should be taken not to approach too closely the often far medially lying carotid or the penetration point of N. opticus. The perforating veins that come from the CSF space, which can reach the basal venous lacunae, are of particular importance. In the middle to upper third of the clivus, Duvernoy describes as "anterior drainage pathway" a connection between the ventrolateral surface of the pons to the dura and Plexus basilaris. The laterally lying connection of V. petrosa sup. and Sinus petrosus sup. between the exit point of N. trigeminus and N. facialis should be mentioned. It is always present and its particular characteristic is its extraordinary variability as regards the calibre and number of its often multiple veins.

Finally there is also a V. petrosa inf., which leads from the region of Polus olivaris sup. into Sinus petrosus inf. These three most important venous connections ventrally and laterally in the middle and caudal brainstem region must be taken into consideration when the brainstem is raised at operation and these vessels are subjected to tension. Their interruption at operation presupposes an adequate drainage by other venous parts (see Chapter 7).

Border Areas Between Fossa cranii ant., Fossa cranii media, Fossa pterygoidea, and Orbita (Figs. 132 and 133)

Tumours of this region may make it necessary to remove all the bones in this area. Figs. 132 and 133 show how by removal of the bone a uniform space is made out of Canalis opticus, Fissura orbitalis sup. Foramen rotundum, Fissura orbit. inf., and Fossa pterygoidea, the roof and side wall of Orbita. It is essential that both Dura and Periorbita are left intact in order to avoid an Enophthalmus or an injury to the contents of Orbita and Fiss. orbit. sup. Such resections are possible with the high-frequency drill. Processus clinoideus ant. should be left intact. If it has to be resected because of tumour invasion, the carotid siphon should be expected to lie medially in the immediate vicinity. Operative interventions in the medial region of Orbita should be made primarily from the nasal approach over the sinuses or from the transfrontal approach. Two-thirds of the orbital funnel are, however, demonstrable laterally: the roof, the side wall, the floor of Orbita up to the roof of Sinus maxillaris, and the area bordering on the middle cranial fossa. Medially from N. maxillaris and Foramen rotundum the dural and periosteal duplications are to be expected. They enclose A. carotis int., laterally to this the cranial nerves, and medially Sinus cavernosus.

G. References

Bedford, M. A.: The "cavernous" sinus. Brit. J. Ophthal. **50**, 41–46 (1966).

Duvernoy, H. M.: The Superficial Veins of the Human Brain. Veins of the Brain Stem and of the Base of the Brain. Berlin–Heidelberg–New York: Springer. 1975.

Friedrich, H., Seeger, W.: Mikrochirurgie der präpontinen Tumoren. Neurochirurgia **19**, 246–260 (1976).

Huang, Y. P., Wolf, B. S.: In: Advances in Cerebral Angiography, edited by Salamon, G., Part I Anatomy: Variations of Basal Cerebral Veins: Embryologic Considerations, p. 82. Berlin–Heidelberg–New York: Springer. 1975.

Martins, L. F., Umbach, W.: Simple determination of the foramen in trigeminus coagulation. Neurochirurgia **18**, 163–166 (1975).

Newton, Th., Potts, D. G.: Radiology of the Skull and Brain Angiography. St. Louis: The C. V. Mosby Company. 1974.

Parkinson, D.: A surgical approach to the cavernous portion of the carotid artery. Anatomical studies and case report. J. Neurosurg. **23**, 474–483 (1965).

Riechert, T.: A new surgical method for treatment of pulsating exophthalmus. Prog. Brain Res. **30,** 445–449 (1968).
Ring, A.: In: The Neglected Cause of Stroke. Occlusion of the Smaller Intracranial Arteries and Their Diagnosis by Cerebral Angiography. St. Louis: Warren H. Green, Inc. 1969.
Tamaki, N., Taomoto, K., Fujiwara, K., Yamashita, H., Matsumoto, S., Takeda, H.: The venous drainage of the tectum mesencephali. Neuroradiology **11,** 151–157 (1976).

Literature for Further Reading

Arutiunov, A. I., Serbinenko, F. A., Shlykov, A. A.: Surgical treatment of carotid-cavernous fistulas. Progr. Brain Res. **30,** 441–444 (1968).
Bergland, R. M., et al.: Anatomical variations in the pituitary gland and adjacent structures in 225 human autopsy cases. J. Neurosurg. **28,** 93–99 (1968).
Bernasconi, V., Cassinari, V.: Un segno carotido grafico tipico di meningioma del tentorio. Chirurgia (Milano) **2,** 286–588 (1956).
Camp, J. D.: 2. The normal and pathologic anatomy of the sella turcica as revealed by roentgenograms. Am. J. Roentgenol. Rad. Ther. Nucl. Med. **12,** 143–156 (1924).
Cushing, H., Eisenhardt, L.: Meningiomas. Their classification, regional behavior, life history and surgical end results, pp. 785. Springfield, Ill.: Ch. C. Thomas. 1938.
Dichiro, G., Nelson, K. B.: The volume of the sella turcica. Am. J. Roentgenol. Rad. Ther. Nucl. Med. **87,** 989–1008 (1962).
Donaghy, R. M. P., Yaşargil, M. G.: Micro-Vascular Surgery. Stuttgart: G. Thieme, St. Louis: C. V. Mosby Co. 1967.
Drake, C. G.: Surgical treatment of ruptured aneurysms of the basilar artery. Experience with 14 cases. J. Neurosurg. **23,** 457–473 (1965).
Drake, C. G.: The surgical treatment of vertebral-basilar aneurysm Clin. Neurosurg. **16,** 114–169 (1969).
Faure, J., Binnert, D., Michotey, P., Salamon, G.: Etude radio-anatomique des branches collatérales de l'artère carotide interne (dans son segment intracaverneux). Neuro-Chirurgie **18,** 561–579 (1971).
Foix, Ch., Hillemand, P.: Les artères de l'axe encéphalique jusqu'au diencéphale inclusivement. Rev. Neuro. **6,** 705–739 (1925).
Hamby, W. B., Dohn, D. F.: Carotid-Cavernous Fistulas: Report of Thirty-Six Cases and Discussion of Their Management. Clin. Neurosurg. **11,** 150–170 (1965).
Hayreh, S. S., Dass, R.: The ophthalmic artery. I. Origin and intracranial and intra-canalicular course. Brit. J. Ophthalm. **46,** 65–98 (1962).
Housepian, M.: Surgical treatment of unilateral optic nerve gliomas. J. Neurosurg. **31,** 604–607 (1969).
Ishimori, S., et al.: Treatment of carotid-cavernous fistula by gelfoam embolization. J. Neurosurg. **27,** 315–319 (1967).
Jacobson, J. H., et al.: Microsurgery as an aid to middle cerebral artery endarterectomy. J. Neurosurg. **19,** 108–114 (1962).
Jefferson, G.: On the saccular aneurysms of the internal carotid artery in the cavernous sinus. Brit. J. Surg. **26,** 267–302 (1938).
Kaplan, H. A.: The transcerebral venous system. An anatomical study. A. M. A. Archives of Neurology **1,** 40/148–44/152 (1959).
Lang, J., Schäfer, K.: Über Ursprung und Versorgungsgebiete der intracavernösen Strecke der A. carotis interna. Gegenbaurs morph. Jahrb., Leipzig **122,** 182–202 (1976).
Lillequist, B.: The subarachnoid cisterns. An anatomic and roentgenologic study. Acta Radiol. **185,** 1–108 (1959).
Meadows, S. P.: Aneurysms of the internal carotid artery. Trans. Ophth. Soc. U. K. 137–155 (1950).
Mittenwallner, F. von: Variationsstatistische Untersuchungen an den basalen Hirngefäßen. Acta anat. **24,** 51–88 (1955).
Monier-Kuhn, A., Bouchet, A., Costaz, G.: Contribution à l'étude anatomique radiologique et chirurgicale de l'artère choroidienne antérieure. Neuro-chir. **1,** 345–370 (1955).
Morello, A., Cooper, I. S.: Arteriographic anatomy of the anterior choriodal artery. Amer. J. Roentgenol. **73,** 748–751 (1955).
Mortara, R., Norrel, H.: Consequences of a deficient sellar diaphragm. J. Neurosurg. **32,** 565–573 (1970).
Nadjmi, M.: Die Radiologie des diencephalo-hypophysären Gebietes als Grundlage für die Stereotaxie. Habilitationsschrift Würzburg 1964.
Otomo, E.: The anterior chorioidal artery. Arch. Neurol. **13,** 656–658 (1965).
Parkinson, D.: The normal anatomy of the cavernous carotid and its surgical signifiance. Presented at meeting of the Harvey Cushing Society, Philadelphia, Pa., April 19, 1963.
Parkinson, D.: Collateral circulation of cavernous carotid artery (anatomy). Canad. J. Surg. **7,** 251–268 (1964).
Pool, J. F., Colton, R. P.: The dissecting microscope for intracranial vascular surgery. J. Neurosurg. **25,** 315–318 (1966).
Rand, R. W., Jannetta, P. J.: Microneurosurgery for aneurysms of the vertebral basilar artery system. J. Neurosurg. **27,** 330–335 (1967).
Rasmussen, A. T.: Proportions of various subdivisions of normal adult human hypophysis cerebri and relative number of different types of cells in pars distalis with biometric evaluation of age and sex differences and special consideration of basophilic invasion into infundibular process. Res. Nerv. Ment. Dis., Proc. **17,** 118–150 (1924).
Renn, H. W., Rhoton, L. A.: Microsurgical anatomy of the sellar region. J. Neurosurg. **43,** 288–298 (1975).
Rothman, S. L. G., Allen, III, W. E., Simeone, J. F.: The medial posterior choroidal artery as an indica of masses at the foramen of Monro. Neuroradiology **11,** 123–129 (1976).
Sindou, M., et al.: Microchirurgie veineuse intracranienne expérimental. Neuro-Chirurgie **21,** N° 3 (1975).
Sjörgren, S. E.: The anterior choroidal artery. Acta radiol. **46,** 143–157 (1956).
Speakman, T. J.: Internal occlusion of a carotid-cavernous fistula. J. Neurosurg. **21,** 303–305 (1964).
Schaefer, J. P.: Some points in the regional anatomy of the optic pathway, with especial reference to tumors of the hypophysis cerebri and resulting ocular changes. Anat. Rec. **28,** 243–279 (1924).
Schnürer, L. B., Stattin, S.: Vascular supply of intra cranial dura from internal carotid artery with special reference to its angiographic significance. Acta radiol. **1,** 441–450 (1963).
Wackenheim, A., Ludwiczak, R., Capesius, P.: The course of the anterior choroidal artery. Neuroradiology **11,** 73–75 (1976).
Wanissorn, R.: Mechanism of experimental muscle embolization of the carotid cavernous fistula and the fate of the emboli. J. Neurosurg. **32,** 344–348 (1970).

Wilson, Ch. B., Sang, H.: Surgical treatment for aneurysms of the upper basilar artery. J. Neurosurg. **44,** 537–543 (1976).

Yaşargil, M. G.: Intracranial microsurgery. Clin. Neurosurg. **17,** 250–255 (1970).

Yaşargil, M. G., Fox, J. L.: The microsurgical approach to intracranial aneurysms. Surg. Neurol. **3,** 7–14 (1975).

Yaşargil, M. G.: Microsurgery Applied to Neurosurgery. Stuttgart: G. Thieme, New York–London: Academic Press. 1969.

Zinn, J. G.: Discriptio anatomica oculi humani, 2nd ed., ed. H. A. Wrisberg, p. 194. Göttingen: Vandenhoeck. 1780. (Cited by Meyer, 1887).

H. Illustrations

(Fig. 93 to 133)

Fig. 93. Lateral and basal superficial relief of temporal lobe. Not.: distance measurements and different planes of curvature
Measurements in millimetres (mm)

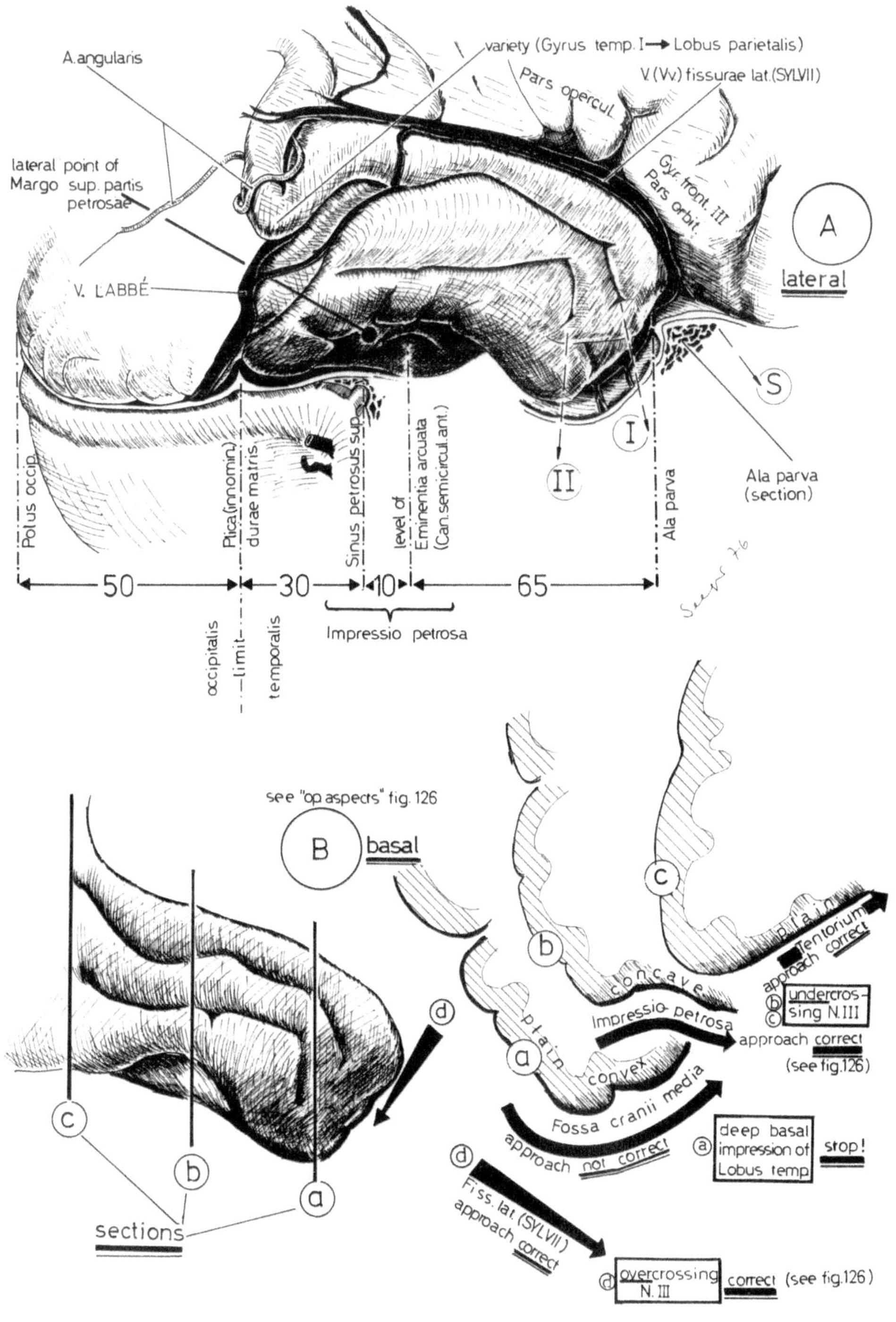
A.angularis
variety (Gyrus temp. I → Lobus parietalis)
Pars opercul.
V.(Vv.) fissurae lat.(SYLVII)
lateral point of
Margo sup. partis
petrosae
Gyr. front. III
Pars orbit.
A
lateral
V. LABBÉ
S
I
II
Ala parva
(section)
Polus occip.
Plica (innomin.)
durae matris
Sinus petrosus sup.
level of
Eminentia arcuata
(Can. semicircul. ant.)
Ala parva
50
30
10
65
Impressio petrosa
occipitalis
limit
temporalis
see "op.aspects" fig. 126
B
basal
c
b
a
d
sections
plain
concave
convex
Impressio petrosa
approach correct
(see fig.126)
Fossa cranii media
approach not correct
tentorium
approach correct
b
c
undercrossing N.III
a
deep basal
impression of
Lobus temp.
stop!
Fiss. lat. (SYLVII)
approach correct
d
overcrossing
N. III
correct (see fig.126)

Fig. 94. A. cerebri media lies with its main trunks adjacent to Insula, the frontal and parietal lobes. Only Aa. temporales bridge Fissura lat. (Sylvii) (obstacle to operative approach!)
Below left: variant of gyri and vascular course

FIG. 94

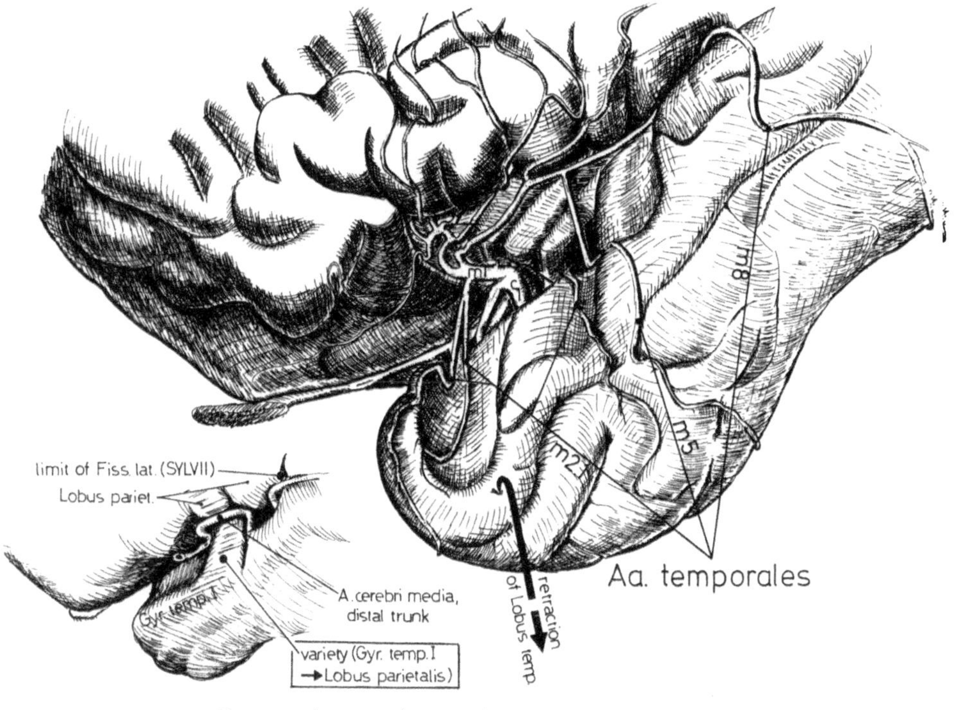
limit of Fiss. lat. (SYLVII)
Lobus pariet.
A. cerebri media, distal trunk
Gyr. temp. I
variety (Gyr. temp. I
→Lobus parietalis)
m1
m23
m5
m8
retraction of Lobus temp.
Aa. temporales

Fig. 95. Schematic frontal section in region of Insula, relations between Insula, inferior surface, to Lobus temporalis and Insula, superior surface, to Pars opercularis with strongly schematized vascular course

Fig. 96. Relations between inferior surface of Insula, Subst. perf. ant., Tractus opt., and tip of Cornu inf. after resection of temporal pole

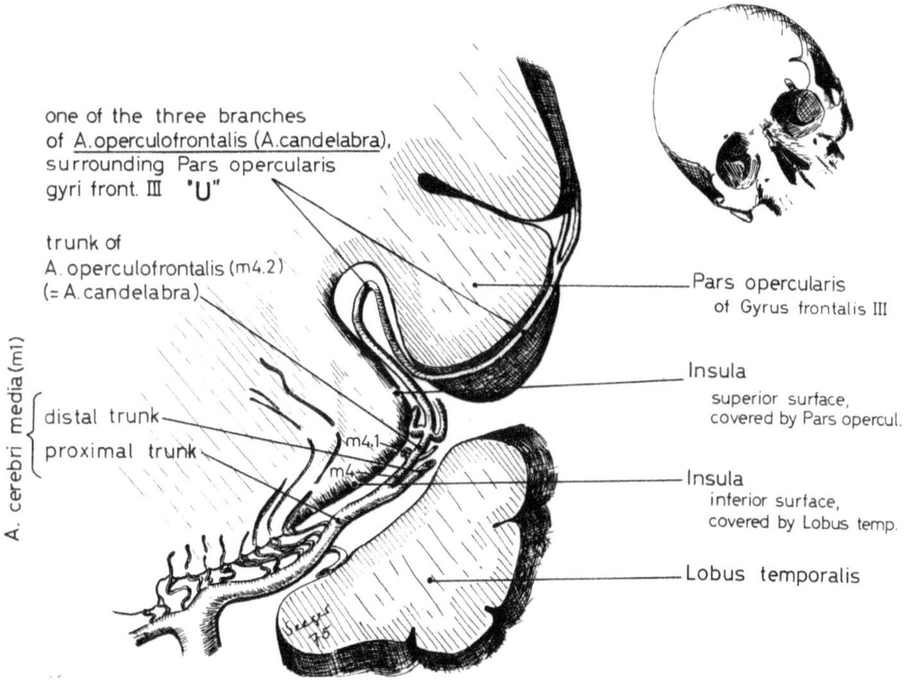
one of the three branches
of A.operculofrontalis (A.candelabra),
surrounding Pars opercularis
gyri front. III "U"
trunk of
A. operculofrontalis (m4.2)
(= A. candelabra)
A. cerebri media (m1)
distal trunk
proximal trunk
m4.1
m4
Pars opercularis
of Gyrus frontalis III
Insula
superior surface,
covered by Pars opercul.
Insula
inferior surface,
covered by Lobus temp.
Lobus temporalis

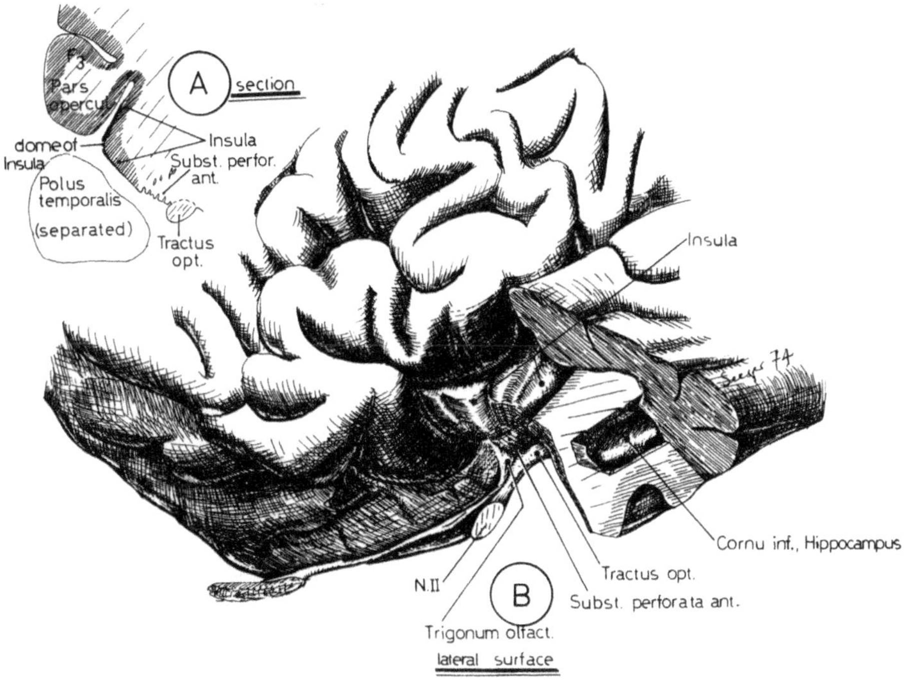
A
section
Pars
opercul.
dome of
Insula
Insula
Subst. perfor.
ant.
Polus
temporalis
(separated)
Tractus
opt.
Insula
Cornu inf., Hippocampus
Tractus opt.
Subst. perforata ant.
N.II
B
Trigonum olfact.
lateral surface

Fig. 97. As Fig. 96, but with arteries; for nomencla ture see Fig. 98. Main trunks of A. cerebri medi over the dome (see Fig. 96 *A*) of Insula. Substanti perforata ant. and Trigonum olfactorium are nearl wholly covered by the carotid bifurcation

FIG. 97

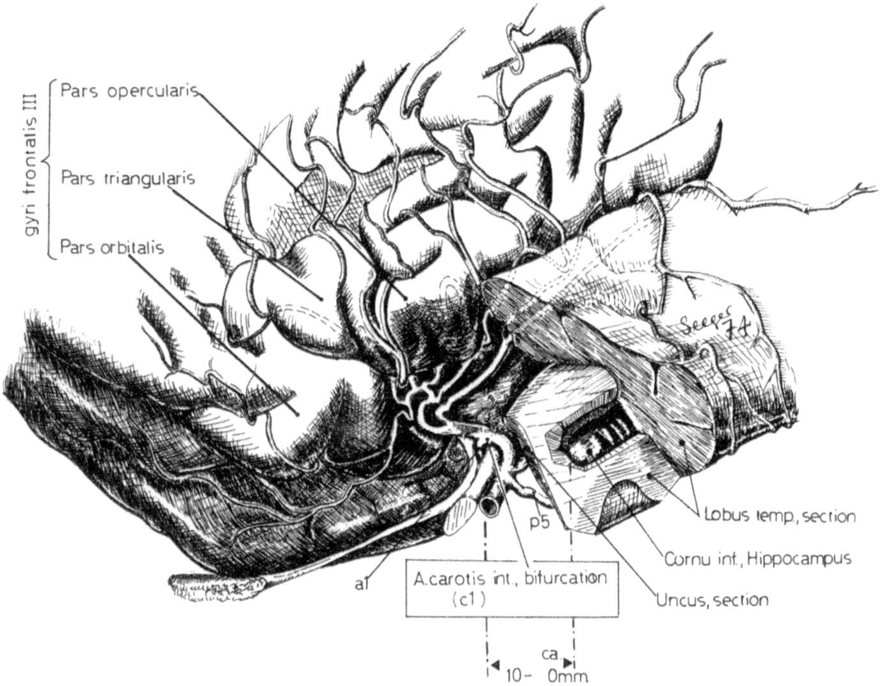
gyri frontalis III
Pars opercularis
Pars triangularis
Pars orbitalis
Seeger 74
Lobus temp, section
Cornu int., Hippocampus
Uncus, section
p5
a1
A.carotis int., bifurcation
(c1)
ca
10- 0mm

Fig. 98. Nomenclature of vessels in Fig. 97. The upper half of Insula with the upper loops of A. frontalis ascendens is overlapped by opercular gyri

Fig. 99. Preparation of Figs. 96–98 after removal of opercular gyri.
A Schematic cross-section at the level of Substantia perf. ant.
B General view showing the upper and lower halves of Insula, whose most anterior part is overlapped by remains of the third frontal gyrus
C Cut surfaces (*c*, *d*) of Pars opercularis of Gyrus frontalis III (foot of the precentral gyrus)

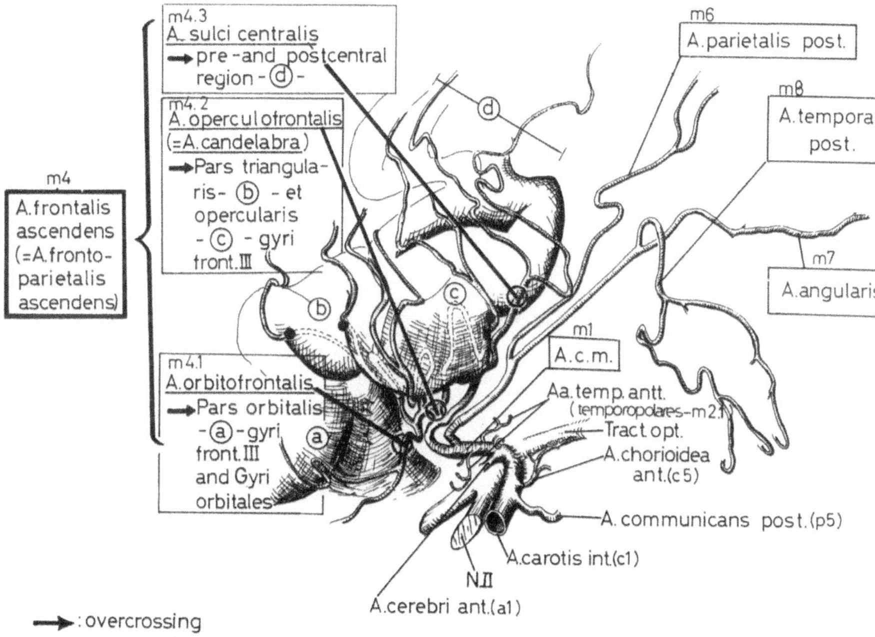

→ : overcrossing

●●● : penetration of branches of A. operculofront. m4.2 between Gyri

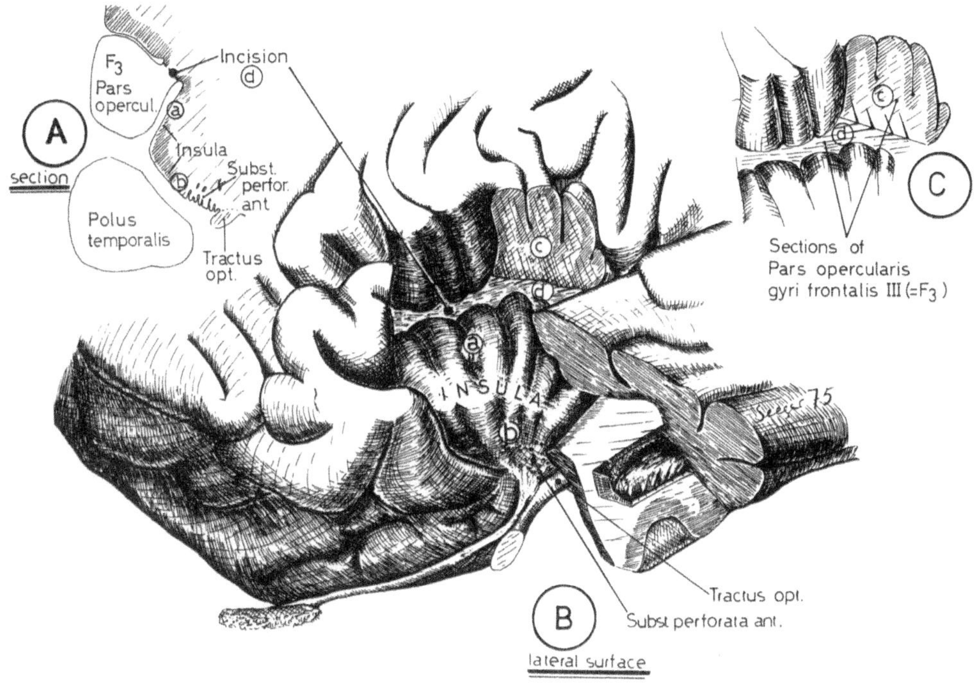

Fig. 100. Preparation of Fig. 99 with vessels sketched in. Only the posterior Sylvian arteries run transversely from depth directly to the surface of the fissure *A*, the branches of A. operculofrontalis *B* dip at first under Pars opercularis, without reaching the highest point of Insula. The tip of Cornu inf. is separated from the bifurcation of A. carotis int. by a zone of white matter at least 10 mm wide (Uncus base)

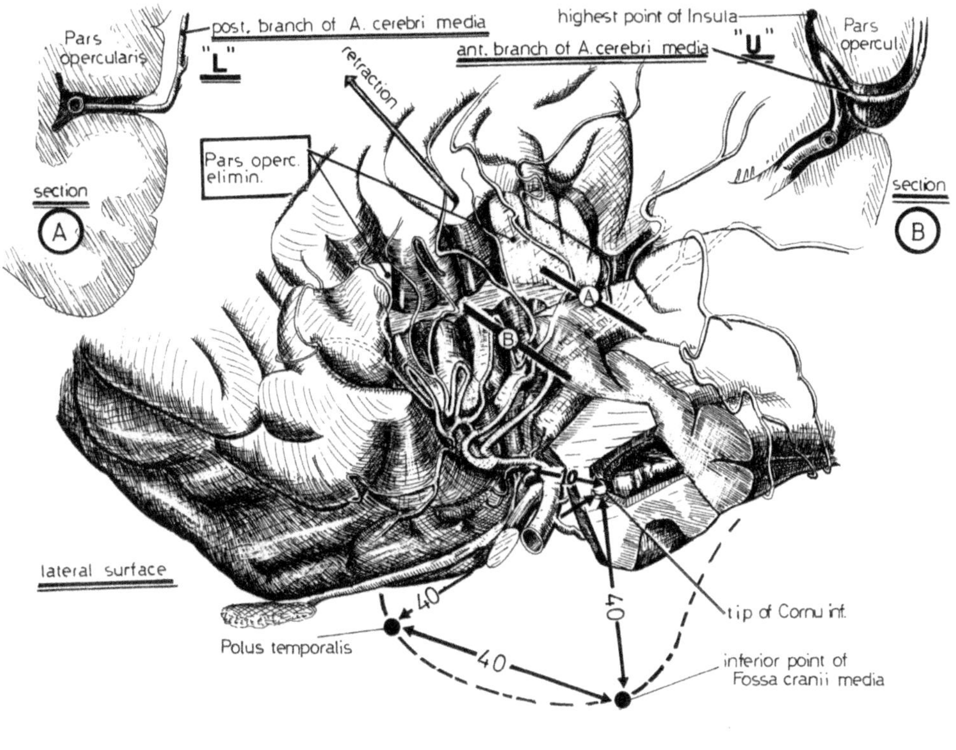
post. branch of A. cerebri media
"L"
Pars opercularis
section
A
retraction
highest point of Insula
ant. branch of A. cerebri media
"U"
Pars opercul.
section
B
Pars operc. elimin.
A
B
10
lateral surface
40
40
40
tip of Cornu inf.
Polus temporalis
inferior point of Fossa cranii media

Fig. 101. Some particularly typical variation A. cerebri media. If a "trifurcation" is present, three trunks may supply different areas. The b cation type consists usually of the two main tr of the vessel

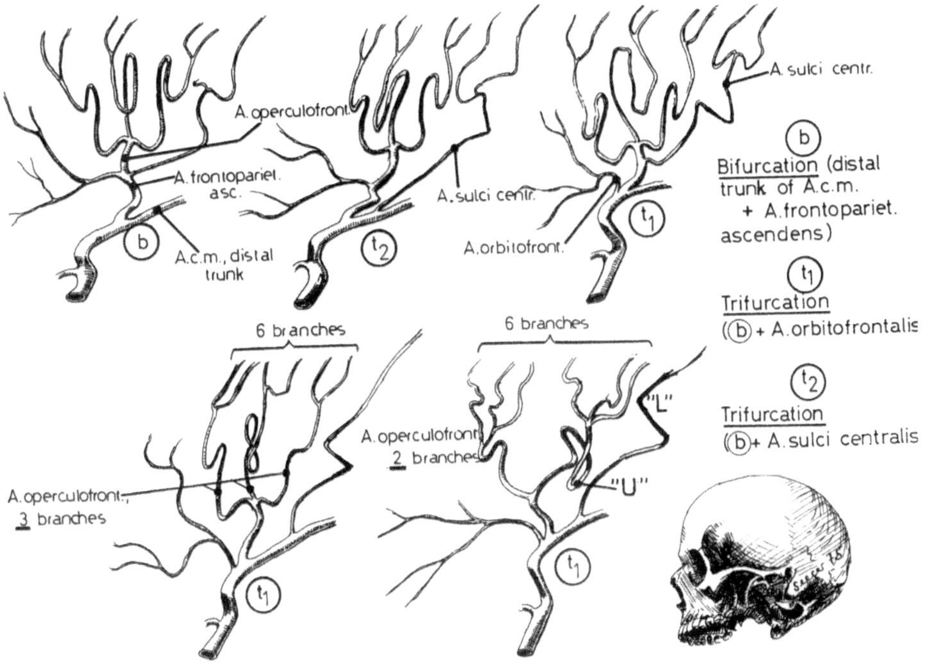
A. operculofront.
A. frontopariet. asc.
A.c.m., distal trunk
b
t2
A. sulci centr.
A. orbitofront.
t1
A. sulci centr.
b
Bifurcation (distal trunk of A.c.m. + A.frontopariet. ascendens)
t1
Trifurcation (b + A.orbitofrontalis
t2
Trifurcation (b + A.sulci centralis
6 branches
A. operculofront., 3 branches
t1
6 branches
"L"
A. operculofront. 2 branches
"U"
t1

Fig. 102.

A Basal view of brain
B View towards base from above; dura (left), bone (right)

Topical relations in the mid-basal region from below and from above (with and without dural covering); distance measurements in millimetres (mm)

Numerical index:

1 Tuberculum sellae
2 Sulcus caroticus
3 Proc. clinoideus ant.
4 Sulcus caroticus
5 Lingula sphenoidalis
6 Foramen lacerum
7 Impressio trigemini
8 Foramen ovale
9 Apex ossis petrosi with small bony process encircling N. abducens
10 Sulcus petrosus sup.
11 Porus acusticus int.
12 Foramen jugulare ant. (for reception of Nn. IX–XI)
13 Foramen jugulare (for reception of Bulbus sup. venae jugularis int.)
14 Tuberculum jugulare
15 Foramen occipitale magnum
16 Dorsum sellae
17 Anterior point of intersection between Tentorium edge and Uncus
18 Infundibulum
19 Diaphragma sellae
20 Beginning of Gyrus parahippocampalis

Measurements in millimetres (mm)

FIG. 102

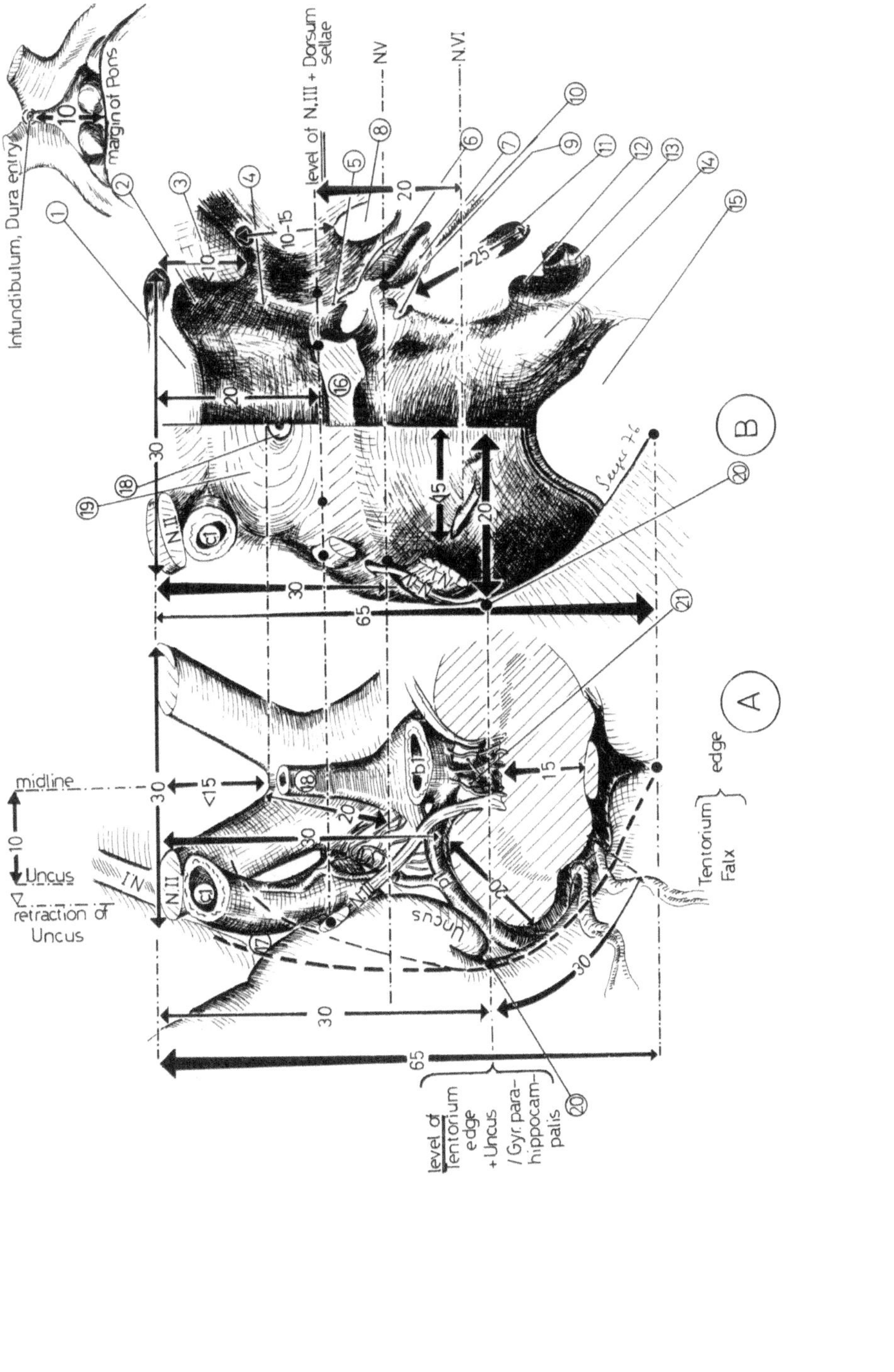
Intundibulum, Dura entry
margin of Pons
level of N.III + Dorsum sellae
N.V
N.VI
midline
Uncus
retraction of Uncus
N.II
Tentorium
Falx
edge
level of Tentorium edge + Uncus / Gyr. para-hippocampalis
A
B

Fig. 103. Preparations of Fig. 102 from oblique view. Nomenclature idem. Measurements in millimetres (mm)

FIG. 103

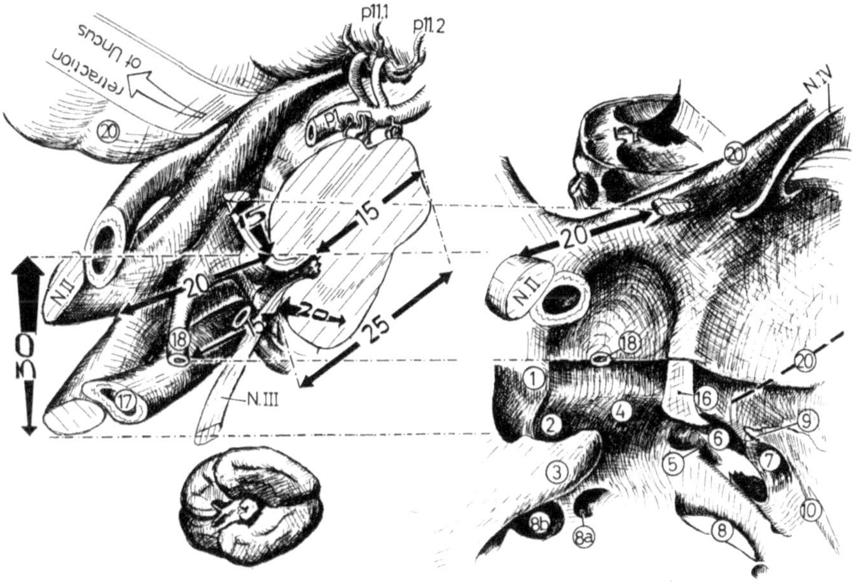
p11.1
p11.2
retraction of Uncus
20
P1
15
15
20
N.II
20
15
25
30
18
17
N.III
N.IV
20
20
N.II
18
20
1
16
2
4
9
6
5
7
3
10
8b
8a
8

Fig. 104. Projection of structures enclosed by the extended tentorial fold under the medially ascending temporobasal dura, somewhat schematized with diminution of trigeminal branches in order to show the underlying structures more clearly
Measurements in millimetres (mm)

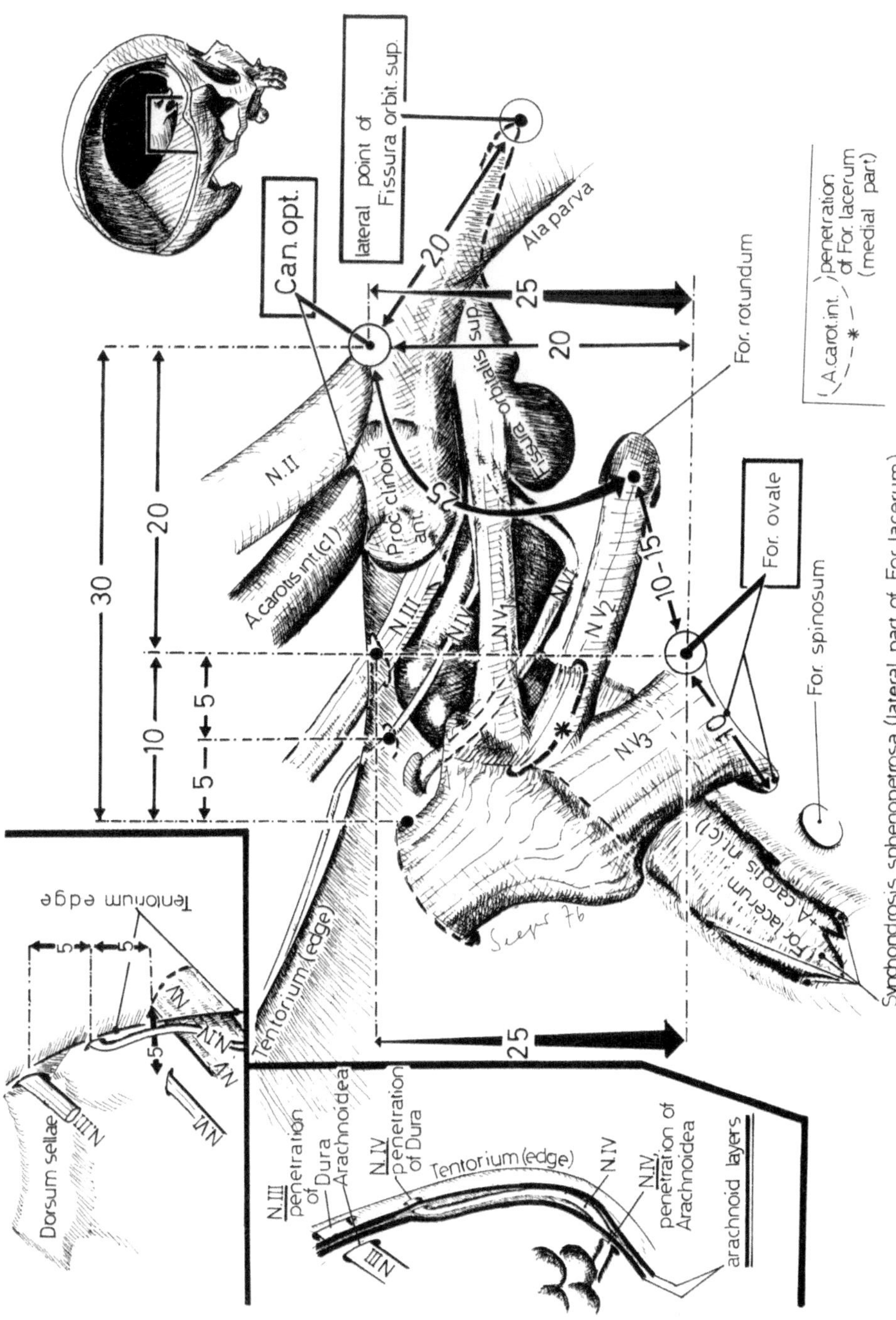
lateral point of Fissura orbit. sup.
Can. opt.
Ala parva
Fissura orbitalis sup.
For. rotundum
For. ovale
For. spinosum
A. carot. int.
penetration of For. lacerum (medial part)
Synchondrosis sphenopetrosa (lateral part of For. lacerum)
Proc. clinoid. ant.
A. carotis int.(c1)
Tentorium (edge)
Tentorium edge
Dorsum sellae
penetration of Dura
Arachnoidea
penetration of Arachnoidea
arachnoid layers
For. lacerum

Fig. 105. Incomplete medial section of Uncus stalk and opening of Fissura chorioidea (arrows). Transverse section of temporal lobe, the anterior part of which is slightly luxated outwards, in order to show a part of Cisterna ambiens

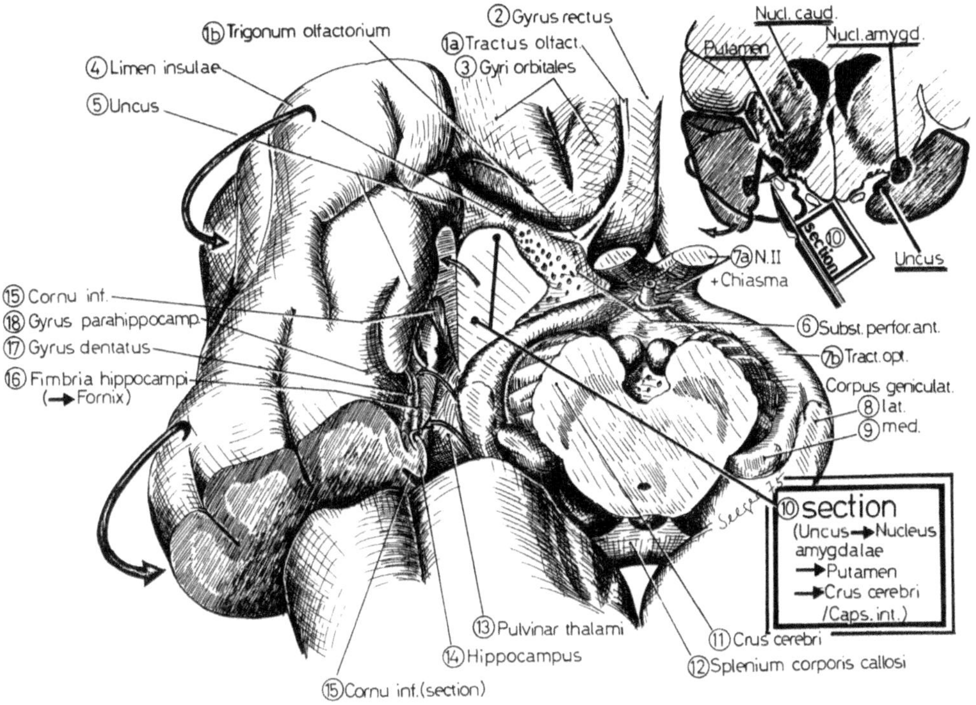

①b Trigonum olfactorium
② Gyrus rectus
①a Tractus olfact.
③ Gyri orbitales
④ Limen insulae
⑤ Uncus
Nucl. caud.
Putamen
Nucl. amygd.
section ⑩
Uncus
⑦a N. II
+Chiasma
⑮ Cornu inf.
⑱ Gyrus parahippocamp.
⑰ Gyrus dentatus
⑯ Fimbria hippocampi
(→Fornix)
⑥ Subst. perfor. ant.
⑦b Tract. opt.
Corpus geniculat.
⑧ lat.
⑨ med.
⑩ section
(Uncus→Nucleus amygdalae
→Putamen
→Crus cerebri
/Caps. int.)
⑬ Pulvinar thalami
⑭ Hippocampus
⑮ Cornu inf. (section)
⑪ Crus cerebri
⑫ Splenium corporis callosi

Fig. 106. Enlarged section of Fig. 105. For numerical index, see Fig. 105

FIG. 106

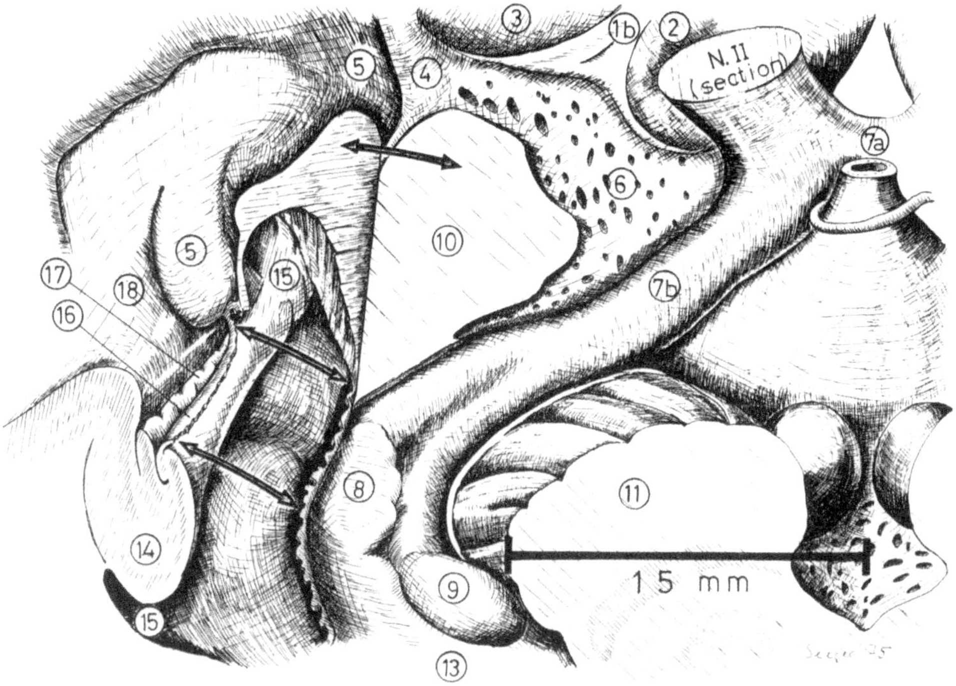

Fig. 107. Preparation of Fig. 106 with arteries. Folding back of the temporal lobe puts tension on A. chorioidea ant. (*c5*) and on the anterior branch of the posterior choroidal group (*p6.1*), as well as on the perforating branches (*c5.2*) from A. chorioidea ant. that run to Crus cerebri, Tractus opticus, and Hypothalamus. The temporopolar branches (*c5.1*) of A. chorioidea ant. that pass to the uncus region had to be previously ligated. See also Fig. 108

FIG. 107

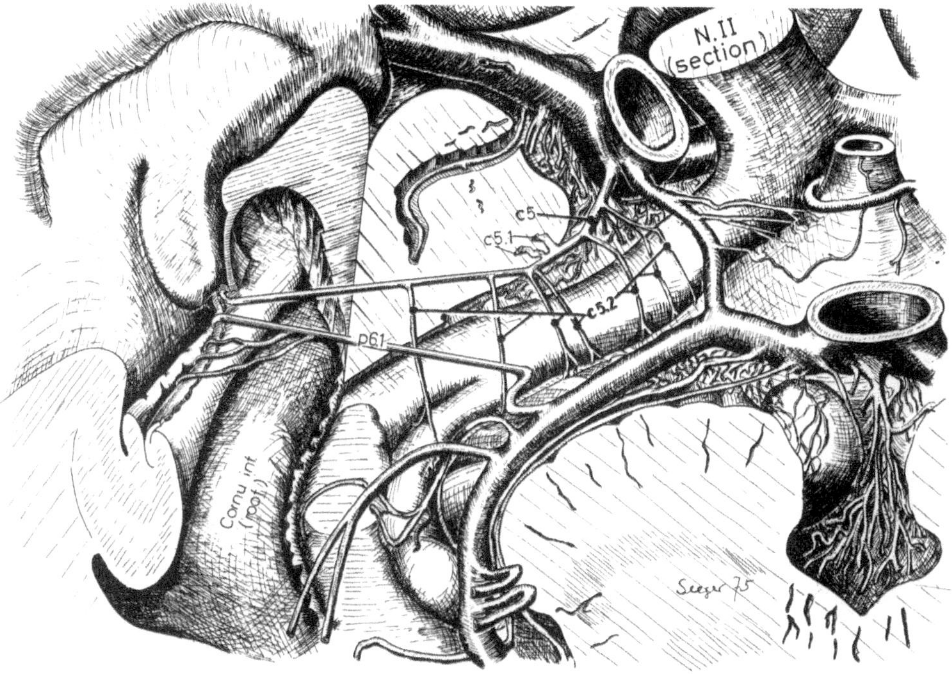

Fig. 108. Nomenclature of vessels in Fig. 107

c1	A. carotis int.
c3	A. hypophys. sup.
c5	A. chorioidea ant.
c5.1	(see Fig. 107) Rami temporales of A. chorioidea ant.
c5.2	Rami perforantes of A. chorioidea ant. to Hypothalamus, Crus cerebri, and Tractus opticus
m1	A. cerebri media, proximal trunk
m2.1	Ramus temporofrontalis
m2.2	Rami perforantes to Substantia perforata ant.
m2.3	Rami perforantes (Aa. lenticulostriatae) to lateral part of Substantia perf. ant. (supply to Put.)
m4	A. frontoparietalis ascendens
p1	A. cerebri post.
p2.1	Aa. thalamoperforantes to Substantia perf. post. (Fossa interpeduncularis)
p2.2	Perforating arteries to the midbrain and Corpora mamillaria
p4	A. quadrigemina
p5	A. communicans post.
p5.1	Perforating arteries from A. communicans post. to Hypothalamus and Tractus opticus
p6.1	Medial anterior branch of posterior choroidal group
p6.2.1, *p6.2.2*	Posterior choroidal group, lateral branches
p7	Branches to Crus cerebri and Tegmentum mesencephali
p8	A. thalamogeniculata
p11.1, *p11.2*	Rami temporales anteriores and posteriores
b1	A. basilaris, bifurcation

FIG. 108

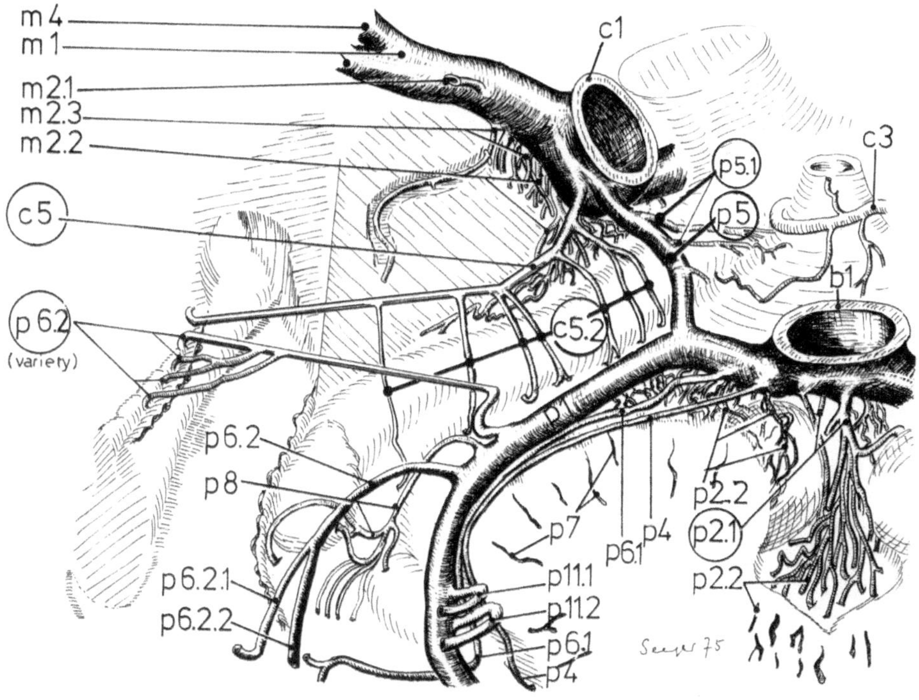
m4
m1
m2.1
m2.3
m2.2
c5
p6.2
(variety)
c1
c3
p5.1
p5
b1
c5.2
p1
p6.2
p8
p7
p6.1
p4
p2.2
p2.1
p2.2
p6.2.1
p6.2.2
p11.1
p11.2
p6.1
p4

Fig. 109

a Chiasma opticum
b Gyrus rectus
c Gyri orbitales
d Tuber cinereum
e Trigonum olfactorium
f Limen insulae
g Cut surface of temporal lobe peduncle (Uncus)
h Insular gyri
i Section of temporal lobe pedicle between Insula and Cisterna ambiens
j Cauda nuclei caudati
k Stria medullaris
l Taenia chorioidea thalami
m Fimbria hippocampi (Crus fornicis)
n Taenia fornicis
o Hippocampus (section)
p Fissura calcarina (section)
q Eminentia collateralis (section)
r Fissura collateralis (section)
s Gyrus occipitotemporalis med. (section)
t Gyrus occipitotemporalis lat.
u Lobulus centralis cerebelli/Ala lobuli centralis
v Cut surface of Lobulus quadrangularis on Brachium pontis (below) and on Culmen (medial)
w Lateral end of Lobulus semilunaris sup.
x Flocculus
y Lobulus biventer
z Tonsilla

Bc Brachium conjunctivum
Bp Brachium pontis
Bqi Brachium quadrigeminum inf.
Bqs Brachium quadrigeminum sup.
Cc Crus cerebri
Cp Corpus pineale
Cm Corpus mamillare
Ci Cornu inf.
Fv Frenulum veli medullaris ant.
Gd Gyrus dentatus (section)
Gl Corpus geniculatum lat.
Gm Corpus geniculatum med.
In Infundibulum
Ol Oliva
Ps Pons
Py Pyramis
Qi Lamina quadrigemina, Colliculus inf.
Qs Lamina quadrigemina, Colliculus sup.
Pt Pulvinar thalami
Tl Trigonum lemnisci
Tr Tractus opticus
Al Ansa lenticularis
N.V
ms N. trigeminus, Portio minor
N. in N. intermedius

Cranial nerve nomenclature: usual abbreviations. Measurements in millimetres (mm)

FIG. 109

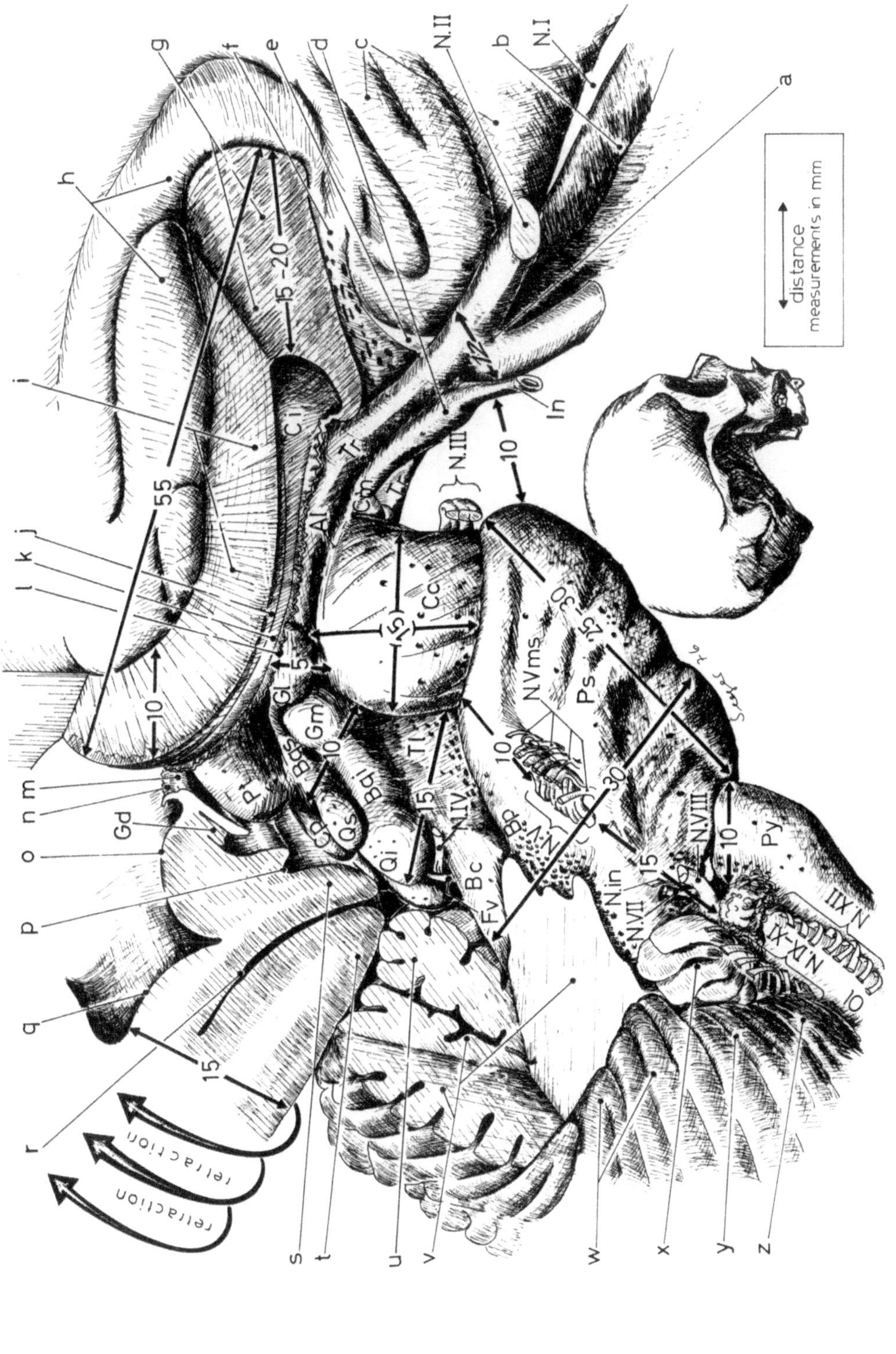
distance
measurements in mm
retraction
retraction
N.I
N.II
N.III
N.IV
N.VII
N.VIII
N.XII
N.in
NVms
Cc
Cl
Cm
Tr
Al
In
Gl
Gm
Gd
Tl
Bc
Fv
Ps
Py
Qi
Qs
10
15
15-20
25
30
55

Fig. 110. Circulation of A. basilaris and neighbouring areas, slightly schematized

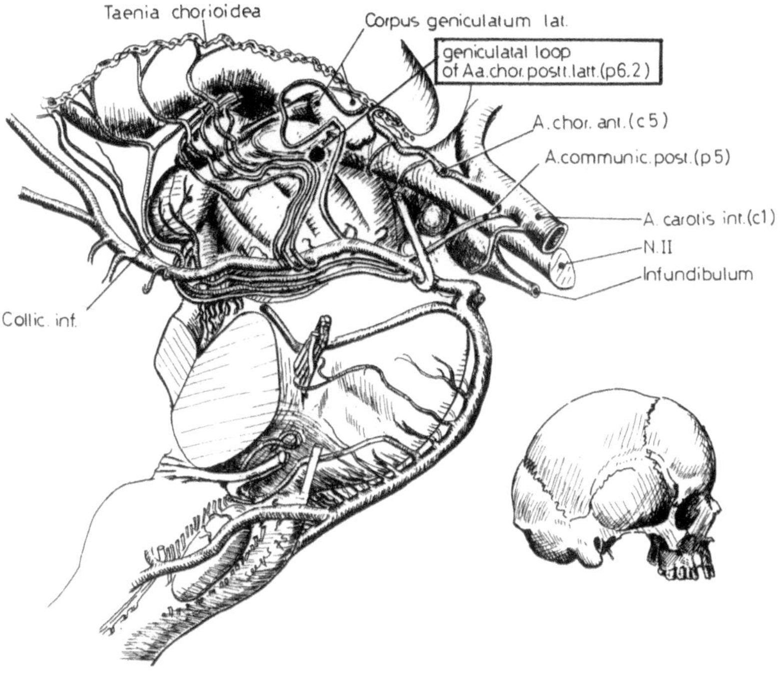
Taenia chorioidea
Corpus geniculatum lat.
geniculatal loop
of Aa.chor.postt.latt.(p6.2)
A.chor. ant.(c5)
A.communic.post.(p5)
A. carotis int.(c1)
N.II
Infundibulum
Collic. inf.

Fig. 111. Nomenclature of arteries for Fig. 110, for explanation see legend to Fig. 108

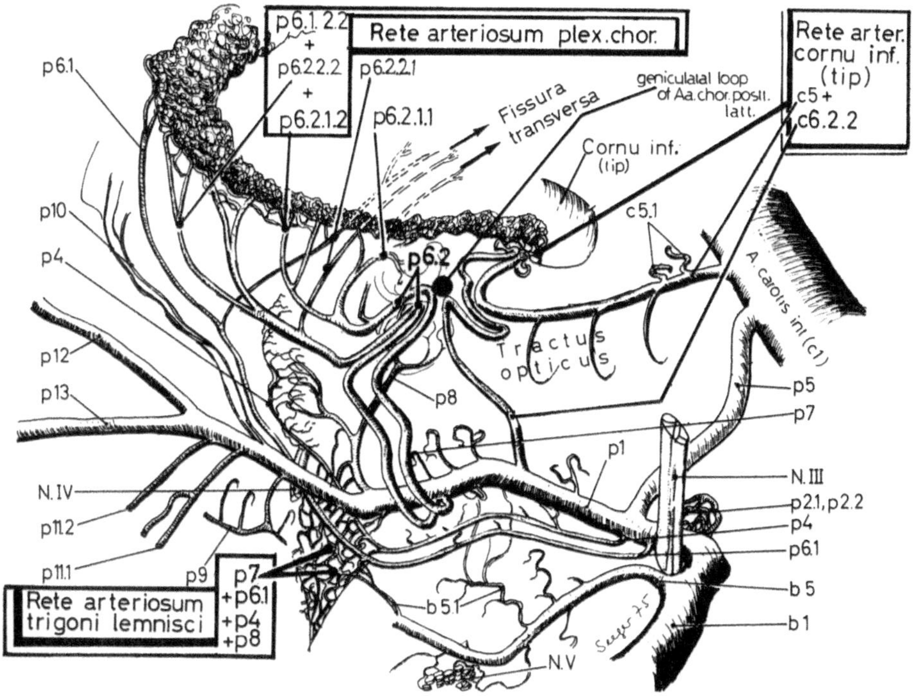
p6.1.2.2
+
p6.2.2.2
+
p6.2.1.2
Rete arteriosum plex.chor.
p6.2.2.1
p6.2.1.1
Fissura transversa
geniculatal loop of Aa.chor.postt. latt.
Rete arter. cornu inf. (tip)
c5 +
c6.2.2
Cornu inf. (tip)
c5.1
A. carotis int.(c1)
p6.1
p10
p4
p6.2
p12
p13
Tractus opticus
p8
p5
p7
p1
N.III
N.IV
p2.1, p2.2
p11.2
p4
p6.1
p11.1
p9
p7
+p6.1
+p4
+p8
Rete arteriosum trigoni lemnisci
b 5
b 5.1
b 1
N.V

Fig. 112. Raising and stretching of A. cerebri post. (arrows) with compression of posterior choroidal group and tension of perforating arteries to the midbrain from the posterior cerebral artery (*p1*), quadrigeminal artery (*p4*), and a medial branch of the posterior choroidal group (*p6.1*). The stretched perforating arteries to Crus cerebri (*B*) are end-arteries, the perforating arteries of Trigonum lemnisci (*A*) are reticulated, those supplying Lamina quadrigemina are end-arteries (*C*)

Fig. 113. Examples of variants of V. basalis (Rosenthal): the inconstantly developed V. cerebri media in the depths of Fissura lat. (Sylvii), which crosses through the perforating arteries, branches of Subst. perforata ant., before Uncus

Below right: Connection to superficial veins of Fissura lat. (Sylvii)

Below left: Hypoplasia of V. basalis (Rosenthal) with dorsally accentuated venous drainage. For veins of the ventricular system see also Chapter 6

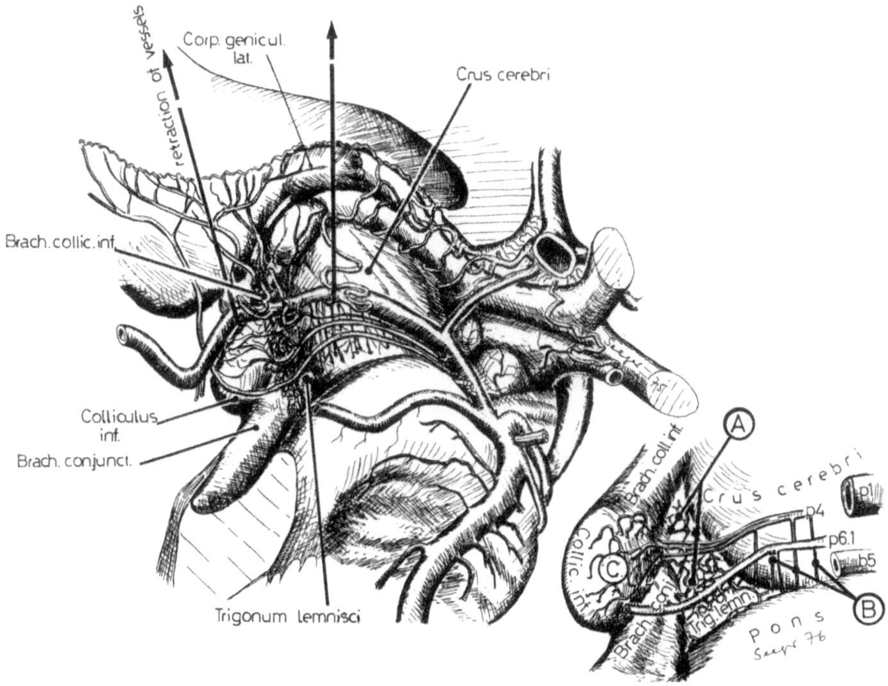
retraction of vessels
Corp. genicul. lat.
Crus cerebri
Brach. collic. inf.
Colliculus inf.
Brach. conjunct.
Trigonum lemnisci
A
Brach. coll. inf.
Crus cerebri
p1
p4
p6.1
b5
Collic. inf.
C
B
Brach. conj.
Trig. lemn.
Pons

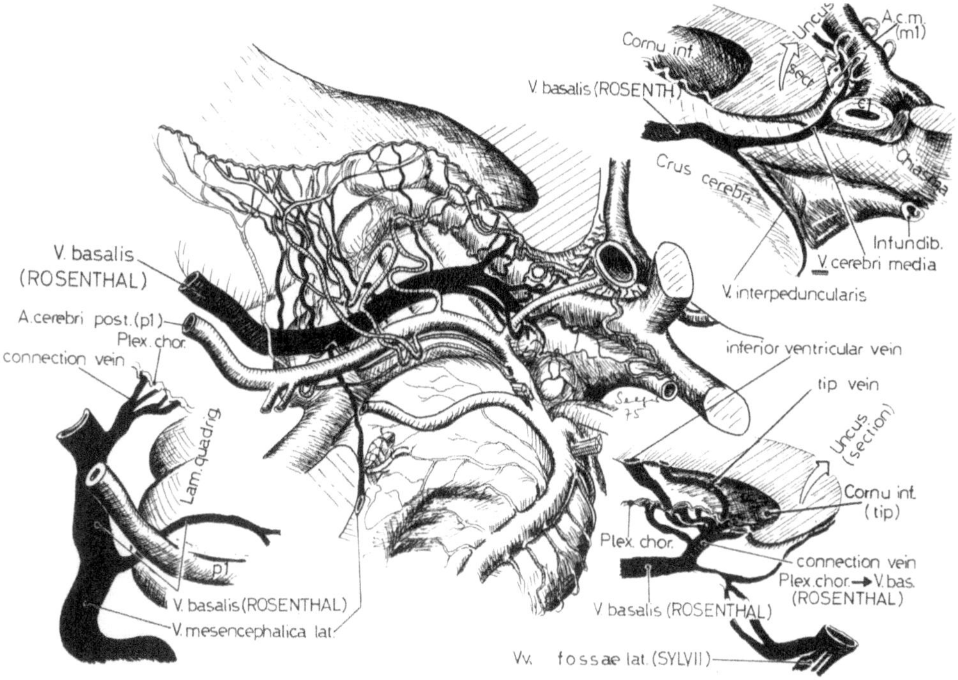
Cornu inf.
Uncus
A.c.m. (m1)
V. basalis (ROSENTH)
Crus cerebri
Infundib.
V. cerebri media
V. interpeduncularis
V. basalis (ROSENTHAL)
A. cerebri post. (p1)
Plex. chor.
connection vein
inferior ventricular vein
tip vein
Lam. quadrig.
p1
V. basalis (ROSENTHAL)
V. mesencephalica lat.
Uncus (section)
Cornu inf. (tip)
Plex. chor.
connection vein Plex. chor. → V. bas. (ROSENTHAL)
V. basalis (ROSENTHAL)
Vv. fossae lat. (SYLVII)

Fig. 114.
Above: Normal findings. Arachnoidal covering structures left out. The trunk of A. cerebri post. often lies higher and may cover V. basalis (Rosenthal). Deepest and most laterally lying: N. trochlearis. The connection between V. basalis (Rosenthal) and the anterior median pontine vein is made by V. interpeduncularis. Veins mostly lying close to the brain surface, arteries freely in arachnoid membranes of Cisterna. Projection from tentorial edge and extradural structures (measurements in millimetres)
For abbreviations in nomenclature of vessels see Fig. 108
Below: Instead of the many possible vascular variants an extreme variant: A. chorioidea ant. unusually strong, with its terminal branch: A. calcarina
A. cerebri post. equal in size, terminal branch A. parietooccipitalis crossing below A. chorioidea ant.
V. mesencephalica lat. not developed
Measurements in millimetres (mm)

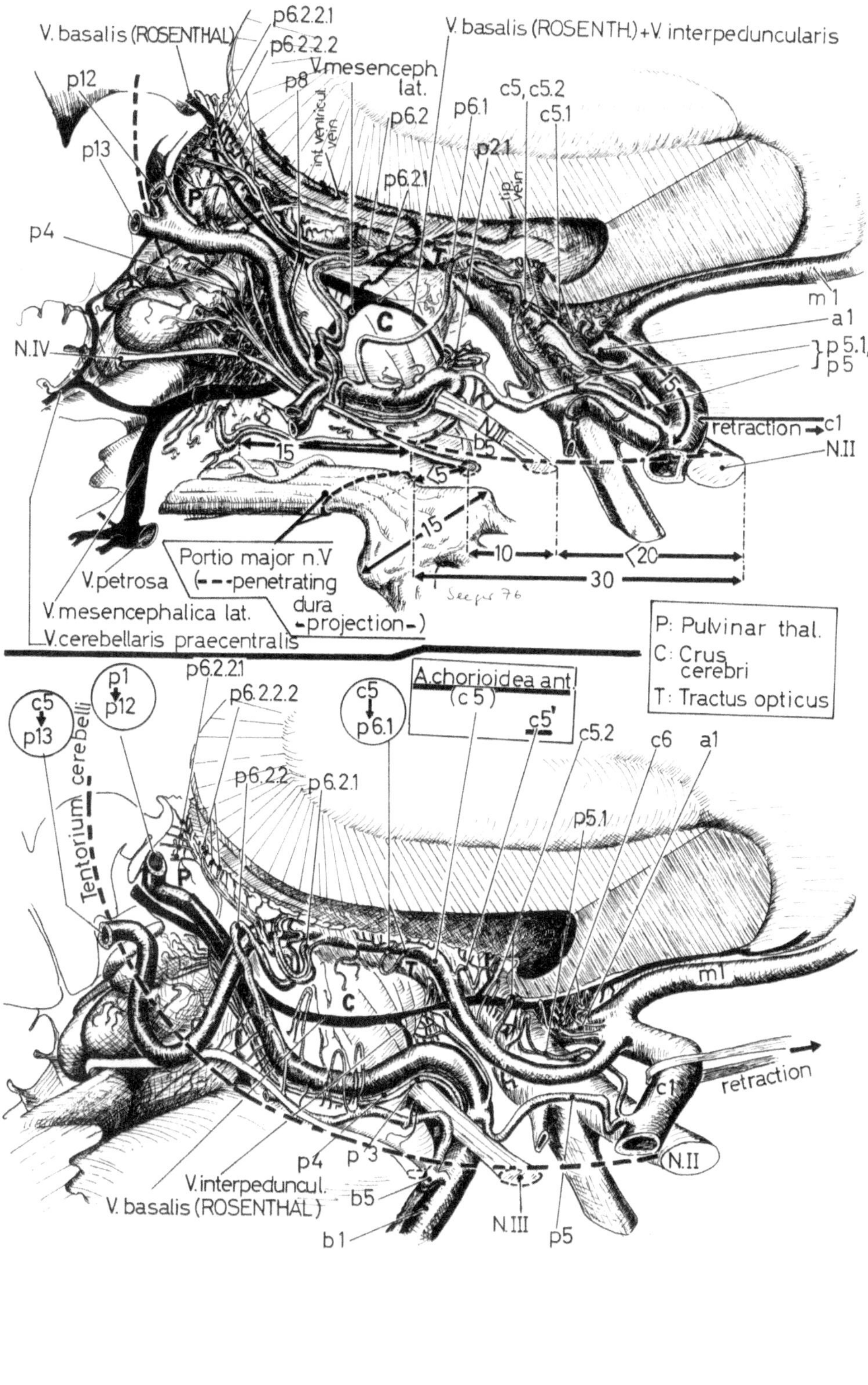
V. basalis (ROSENTHAL)
p6.2.2.1
p6.2.2.2
V. basalis (ROSENTH.)+V. interpeduncularis
V. mesenceph lat.
p12
p8
int. ventricul. vein
c5, c5.2
p6.2
p6.1
c5.1
p13
p2.1
p6.2.1
P
T
C
p4
m1
a1
N.IV
p5.1,
p5
retraction → c1
N.III
b5
N.II
15
5
15
10
20
30
Portio major n.V
(- - -penetrating dura -projection-)
V. petrosa
V. mesencephalica lat.
V. cerebellaris praecentralis
P: Pulvinar thal.
C: Crus cerebri
T: Tractus opticus
c5 → p13
p1 → p12
p6.2.2.1
p6.2.2.2
A. chorioidea ant. (c5)
c5'
c5 → p6.1
c5.2
c6
a1
Tentorium cerebelli
p6.2.2
p6.2.1
p5.1
P
C
T
m1
retraction
c1
N.II
p4
p3
V. interpeduncul.
V. basalis (ROSENTHAL)
b5
b1
N.III
p5

Fig. 115. Drawn from a ventriculogram; a-p film somewhat distorted
Lower picture: Shorter distance to x-ray tube
The floor of the middle cranial fossa (see upper picture) projects between Porus acusticus int. and ext.
Polus temporalis, the inferior point of Fossa cranii media, and tip of Cornu inf. form an almost equilateral triangle in lateral projection
Measurements in millimetres (mm)

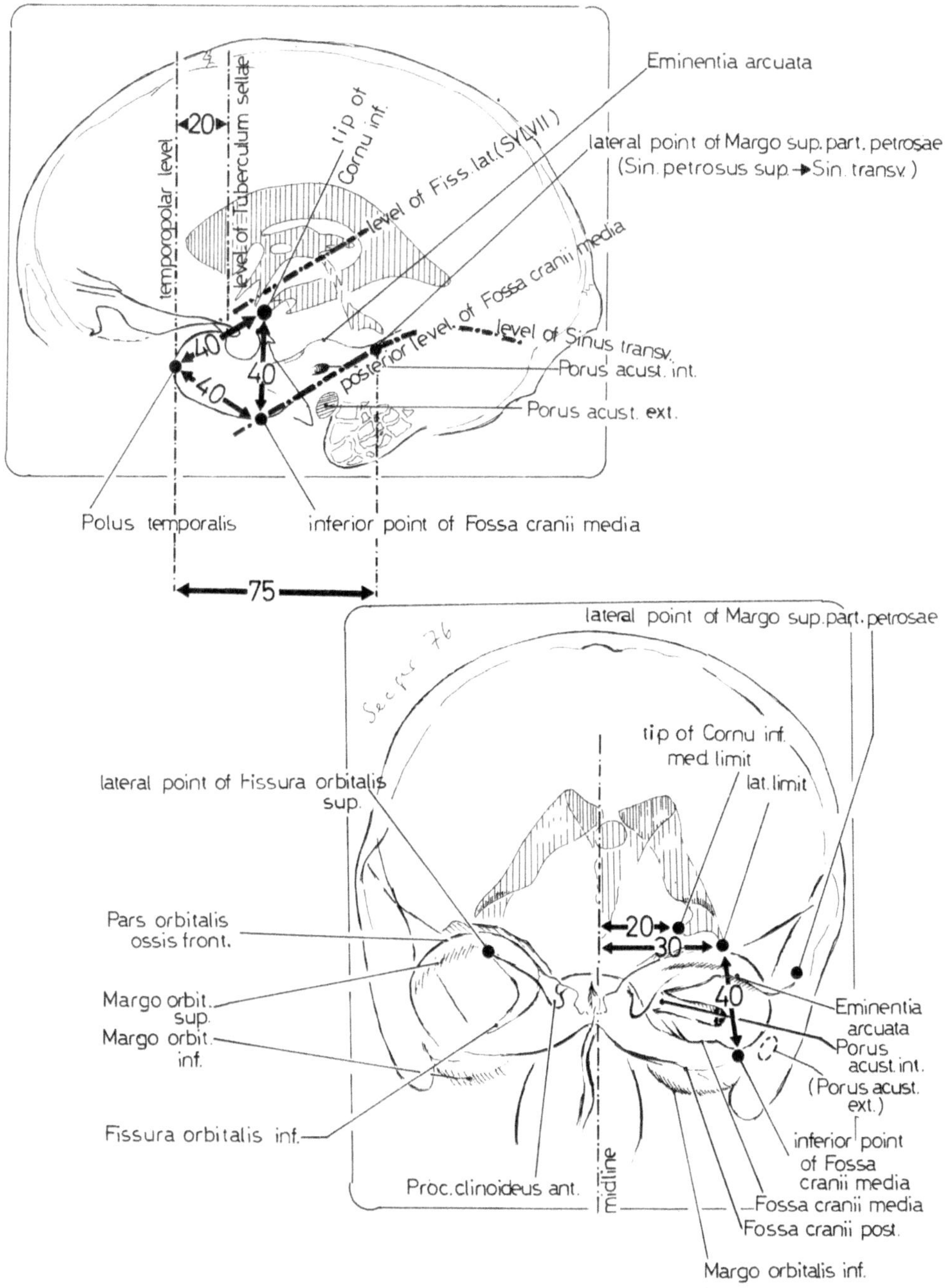
Eminentia arcuata
lateral point of Margo sup. part. petrosae
(Sin. petrosus sup. → Sin. transv.)
temporopolar level
level of Tuberculum sellae
20
tip of Cornu inf.
level of Fiss. lat. (SYLVII)
posterior level of Fossa cranii media
level of Sinus transv.
Porus acust. int.
Porus acust. ext.
40
40
40
Polus temporalis
inferior point of Fossa cranii media
75
lateral point of Margo sup. part. petrosae
tip of Cornu inf.
med. limit
lat. limit
lateral point of Fissura orbitalis sup.
Pars orbitalis ossis front.
Margo orbit. sup.
Margo orbit. inf.
Fissura orbitalis inf.
Proc. clinoideus ant.
midline
20
30
40
Eminentia arcuata
Porus acust. int.
(Porus acust. ext.)
inferior point of Fossa cranii media
Fossa cranii media
Fossa cranii post.
Margo orbitalis inf.

Fig. 116. In contrast to the deep frontal to occipital processes, in deep temporal processes the projection on to the surface of the skull is of less importance than the exact determination of the neighbourhood relationships to vessels and bony structures and to the CSF spaces

A1 and *B1*: In the horizontal planes of both pictures Bregma – Lambda – level of petrous bone, etc. correspond. Position of Cornu inf. (*A1*) marked by end of A. chorioidea ant. (cf. Fig. 115); superficial Sylvian veins (*A1*, *A4*, and *A5*) mark only inexactly the outer border of Fissura lat. (Sylvii), depth of the fissure marked by main trunks of A. cerebri media

A2 and *A3*: Proximal dural (*A2*) and distal dural (*A3*) exit of A. communicans post. Rami perforantes (*p5.1*) endangered – e.g., by application of clips to A. carotis int. in *A2*

B2 and *B3*: Varying distance between carotids

Enlargement of this distance in the presence of space-occupying processes (*B3*) supplemented by basal projections of angiograms

Measurements in millimetres (mm)

FIG. 116

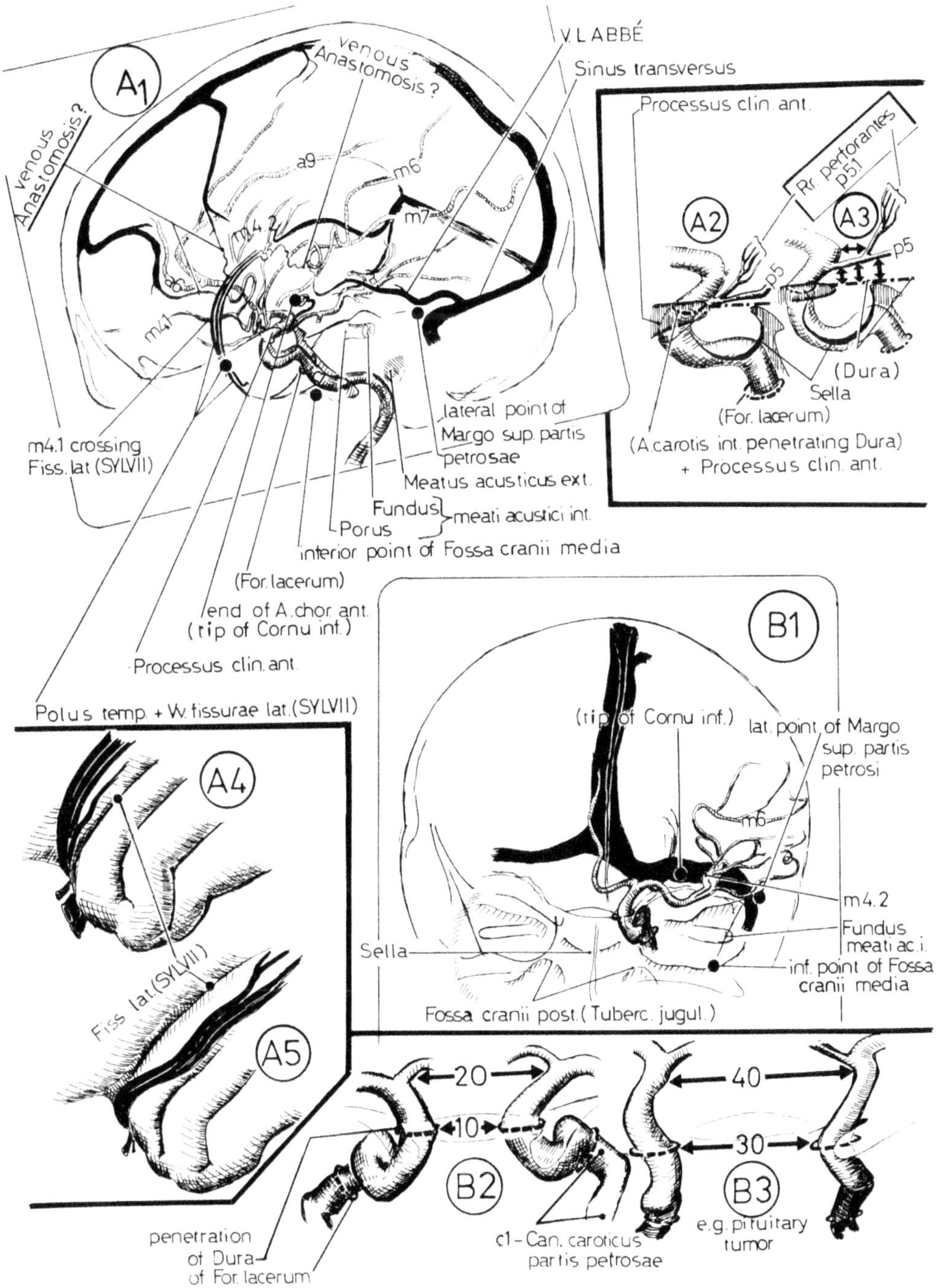
A1
venous Anastomosis?
venous Anastomosis?
V. LABBÉ
Sinus transversus
a9
m6
m7
m4.2
a6
m4.1
lateral point of Margo sup. partis petrosae
Meatus acusticus ext.
Fundus
Porus
meati acustici int.
interior point of Fossa cranii media
(For. lacerum)
end of A. chor. ant. (tip of Cornu inf.)
Processus clin. ant.
Polus temp. + Vv. fissurae lat. (SYLVII)
m4.1 crossing Fiss. lat (SYLVII)
Processus clin. ant.
Rr. perforantes p5.1
A2
A3
p5
p5
(Dura)
Sella
(For. lacerum)
(A. carotis int. penetrating Dura) + Processus clin. ant.
A4
A5
Fiss. lat. (SYLVII)
B1
(tip of Cornu inf.)
lat. point of Margo sup. partis petrosi
m6
m4.2
Fundus meati ac. i.
inf. point of Fossa cranii media
Sella
Fossa cranii post. (Tuberc. jugul.)
20
10
40
30
B2
B3
penetration of Dura of For. lacerum
c1 - Can. caroticus partis petrosae
e.g. pituitary tumor

Fig. 117. Course of A. cerebri post. (*p1*) and projection of a midbrain horizontal section from half-axial view (left) and with inadequate projection (right)

FIG. 117

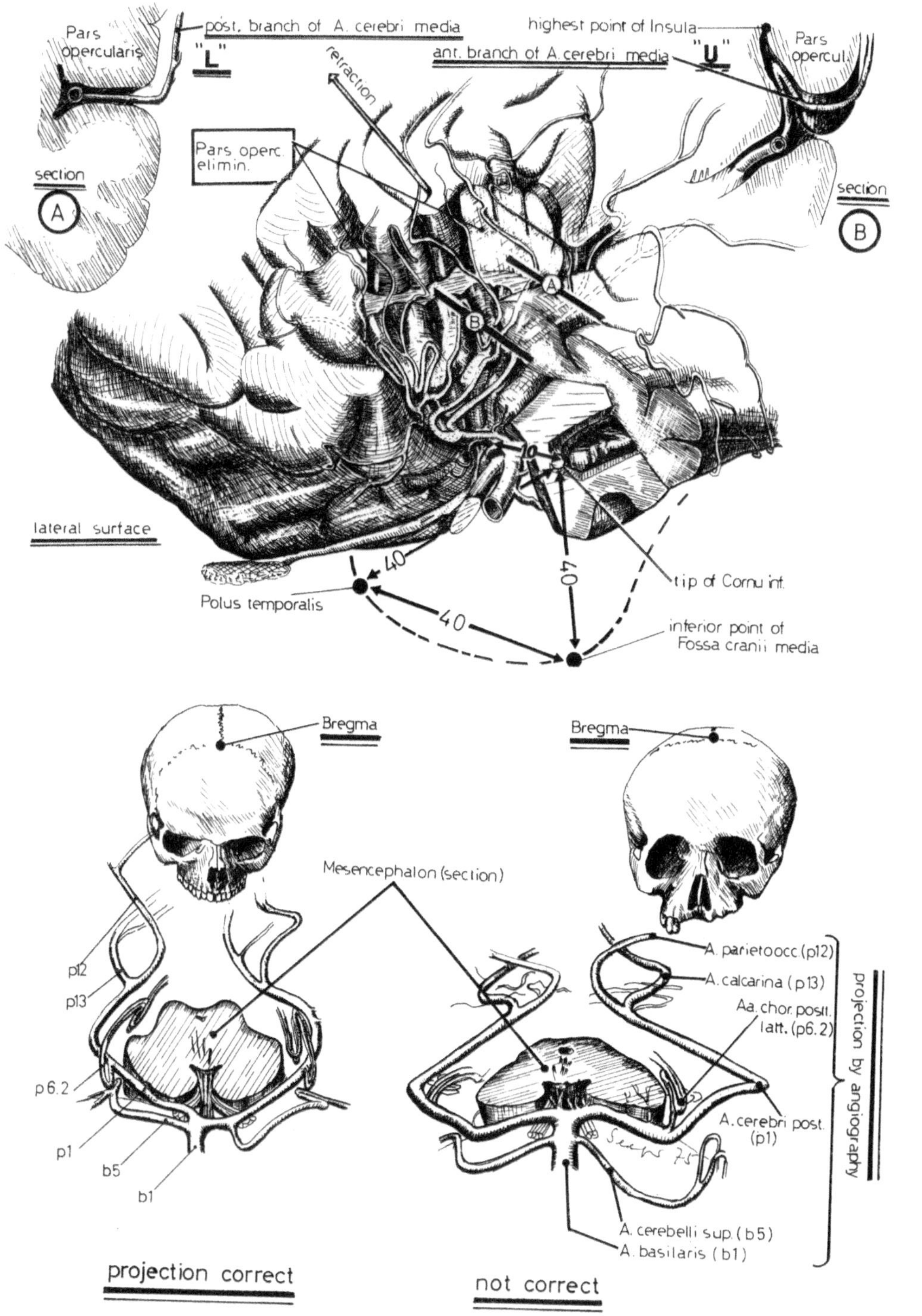
Pars opercularis
post. branch of A. cerebri media
"L"
retraction
highest point of Insula
ant. branch of A. cerebri media
"U"
Pars opercul.
Pars operc. elimin.
section
A
section
B
lateral surface
40
40
40
Polus temporalis
tip of Cornu inf.
inferior point of Fossa cranii media
Bregma
Bregma
Mesencephalon (section)
p12
p13
p6.2
p1
b5
b1
A. parietoocc. (p12)
A. calcarina (p13)
Aa. chor. postt. latt. (p6.2)
A. cerebri post. (p1)
A. cerebelli sup. (b5)
A. basilaris (b1)
projection by angiography
projection correct
not correct

Fig. 118. Indian ink copy of angiogram with correct projection (see also Fig. 117)*

* Thanks are due to Prof. Lüttcke, University Hospital for Nervous Diseases, Marburg, for providing the angiograms.

Fig. 119. Lateral projection of the case in Fig. 118 with slight tilting, with venous phase drawn in
Arrow: Normal swing of A. cerebri post. diagonal to upper area of Crus cerebri. Tip of Cornu inf. marked by the end of A. chorioidea ant. Variant of A. cerebelli sup. [exit from A. cerebri post. left (frequent variant)].
Probable course of N. oculomotorius in this variant

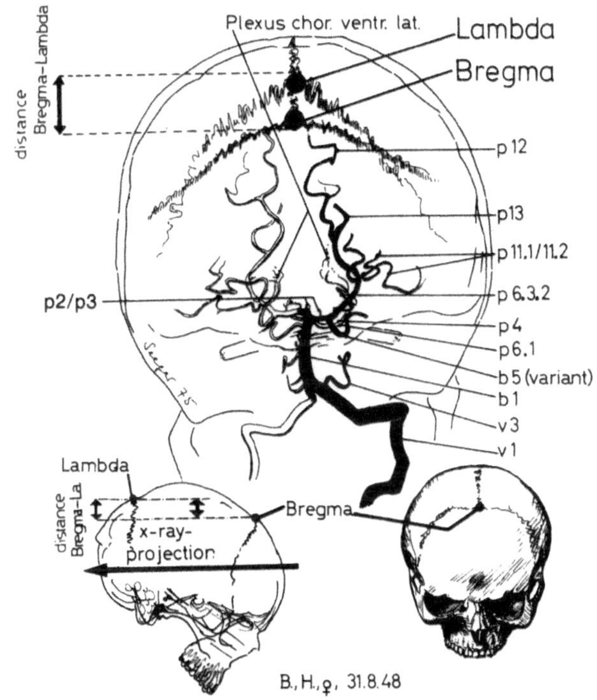

B., H., ♀, 31.8.48

University Hospital for Nervous Diseases, Marburg/L.

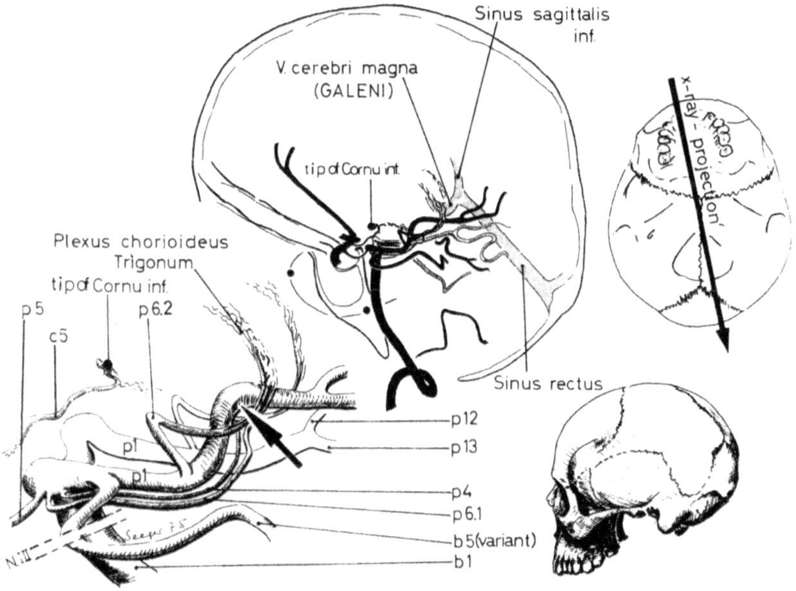

Fig. 120. Too flat projection in an older person with stiff cervical spine

Fig. 121. Case of Fig. 120 with ventriculogram drawn in (tumour of 4th ventricle: see arrow). Despite obstructive Hydrocephalus the vessels are still strongly coiled as is common in senile atrophy. The marking of the tip of Cornu inf. (*c5* = A. chor. ant., see Fig. 119) is of little use if the ventricle is distended. Shortening of distance between tip of Cornu inf. and A. carotis int. (narrowing of Uncus insertion)
For nomenclature of vessels see catalogue of arteries, pages 3–4

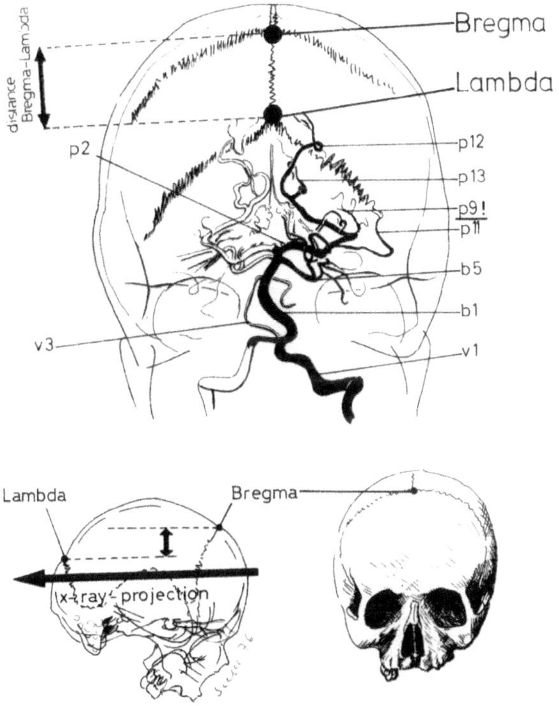
Bregma
Lambda
distance Bregma-Lambda
p2
p12
p13
p9!
p11
b5
b1
v3
v1
Lambda
Bregma
x-ray projection

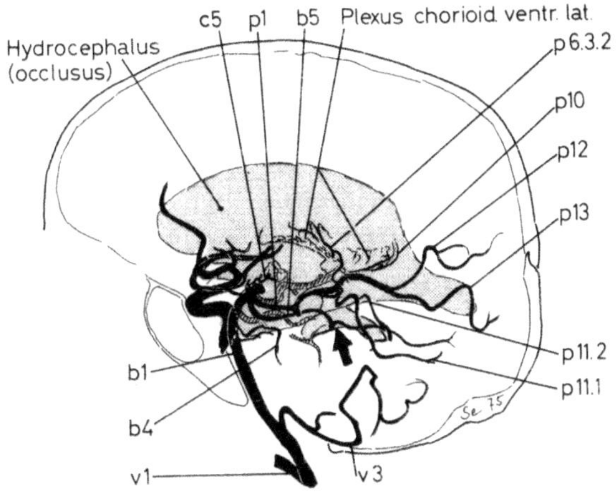
c5
p1
b5
Plexus chorioid. ventr. lat.
Hydrocephalus (occlusus)
p6.3.2
p10
p12
p13
p11.2
p11.1
b1
b4
v1
v3

Fig. 122. Example of temporal approach:
Subperiosteal removal of temporal muscle (*1*), correct position of burrhole outside Orbita (*2*), incision of the temporal muscle basal (*3*), avoidance of injury in the region of Sinus transversus or Tegmen tympani (*4*), limitation of trepanation of the temporal region (*5*), secondary osteoclastic extension towards the base (*6*)

FIG. 122

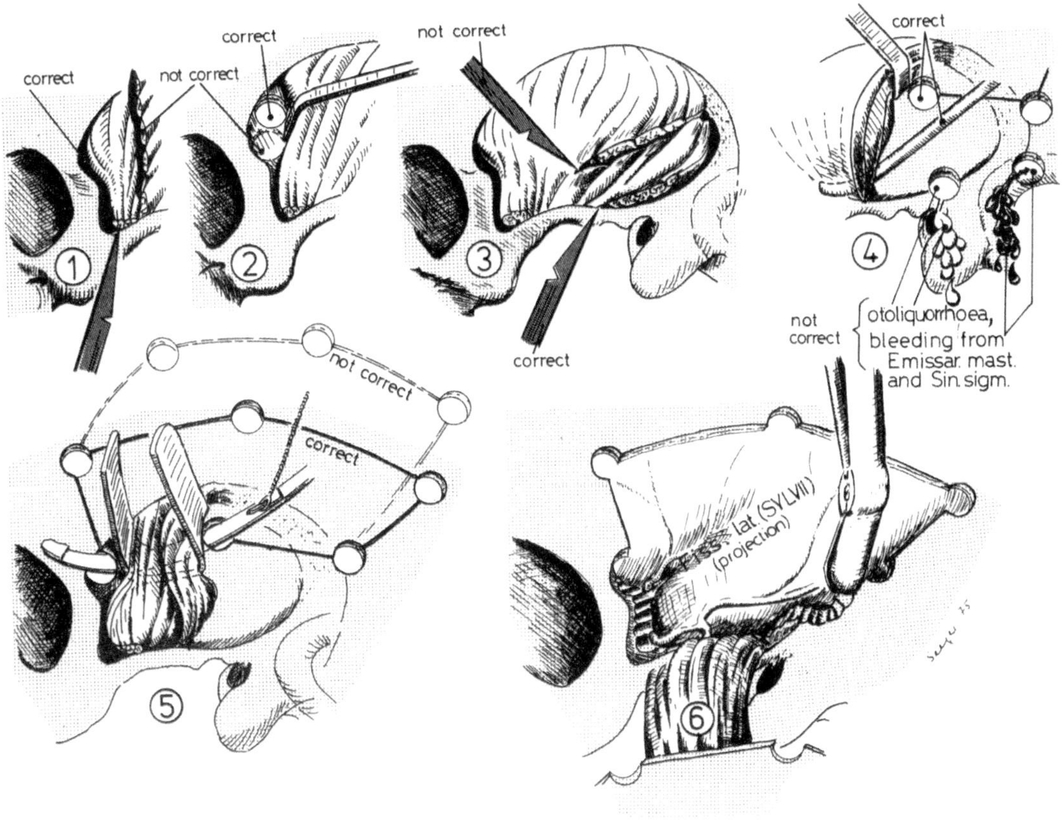
correct
not correct
correct
not correct
correct
correct
not correct
correct
otoliquorrhoea,
bleeding from
Emissar. mast.
and Sin. sigm.
not correct
correct
Fiss. lat. (SYLVII)
(projection)
1
2
3
4
5
6

Fig. 123 a.
A Anatomical layers of the temporal region
B Significance of Linea temporalis superior and inferior
C Principles of resection of Arcus zygomaticus with temporobasal trepanation

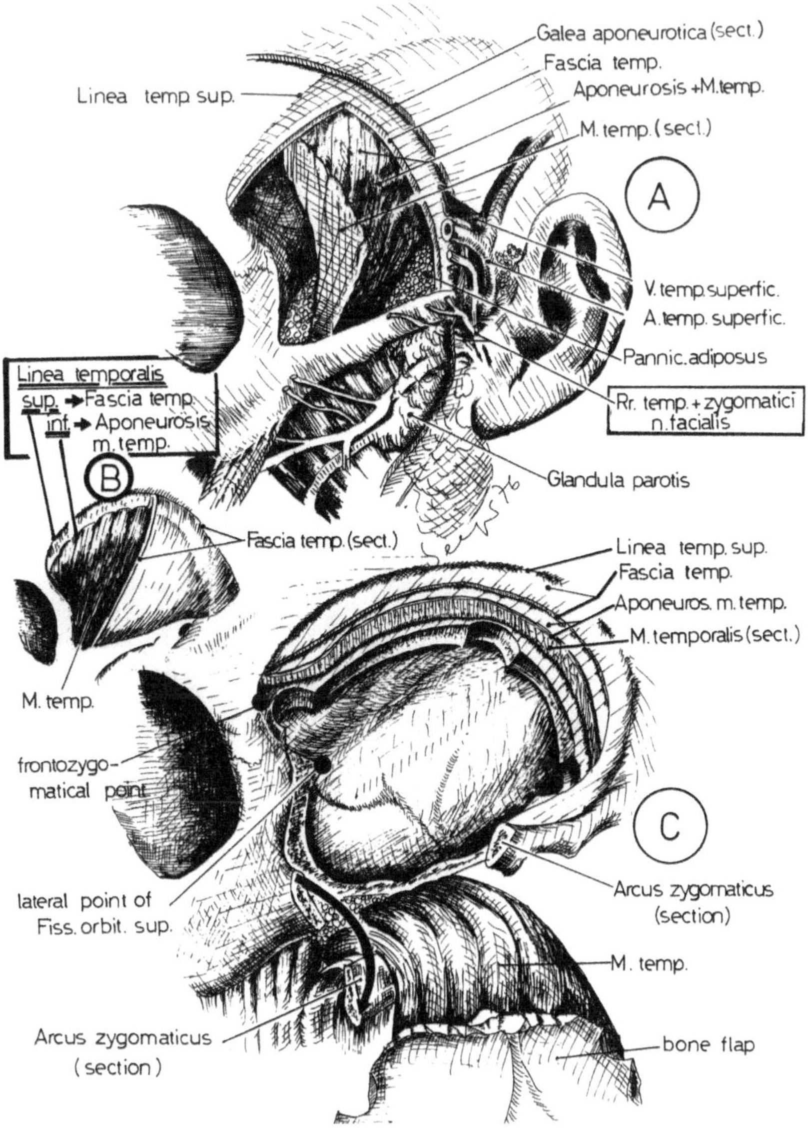
Galea aponeurotica (sect.)
Fascia temp.
Linea temp. sup.
Aponeurosis +M.temp.
M. temp. (sect.)
A
V. temp. superfic.
A. temp. superfic.
Pannic. adiposus
Linea temporalis
sup. → Fascia temp.
inf. → Aponeurosis m. temp.
Rr. temp. + zygomatici n. facialis
Glandula parotis
B
Fascia temp. (sect.)
Linea temp. sup.
Fascia temp.
Aponeuros. m. temp.
M. temporalis (sect.)
M. temp.
frontozygomatical point
C
Arcus zygomaticus (section)
lateral point of Fiss. orbit. sup.
M. temp.
Arcus zygomaticus (section)
bone flap

Fig. 123 b. Subperiostal resection of Arcus zygomaticus, modified after Gilsbach: oblique bone resection prevents dislocation in a caudal direction

FIG. 123 b

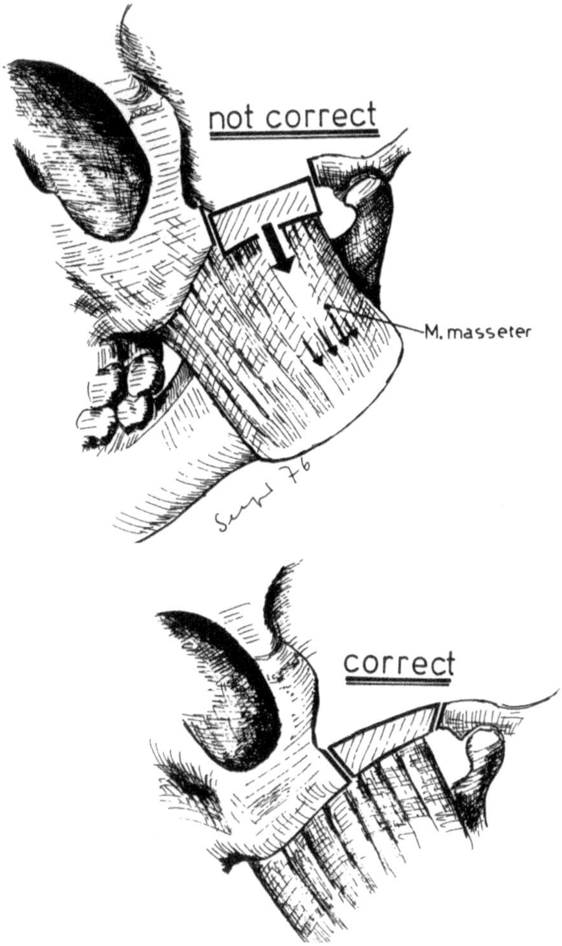

Fig. 123 c. Avoidance of dural injury at the insertion of Ala parva. The trepanation must not be made too far in a basal direction, in order to avoid deviation of the dural protector (above left). Determination of the burrhole localization (below right)
Measurements in millimetres (mm)

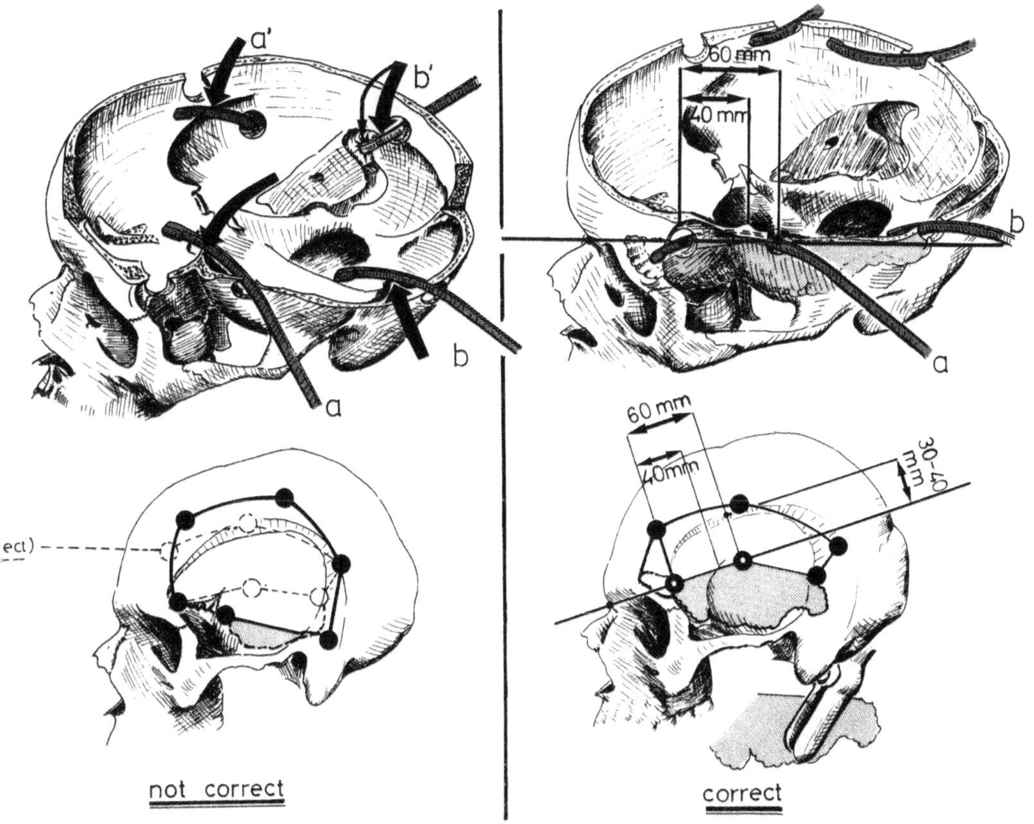
a'
b'
b
a
60 mm
40 mm
b
a
60 mm
40mm
30-40 mm
ect)
not correct
correct

Fig. 124. Position of Vv. ophthalmicae superiores in Fissura orbitalis superior
A Sagittal section at level of the lateral point of Fissura orbitalis sup.
B Sagittal section through the lateral part of the fissure outside Anulus tendineus (Zinii)
C Dural fold in the region of the fissure, which encloses V. (Vv.) ophthalmica sup. and the nerves passing outside Anulus tendineus (Zinii). The fold merges into Periorbita in the orbital funnel and is covered by the spur-shaped remnant of Ala parva protruding at resection, penetrated by R. frontalis a. meningeae mediae
This dural fold must not be coagulated

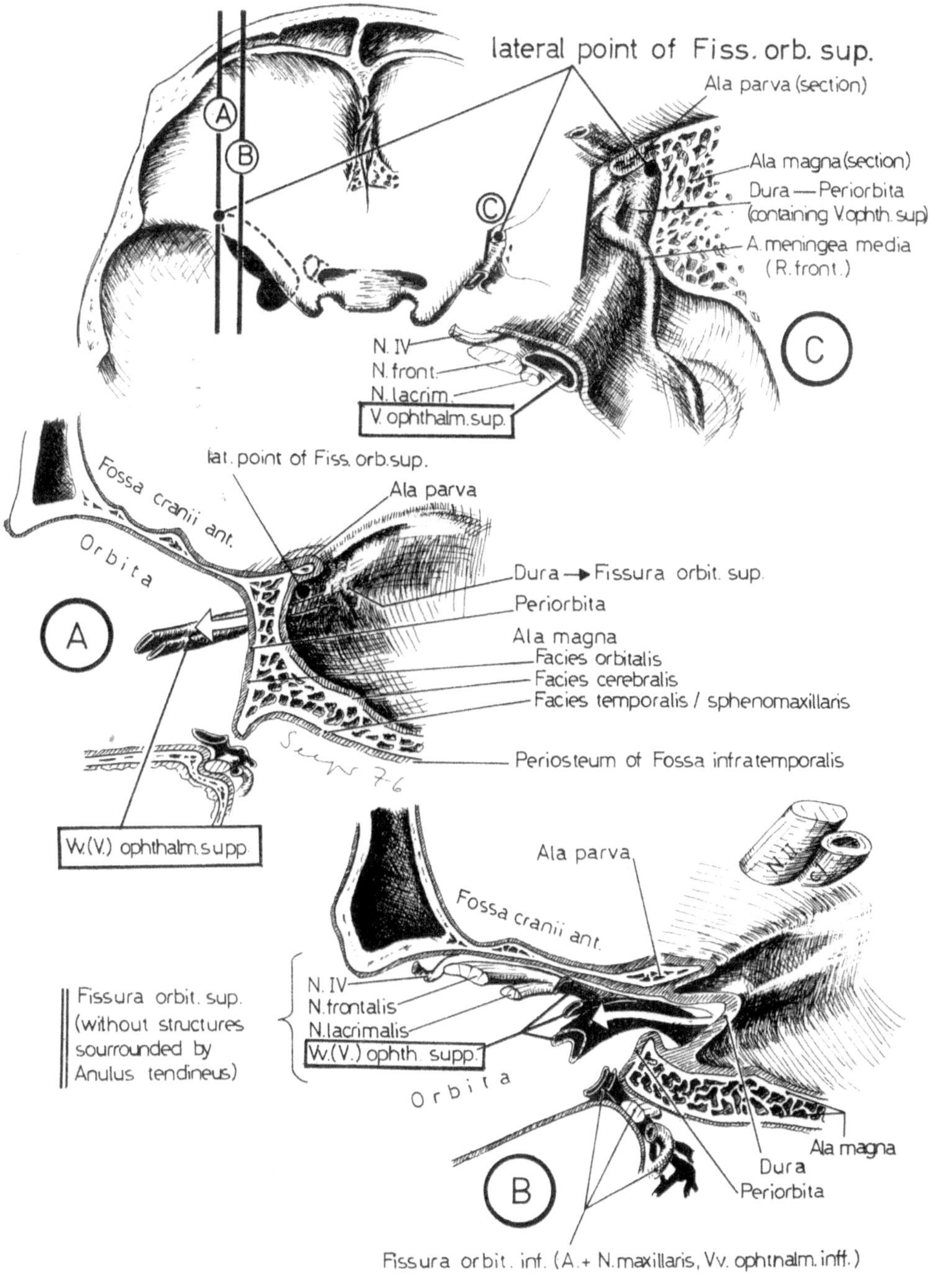
lateral point of Fiss. orb. sup.
Ala parva (section)
Ala magna (section)
Dura — Periorbita
(containing V.ophth. sup)
A. meningea media
(R. front.)
A
B
C
N. IV
N. front.
N. lacrim.
V. ophthalm. sup.
lat. point of Fiss. orb. sup.
Fossa cranii ant.
Ala parva
Orbita
Dura → Fissura orbit. sup.
Periorbita
Ala magna
Facies orbitalis
Facies cerebralis
Facies temporalis / sphenomaxillaris
Periosteum of Fossa infratemporalis
Vv.(V.) ophthalm. supp.
Ala parva
Fossa cranii ant.
Fissura orbit. sup.
(without structures
sourrounded by
Anulus tendineus)
N. IV
N. frontalis
N. lacrimalis
Vv.(V.) ophth. supp.
Orbita
Ala magna
Dura
Periorbita
Fissura orbit. inf. (A.+ N. maxillaris, Vv. ophthalm. inff.)

Fig. 125. Resection of Ala parva up to the lateral point of Fissura orbitalis sup. Search for N. opticus above this measuring point. Coagulations at the lateral point of Fissura orbitalis sup. must not be carried out (see Fig. 124)
Measurements in millimetres (mm)

FIG. 125

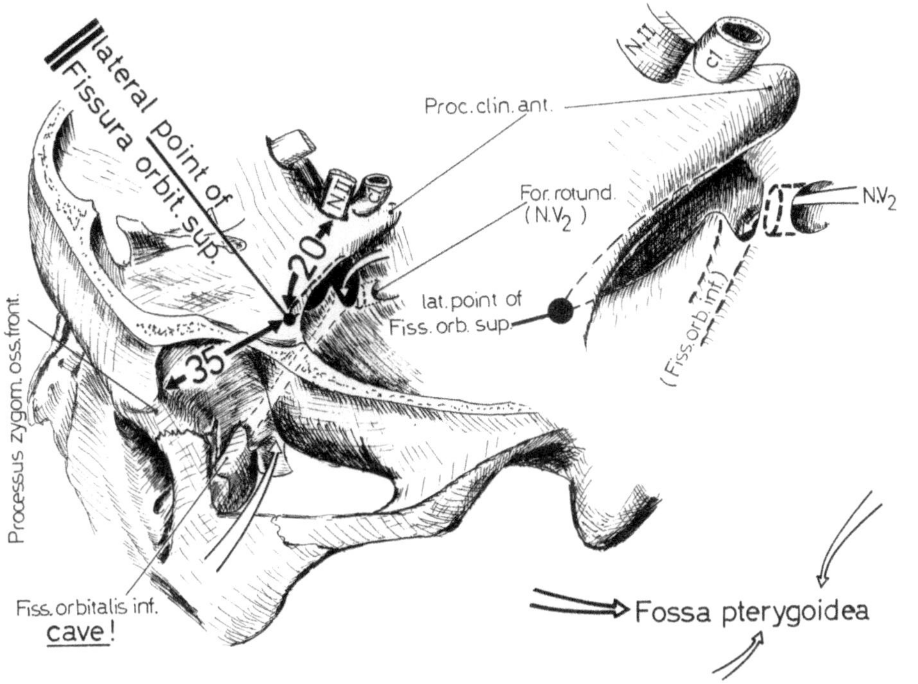
lateral point of
Fissura orbit. sup.
N.II
C.I
Proc. clin. ant.
For. rotund.
(N.V2)
N.V2
20
35
lat. point of
Fiss. orb. sup.
(Fiss. orb. inf.)
Processus zygom. oss. front.
Fiss. orbitalis inf.
cave!
Fossa pterygoidea

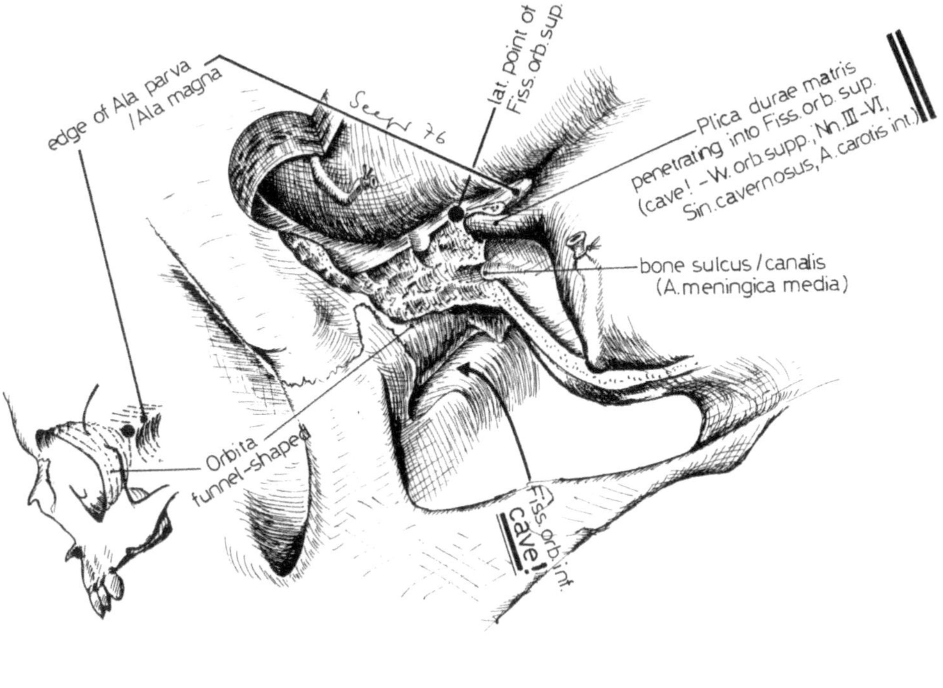
lat. point of
Fiss. orb. sup.
edge of Ala parva
/Ala magna
Plica durae matris
penetrating into Fiss. orb. sup.
(cave! - W. orb. supp., Nn. III-VI,
Sin. cavernosus, A. carotis int.)
bone sulcus / canalis
(A. meningica media)
Orbita
funnel-shaped
Fiss. orb. inf.
cave!

Fig. 126. Temporal right approach to Cisterna ambiens and Fissura lat. (Sylvii) drawn after operation. All areas shown must never be viewed simultaneously, but always stepwise one after the other, in order to avoid injury due to stretching and compression. For technique see lower half of picture
Preparation:
1) Opening of Arachnoidea between the edge of Tentorium and Uncus or Gyri orbitales ·
2) Preparation on the arachnoidal covering of *N. IV*, which overlaps onto A. cerebri post. and its accompanying vessels. Cisterna chiasmatis accessible between N. opticus and A. carotis int., Cisterna praepontina between A. carotis int. and A. basilaris. Between N. oculomotorius and A. carotis int. the perforating arteries can be exposed and isolated
Beware of opaque thickened Arachnoidea! If Infundibulum is not exposed, A. hypophysea sup. cannot be identified; it is only one of the many perforating arteries passing to Hypothalamus region

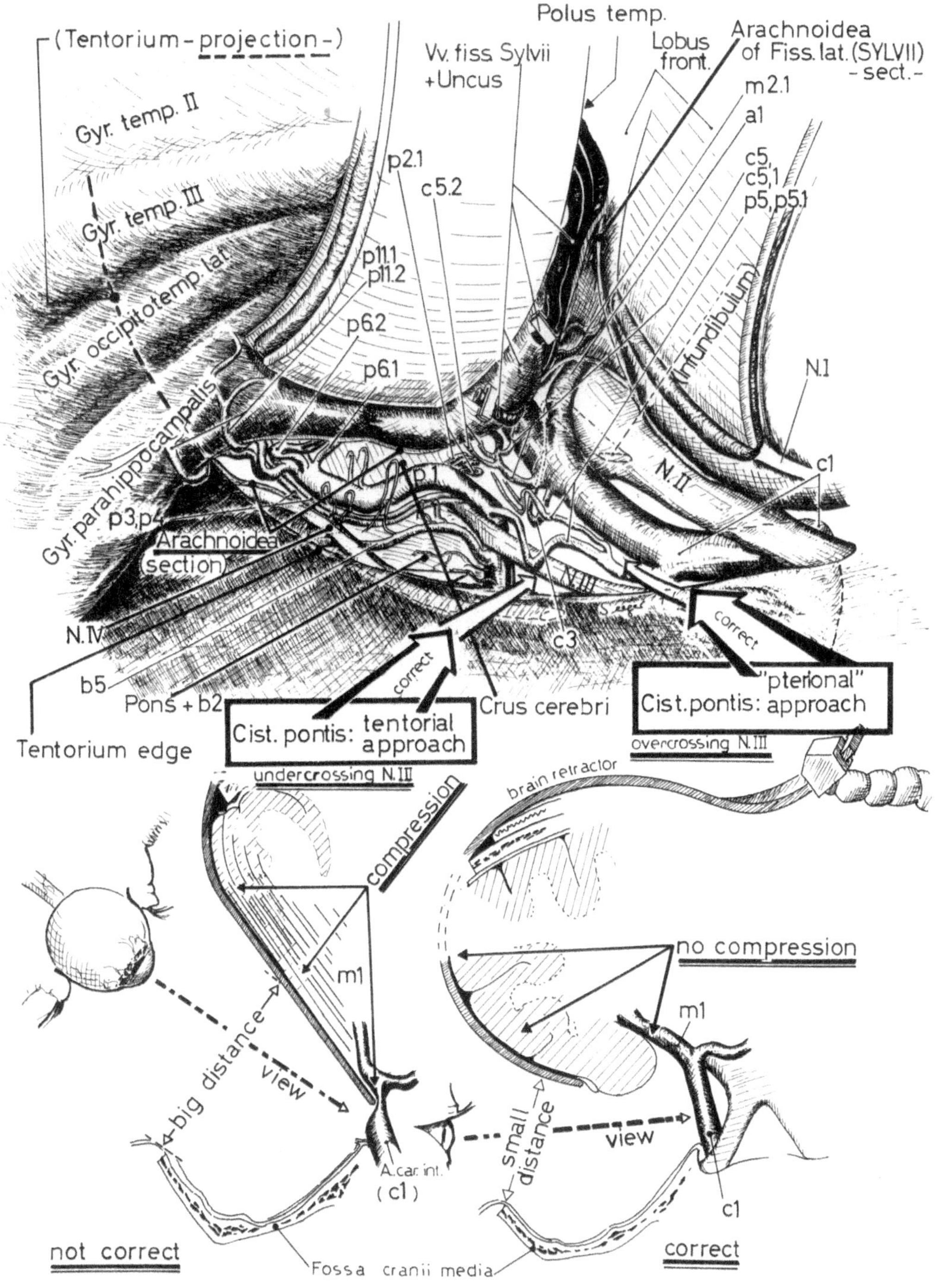
(Tentorium - projection -)
Polus temp.
Vv. fiss. Sylvii + Uncus
Lobus front.
Arachnoidea of Fiss. lat. (SYLVII) - sect. -
m2.1
a1
c5, c5,1
p5, p5.1
Gyr. temp. II
Gyr. temp. III
Gyr. occipitotemp. lat.
Gyr. parahippocampalis
p2.1
c5.2
p11.1
p11.2
p6.2
p6.1
(Infundibulum)
N.I
N.II
c1
p1
p3, p4
Arachnoidea section
N.IV
b5
Pons + b2
Tentorium edge
N.III
c3
correct
Crus cerebri
"pterional" Cist. pontis: approach
Cist. pontis: tentorial approach
undercrossing N.III
overcrossing N.III
brain retractor
compression
no compression
m1
big distance
view
small distance
A. car. int. (c1)
not correct
correct
Fossa cranii media

Fig. 127. Thicker arachnoid membranes at tentorial edge. N. opticus and A. carotis int. easy to visualize. Caution in detaching the arachnoid membrane of Uncus – risk of injury to N. oculomotorius and N. trochlearis. Tentorium begins only beyond Sinus petrosus sup. (more than 30 mm behind *N. II*). Incisions farther forward endanger A. carotis int., Sinus cavernosus, N. trigeminus, and other cranial nerves

Above left: View of Cisterna chiasmatis after removal of tumour, which has pushed N. opticus apart from A. carotis int.

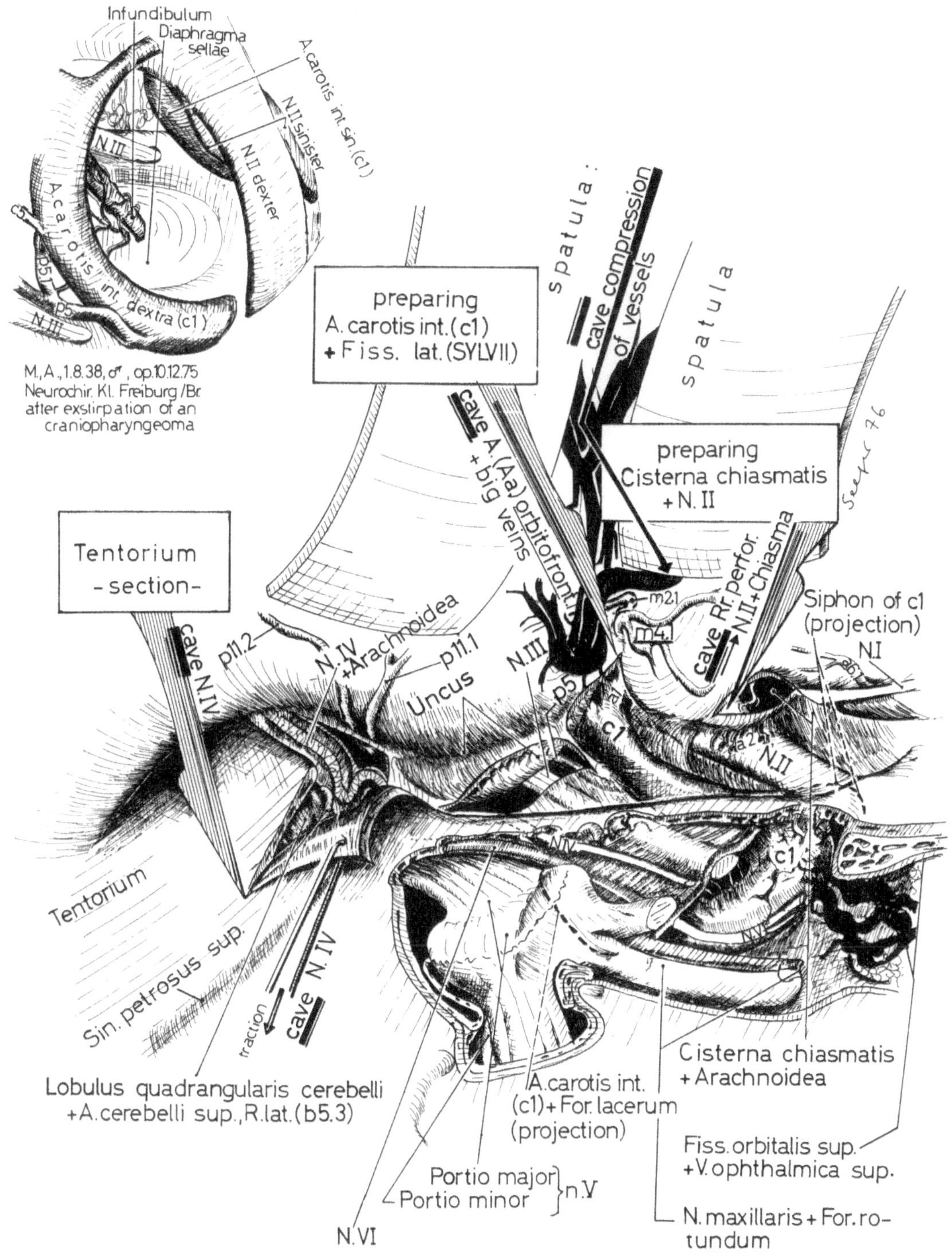
Infundibulum
Diaphragma sellae
A. carotis int. sin. (c1)
N.II sinister
N.III
N.II dexter
A. carotis int. dextra (c1)
p5
N.III
M., A., 1.8.38, ♂, op. 10.12.75
Neurochir. Kl. Freiburg /Br.
after exstirpation of an craniopharyngeoma
preparing
A. carotis int. (c1)
+ Fiss. lat. (SYLVII)
spatula:
cave compression of vessels
spatula
cave A. (Aa) orbitofront.
+ big veins
preparing
Cisterna chiasmatis
+ N. II
Tentorium
-section-
cave N.IV
p11.2
N.IV
+Arachnoidea
p11.1
Uncus
N.III
p5
m2.1
m4.1
cave Rr. perfor.
N.II + Chiasma
Siphon of c1
(projection)
N.I
c1
N.II
c1
Tentorium
Sin. petrosus sup.
traction
cave N.IV
Lobulus quadrangularis cerebelli
+A. cerebelli sup., R. lat. (b5.3)
A. carotis int.
(c1) + For. lacerum
(projection)
Cisterna chiasmatis
+ Arachnoidea
Fiss. orbitalis sup.
+V. ophthalmica sup.
Portio major
Portio minor
n.V
N.VI
N. maxillaris + For. rotundum

Figs. 128 to 130. Parasellar and Sella region

Fig. 128. Points of dural penetration (upper picture) and intradural course of cranial nerves III-VI

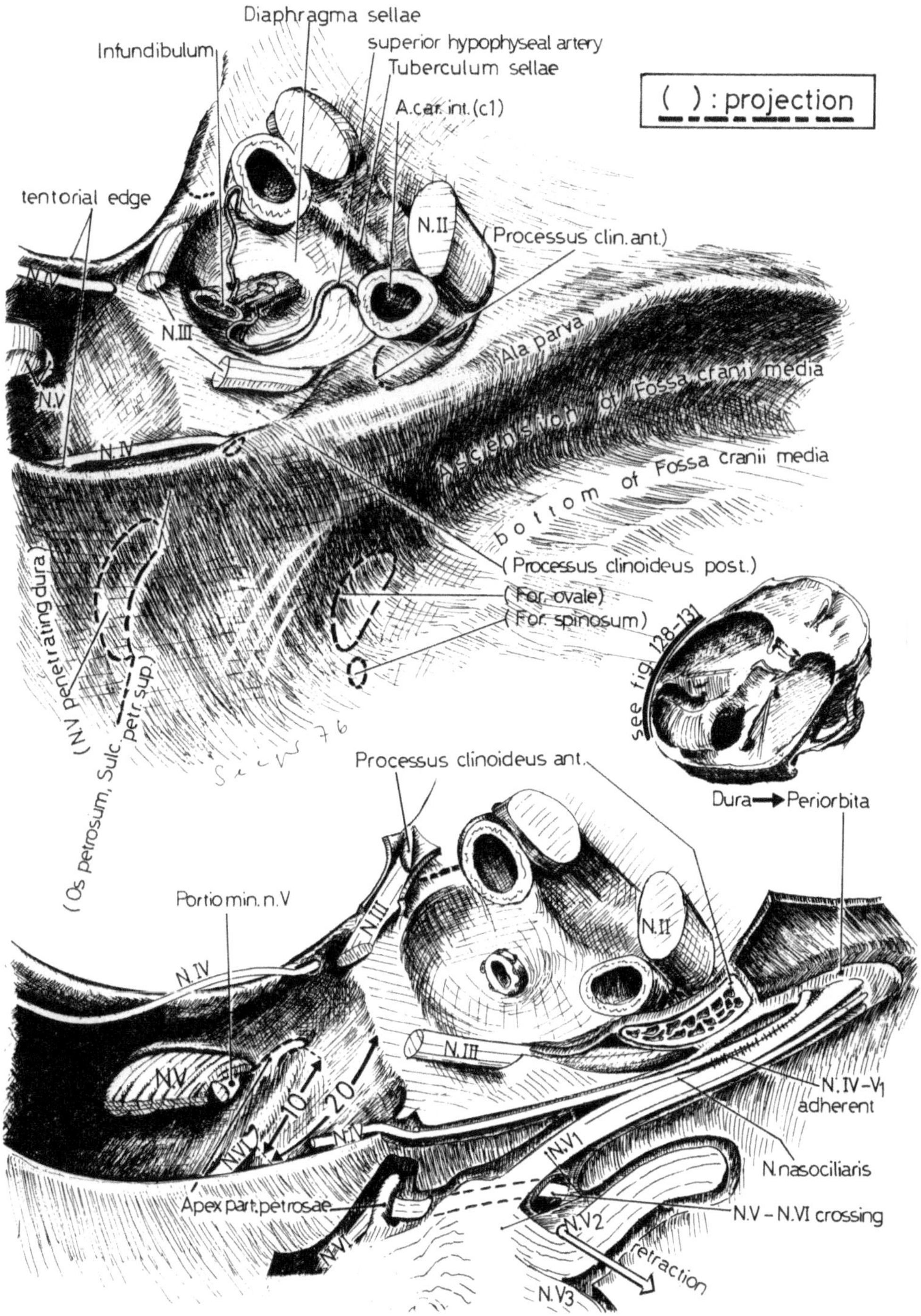
Diaphragma sellae
Infundibulum
superior hypophyseal artery
Tuberculum sellae
( ) : projection
A.car. int.(c1)
tentorial edge
N.II
(Processus clin. ant.)
N.V
N.III
Ala parva
Ascension of Fossa cranii media
N.V
N.IV
bottom of Fossa cranii media
(Processus clinoideus post.)
(For. ovale)
(For. spinosum)
(N.V penetrating dura)
(Os petrosum, Sulc. petr. sup.)
see fig. 128–131
Processus clinoideus ant.
Dura → Periorbita
Portio min. n.V
N.III
N.II
N.IV
N.III
N.V
10
20
N.IV–V1 adherent
N.VI
N.V
N.V1
N.nasociliaris
Apex part. petrosae
N.V – N.VI crossing
N.VI
N.V2
retraction
N.V3

Fig. 129. Lateral exposure of the deeper structures enclosed by the tentorial fold. Cranial nerves and vessels enclosed by Anulus tendineus, and those that pass outside Anulus tend. laterally (cf. Fig. 124)

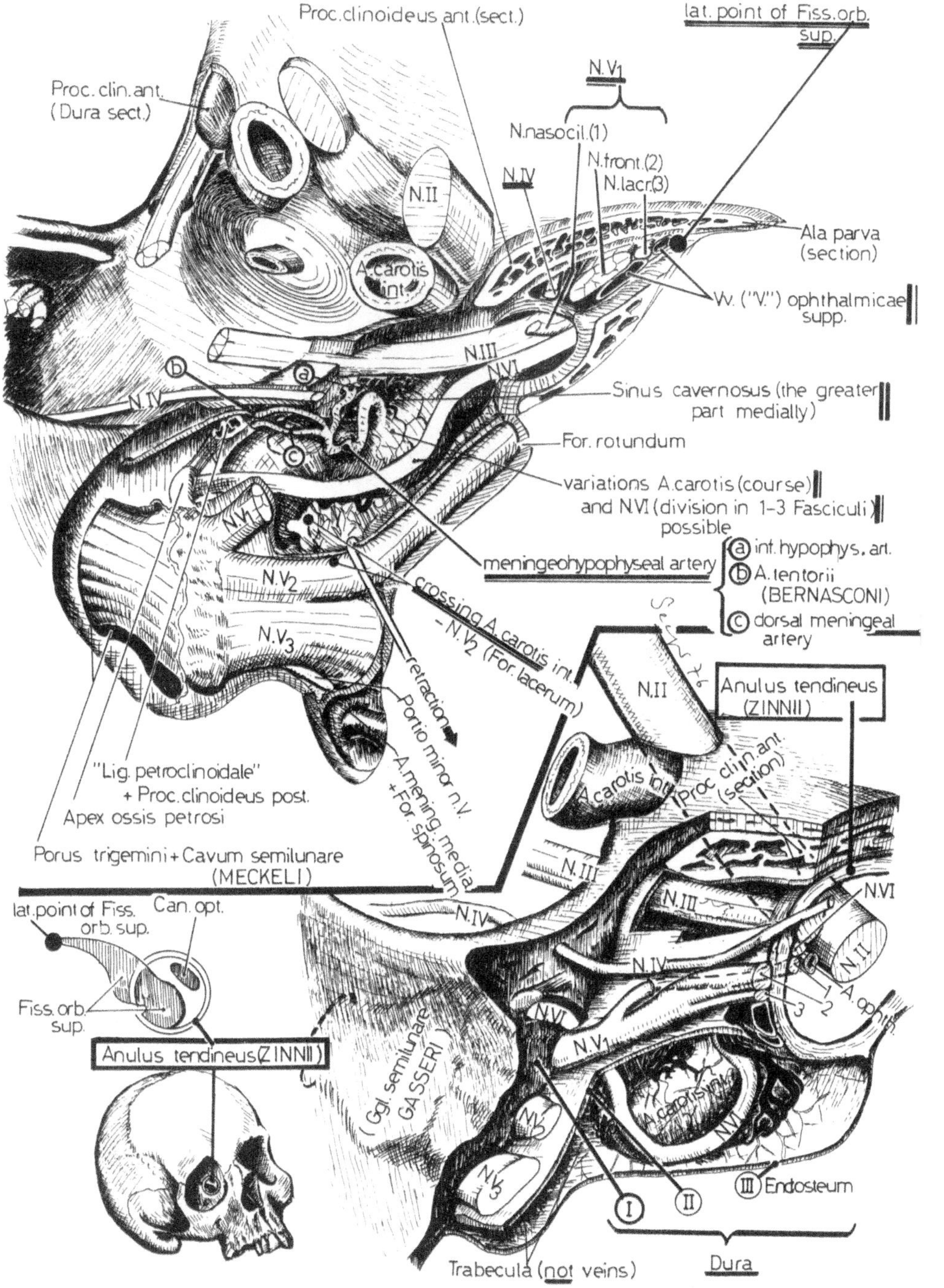

Proc. clinoideus ant. (sect.)
lat. point of Fiss. orb. sup.
Proc. clin. ant. (Dura sect.)
N.V1
N. nasocil. (1)
N. front. (2)
N. lacr. (3)
N.IV
N.II
A. carotis int.
Ala parva (section)
Vv. ("V.") ophthalmicae supp.
N.III
N.VI
N.IV
Sinus cavernosus (the greater part medially)
For. rotundum
variations A. carotis (course) and N.VI (division in 1–3 Fasciculi) possible
meningeohypophyseal artery
(a) int. hypophys. art.
(b) A. tentorii (BERNASCONI)
(c) dorsal meningeal artery
N.V1
N.V2
N.V3
crossing A. carotis int. – N.V2 (For. lacerum)
retraction
Portio minor n.V.
A. mening. media + For. spinosum
"Lig. petroclinoidale" + Proc. clinoideus post.
Apex ossis petrosi
Porus trigemini + Cavum semilunare (MECKELI)
N.II
Anulus tendineus (ZINNII)
A. carotis int.
Proc. clin. ant. (section)
N.III
N.VI
N.IV
N.II
A. ophth.
1
2
3
N.VI
N.V1
A. carotis int.
N.V2
N.V3
Ggl. semilunare GASSERI
lat. point of Fiss. orb. sup.
Can. opt.
Fiss. orb. sup.
Anulus tendineus (ZINNII)
I
II
III Endosteum
Dura
Trabecula (not veins)

Fig. 130. Partial removal of the dura including its deepest – periosteal – layer.
A General view (senile atrophic enlargement of Fissura orbit. sup.)
spl. Border zone at which the dura splits into several layers
Arterial nomenclature from Renn and Rhoton (1975)
B Fissura orbit. sup. in childhood
C Schematic section at the level of Foramen lacerum and ovale
D Section plane of illustrations *B* and *C*
Measurements in millimetres (mm)

FIG. 130

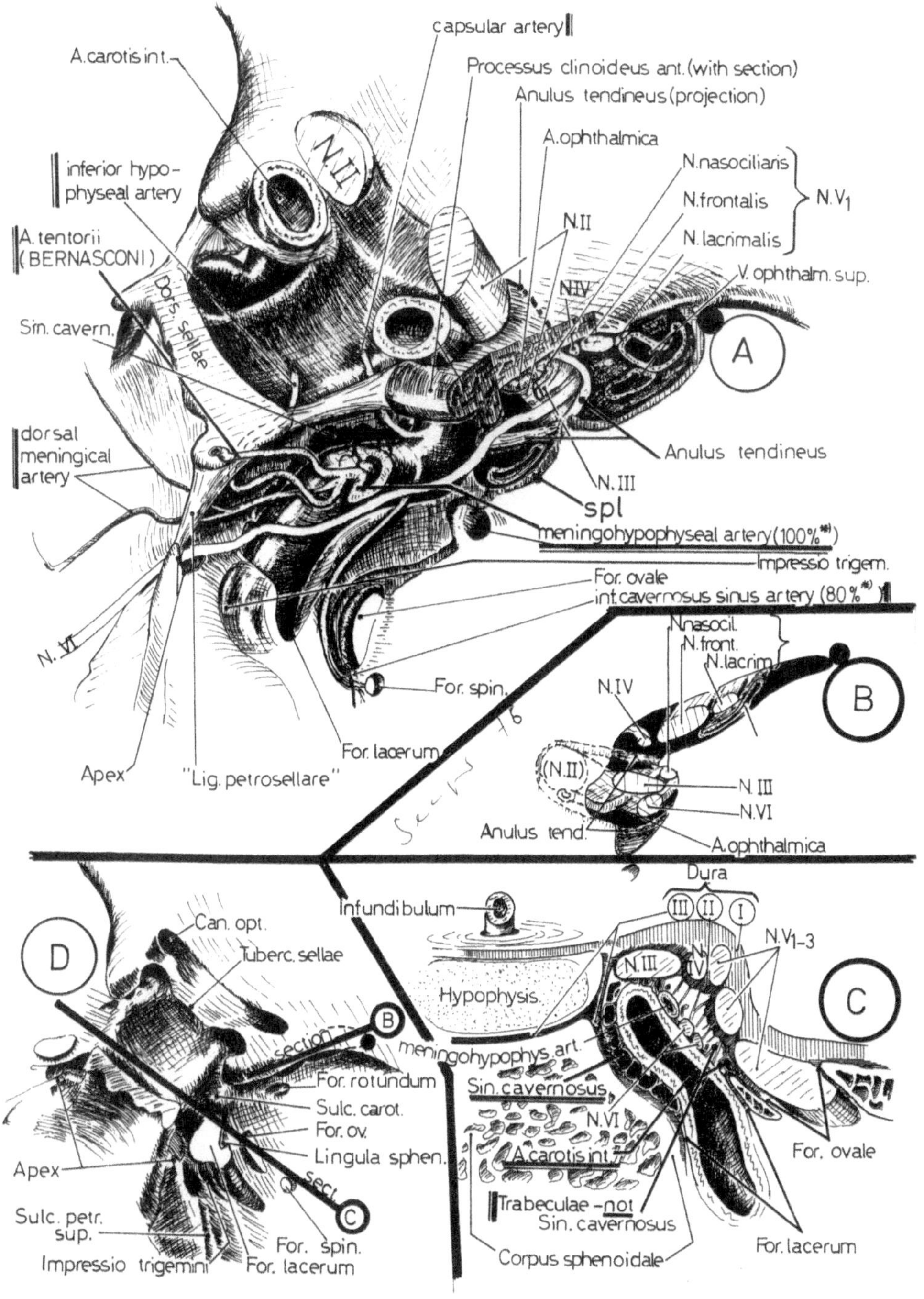

A.carotis int.
capsular artery
Processus clinoideus ant.(with section)
Anulus tendineus (projection)
A.ophthalmica
inferior hypophyseal artery
N.II
N.nasociliaris
N.frontalis
N.lacrimalis
N.V1
A.tentorii (BERNASCONI)
Dors. sellae
N.IV
V. ophthalm. sup.
Sin. cavern.
A
dorsal meningical artery
Anulus tendineus
N.III
spl
meningohypophyseal artery (100%**)
Impressio trigem.
For. ovale
int.cavernosus sinus artery (80%**)
N. VI
For. spin.
For. lacerum
Apex
"Lig. petrosellare"
N.nasocil.
N.front.
N.lacrim.
B
N.IV
(N.II)
N. III
N.VI
Anulus tend.
A.ophthalmica
D
Can. opt.
Tuberc. sellae
section
For. rotundum
Sulc. carot.
For. ov.
Lingula sphen.
Apex
Sulc. petr. sup.
sect.
For. spin.
Impressio trigemini
For. lacerum
Infundibulum
Dura
III II I
N.V1-3
N.III
IV
Hypophysis
C
meningohypophys.art.
Sin.cavernosus
N.VI
A.carotis int.
For. ovale
Trabeculae - not Sin. cavernosus
Corpus sphenoidale
For. lacerum

Fig. 131. The sinuses at the base of the brain lying between the dural layers are dense zones of an overall venous network. Dorsum sellae is almost completely bypassed. Veins projected onto the base of the skull. Sinus cavernosus is almost exclusively adjacent only to the medial wall of A. carotis int.

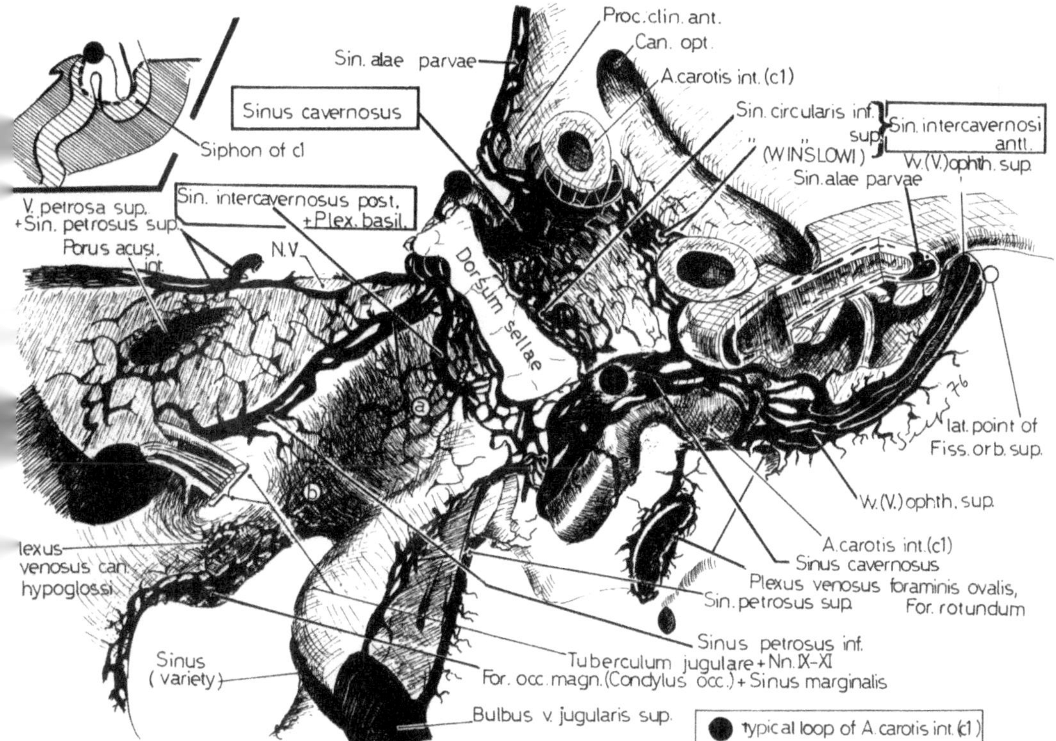
Proc. clin. ant.
Can. opt.
Sin. alae parvae
A. carotis int. (c1)
Sinus cavernosus
Sin. circularis inf.
sup.
" " (WINSLOWI)
Sin. intercavernosi antt.
W. (V.) ophth. sup.
Sin. alae parvae
Siphon of c1
Sin. intercavernosus post. + Plex. basil.
V. petrosa sup. + Sin. petrosus sup.
Porus acust. int.
N. V.
Dorsum sellae
lat. point of Fiss. orb. sup.
W. (V.) ophth. sup.
A. carotis int. (c1)
Sinus cavernosus
Plexus venosus foraminis ovalis, For. rotundum
Sin. petrosus sup.
lexus venosus can. hypoglossi
Sinus petrosus inf.
Tuberculum jugulare + Nn. IX–XI
For. occ. magn. (Condylus occ.) + Sinus marginalis
Sinus (variety)
Bulbus v. jugularis sup.
typical loop of A. carotis int. (c1)

Fig. 132. Bony resection with transformation of Canalis opticus, Fissura · orbitalis sup., Foramen rotundum, and Fissura orbit. inf. into a common space. Only medially in the carotid region is the dura more closely attached to the bone. Processus clin. ant. is left in situ in order not to endanger A. carotis int.

A Transition of the dura into the periosteal sheath of Canalis opticus and into Periorbita

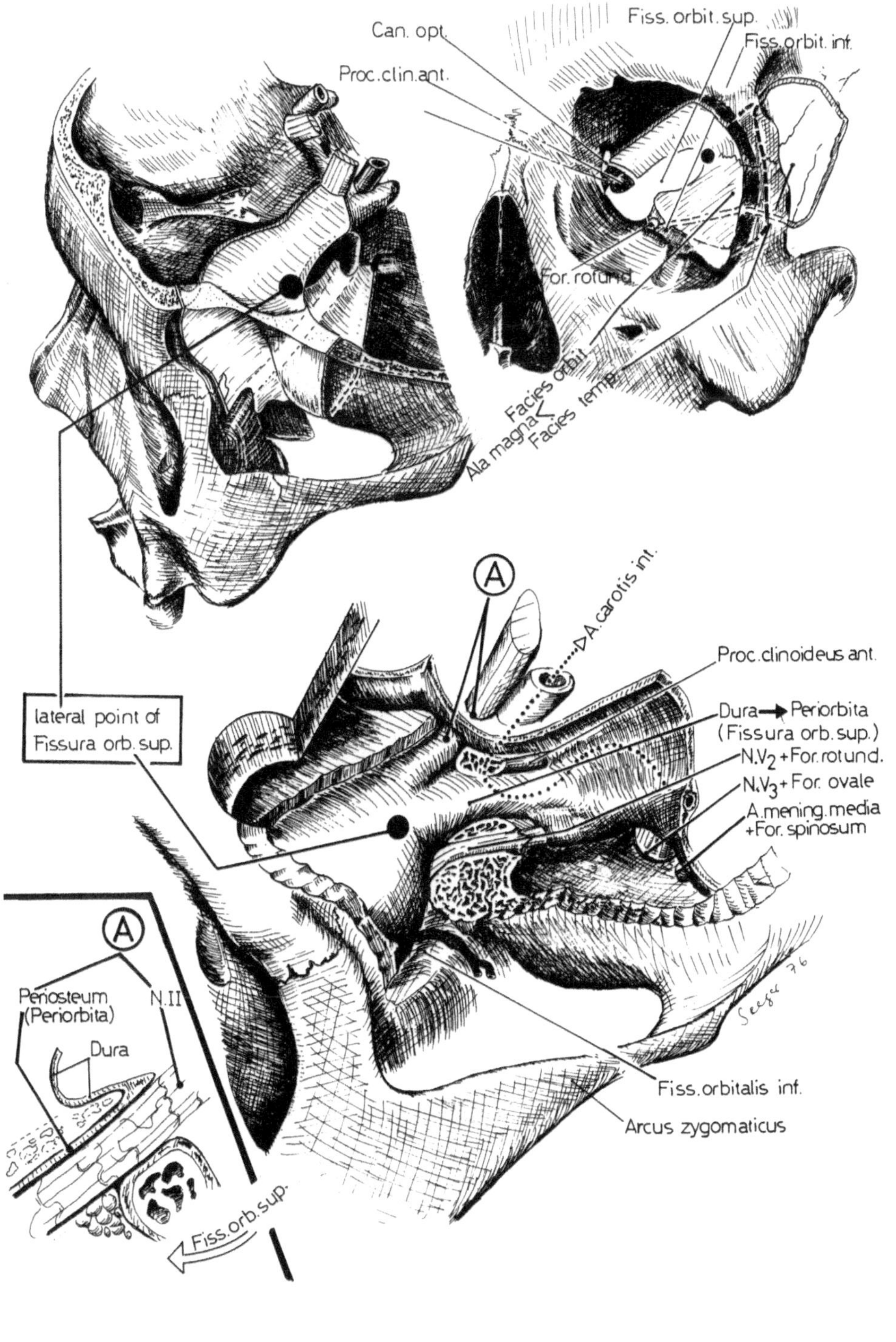
Can. opt.
Proc. clin. ant.
Fiss. orbit. sup.
Fiss. orbit. inf.
For. rotund.
Facies orbit.
Ala magna
Facies temp.
lateral point of Fissura orb. sup.
A
A. carotis int.
Proc. clinoideus ant.
Dura → Periorbita (Fissura orb. sup.)
N. V2 + For. rotund.
N. V3 + For. ovale
A. mening. media + For. spinosum
Periosteum (Periorbita)
N. II
Dura
Fiss. orb. sup.
Fiss. orbitalis inf.
Arcus zygomaticus

Fig. 133. Supplement to Fig. 132. Limits of resection:

a, b lateral orbital region
c Ala parva to Canalis opticus
d Canalis opticus to Fissura orbit. sup.
e Fissura orbit. sup. to Foramen rotundum/Fossa pterygoidea
f Fossa pterygoidea to lateral limit of Fissura orbit. inf.
g Fissura orbit. inf. to squamous part of temporal bone and Ala magna

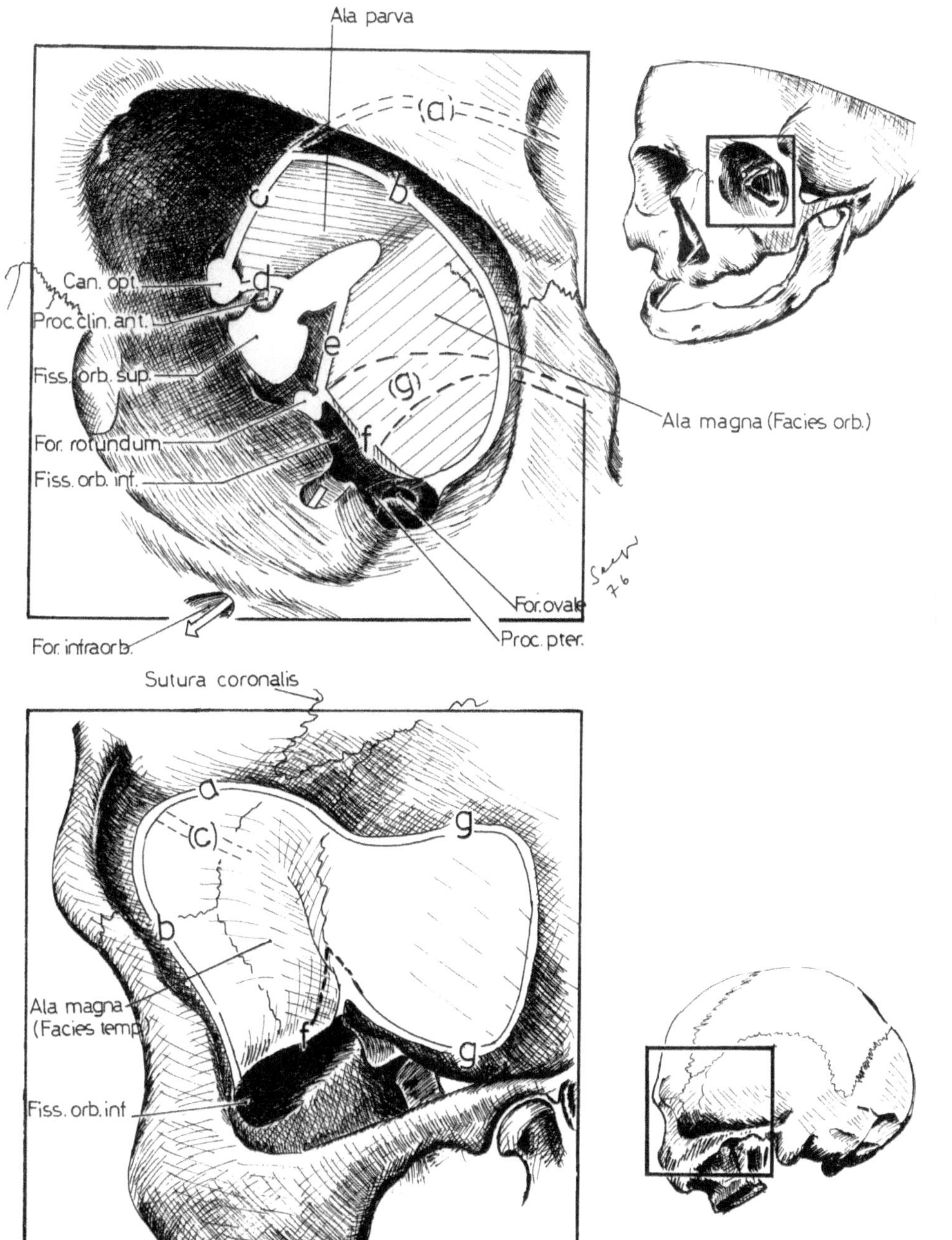
Ala parva
(a)
c
b
Can. opt.
d
Proc. clin. ant.
e
Fiss. orb. sup.
(g)
For. rotundum
f
Fiss. orb. inf.
Ala magna (Facies orb.)
For. ovale
For. infraorb.
Proc. pter.
Sutura coronalis
a
(c)
g
b
Ala magna
(Facies temp.)
f
g
Fiss. orb. inf.

Chapter 4
Parietal Lobe

A. Surface

Beginning anteriorly at Sulcus centralis and ending posteriorly and medially at Fissura parietooccipitalis, the region extends at Fissura longitudinalis as far as Corpus callosum, and at the outer surface as far as the Sylvian fissure (from Pars opercularis gyri front. III to the curved-up end of Fissura lat. [Sylvii]). Anteriorly the border is clearly defined, but posteriorly the borders are not sufficiently definable for practical purposes, owing to variations in the length of the Sylvian fissure and its difficult identification in this area, as well as the medially concealed site of Fissura parietooccipitalis. Orientation is easier from the surface of the skull (see Fig. 134): the precentral region begins 10 to 30 mm behind Bregma, and Fissura parietooccipitalis ends in the vicinity of Lambda. The parietal bone thus covers posteriorly the parietal lobe and anteriorly also part of the frontal lobe. The squamous part of the temporal bone also covers the portion of the parietal lobe lying over Fissura lat. (Sylvii). At the outer surface of the brain the limits of the precentral region can only be defined if the neighbouring frontal gyri take a mainly sagittal course and are demarcated from the obliquely lying precentral and postcentral regions. Behind this the relief is so irregular, and its form so masked by the leptomeninges and vessels, that it is usually better to take orientation from the course of the vessels (comparison with the angiogram, especially the superficial cerebral veins).
On the other hand in Fissura longitudinalis the meandering first frontal gyrus can be demarcated from the broad-surfaced, poorly convoluted, block of Lobulus paracentralis, as far as the narrow approach allows this. Marking of Bregma is more important. The position of the precentral region and the paracentral region in relation to Bregma is, however, also variable (see Fig. 134).
In contrast to the more irregular structure of the first frontal gyrus and Lobulus paracentralis, Gyrus cinguli can be identified, also at depth, by its regular course and its proximity to Corpus callosum.
In the roof of Fissura lat. (Sylvii) transversely running gyri roll up and lie in parallel fashion in columnar formation above Heschl's gyrus, behind which the transverse gyri of the temporal lobe pass. Gyri of the parietal and temporal lobes may merge with one another in the fissure (see Chapter 3, Fig. 94, behind), and thus interrupt the Sylvian fissure with lateral displacement of the vessels contained in the fissure.

B. Deep Structures and Vessels

In accordance with the mainly triangular cross-section of Sinus sagittalis sup., the edge of Pallium is slightly sloped, so that the sinus has to be undermined during operation in order to reach Fissura longitudinalis. The main problem in exposing this is presented by the cerebral veins entering the sinus (see Fig. 137, a-d). Extensive widely spread adhesions of the leptomeninges to the wall of the sinus are possible. The relief in Fissura longitudinalis is flat. Corpus callosum is reached at a depth of 40 to 50 mm (Fig. 94 in Chapter 3). Between the edge of Falx and Corpus callosum there is only a few millimetres' space, and this practically disappears in the occipital direction, so that Corpus callosum and the lower edge of Falx touch there.
It is important that beyond the 20 mm-wide ventricle (Fig. 135, above) the white matter between the lateral ventricle wall and the floor of Fissura lat. (Sylvii) is only 15 to 20 mm wide. The fibres of Corona radiata lie in this region. Laterally situated to the ventricular system at this level, even small lesions may be expected to result in sensory and motor dificits (Fig. 135). This zone can hardly be reached from the lateral direction, since the distance between the surface of Fissura lat. (Sylvii) and its floor measures 40 mm and the approach is hindered by the vessels of the fissure. A strictly medial resection may initially be expected to result in destruc-

tion of pyramidal tracts to lower limbs only. The more deeply the white matter is penetrated, the more likelihood there is that the medially radiating tracts for arms and face will be reached in the medial parts of Corona radiata (Fig. 73, upper picture, Chapter 2).

In opening the ventricle, attention should be paid to the reference structures which facilitate the search for Foramen interventriculare (Monroi) – in particular, the course of Plexus chorioideus, V. thalamostriata (extremely variable!) and Stria terminalis (see Fig. 136). Thalamus arches forward and upwards, so that a view into Foramen interventriculare (Monroi) is only possible from the mid – and anterior parietal or from the frontal region.

Arteries:
At the side of the edge of Pallium lies the border area between branches of the anterior and posterior cerebral artery. An incision in the sagittal direction, carried out not directly at the edge of Pallium but somewhat to the side, would not lead to encephalomalacia because endarteries overlap. The variants of A. cerebri media described by Ring in 1969 refer mainly to the calibre of the branches and their different sites of origin from the main trunk in Fissura lat. (Sylvii). In accordance with the general rule in the convexity, they start mediobasally and run in an upward lateral direction. The anastomoses familiar from neuroradiology in the vicinity of the edge of Pallium to A. cerebri ant. are fine, and even in injection preparations under the microscope are only occasionally recognizable up to the precapillary level. The posteriorly lying branches of A. cerebri ant. in Fissura longitudinalis – A. paracentralis, A. pericallosa, and its end branch, A. praecunealis – supply exclusively the functional cortical areas in the region of Fissura longitudinalis.

Two different types of arterial courses in the region of Fissura lat. (Sylvii) can be differentiated: anteriorly in the arborization of A. frontoparietalis ascendens they swing up S-shaped over the surface of Insula and do not quite return to the surface of Fissura lat. (Sylvii), but penetrate the surface of the brain in the transverse sulci of the opercular gyri. Farther back, the arteries run transversely ("L-shaped"), in accordance with the direction of Fissura lat. (Sylvii) from mediobasally to upwards laterally, and here they show a tendency to reach directly through the fissure to the surface of the brain (Figs. 7 and 8, Chapter 1).

Veins:
The venous system of the superficial cortex has been repeatedly investigated in recent years by Kaplan et al., and the connection to the deep Sylvian vein, the so-called V. (Vv.) cerebri media (Duvernoy) demonstrated. This vein is connected via superficial cerebral veins with Sinus sagittalis sup., and is connected basally with V. basalis (Rosenthal). In addition, Kaplan investigated venous connections between Cortex and ventricle wall. In contrast to the arterial arborization, numerous minute venous anastomoses are to be expected in the parietal region, as in other parts of the brain, this being particularly well-known in regard to the inner cerebral veins (Lin et al., 1955).
With the extremely variable types of entry of superficial cerebral veins into Sinus sagittalis sup., it is important that their last stretch is situated between the dural layers before Sinus sagittalis sup. is reached (Fig. 137). Pacchioni's granulations may indicate this type of course. In this part of their course the veins show connections to branched venous lacunae, which are particularly prominent in the parietal region. The sinus wall varies in strength; although thickwalled on the surface, it is penetrated by numerous Pacchioni's granulations. The sidewall is very thin in some places (Fig. 137).
Kaplan and co-workers have described the variants of Sinus sagittalis sup. and have proved that it may in some cases show an atresia during the first 3 to 5 cm of its course. Vesalius and his draughtsman, Jan Kalkar (1543), already recognized the irregularity in the course of the sinus in the frontal region (Fig. 138).
A modern injection preparation by Stephens and Stilwell (1969) shows the entrance of a frontal bridging vein crossing over the sinus into the contralateral half of the bipartite sinus (Fig. 139). Here the lateral deviation of the left half of the sinus can be recognized.
The course of the sinus is particularly irregular in the vicinity of the always widely spread parietal Sinus lacunae, which reach far laterally. In the preparation of Stephens and Stilwell they are connected to a stenosis of the middle to posterior third of the sinus, which branch out centrally several times, so that the bloodstream is diverted laterally into Lacunae. In vivo the lumen of the sinus (whose width is constant) and of cerebral veins varies according to the venous pressure depending on the sitting or lying position of the patient. In the sitting

position the veins and Villi arachnoidales may collapse, as in the cadaver (Fig. 138, a fresh preparation after decapitation and opening of Sinus sagittalis sup). The considerable increase in volume is reproduced in the injection preparation (Fig. 139).

C. Preoperative Radiology – Some Aspects

Fig. 140 presents localization in relation to tilted projections, also a-p and lateral views are correctly compared. On these views depends the exact localization of intracranial processes (Fig. 140, *B* and *C*). In the projection of deep-seated processes on to the surface of the skull the shallow convexity high parietally must be taken into account. This appears considerably foreshortened from the lateral view (*C* in Fig. 140).

Because of the importance of the parietal functional (cortical) areas and projection pathways it is often necessary to make a frontal approach for frontoparietal processes, and a occipitoparietal approach for processes lying farther back. In the preoperative radiological projection of the process onto the frontal (see Fig. 143) or parietooccipital (see Fig. 144) surface of the skull, the probable displacement of the fibres of Corona radiata must be taken into account. Furthermore in making the approach the position of the cerebral veins should be kept in mind, since larger cerebral veins must not be damaged. The knowledge of localization of arteries is not so important for white matter processes. For extracerebral processes they must be exactly localized before operation. On lateral projection in the upper parietal region not only the vault of the skull but also the cerebral veins flowing into the sinus are foreshortened (Fig. 141). Several centimetres of the course of the veins before their junction with the sinus cannot be identified in the angiogram if they are superimposed on Sinus sagittalis sup. Just as Jan Kalkar in 1543 chose an oblique projection to obtain a better presentation, in the modern angiogram, too, oblique pictures should be used for the localization of the position of the junction. The frequently alleged acute-angled counterflow entry of the cerebral veins into the sinus is an exception (see injection preparation of Fig. 139). The veins enter mainly in the direction of flow or rectangularly, even if they have previously taken an oblique course over the convexity against the direction of flow of the sinus. Andreas Vesalius and Jan Kalkar had already seen this course correctly (Fig. 138). If cerebral veins run for a longer stretch between the dural layers, however, their entry into the dura in a forward direction is not unusual.

Pacchioni's granulations are most pronounced in the region of the parietal lacunae. Well-developed Pacchioni's granulations should be taken to indicate the possibility of larger cerebral veins or lacunae and stenoses of the sinus. Since the interruption of the lacunae in cases of constriction of the sinus stream may possibly endanger the venous circulation (see Fig. 142), it should be determined from the recommended oblique films whether Sinus sagittalis sup. in the posterior parietal region has a wide lumen or is flatly branched.

D. Operative Techniques – Some Aspects

A dogmatic ruling for the customary incision (temporal flap, occipital or parietal flap) is not convenient.

It should, however, be attempted to protect the temporal branch of N. facialis. It runs under the main frontal branch of A. temporalis superficialis. Some possibilities of avoiding damage to it are given in Fig. 145.

The type of trepanation illustrated in Fig. 146 (above) is customary for many processes localized extracerebrally, but is impracticable for processes near the midline. Here Fissura longitudinalis should be exposed over a stretch as extended as possible (Fig. 146, below).

Wide spread processes of Fissura longitudinalis should on occasion be approached bilaterally (Fig. 147), in which case the displacement syndrome of the arteries is the criterion for the exact determination of the trepanation area, and the angiographically localized course of the veins (see Fig. 147 *B*) is important for orientation during operation. Extracerebral processes may begin primarily near the surface and are more easily accessible; the difference in deep-seated processes is that a compressed zone of Gyrus cinguli lies between the floor of the process and the vessels of Corpus callosum (Fig. 148). In everting the dura in the parietal region the stretch of cerebral veins lying between the dural layers is particularly at risk (Figs. 149 and 150). If the process lies in the brain substance itself (Fig. 149 *C*, *D*) it is important to make a subpial approach from the frontal lobe, avoiding damage to Aa. frontales internae and especially to A. paracentralis. Also, frontally larger cerebral veins should be spared (Fig. 150 *D*).

Extremely deep-seated processes – e.g., angiomas of A. pericallosa, ventricular or Corpus callosum or tumours – demand a deep approach into Fissura longitudinalis. It is important here to pay attention to the frequent venous connections between the falx and the medial surface of the parietal lobe (Fig. 151). If, due to fear of injury to the sinus, the midline is not approached closely enough, the edge of Pallium will be crushed during undermining of the dura and veins, and be torn out of the falx or the laterally thin-walled Sinus sagittalis sup. (Fig. 151, above).

If, on the other hand, the trepanation is made too near the midline or even towards the opposite side, eversion of the dura may lead to compression of the sinus, which if thin-walled may likewise rupture (Fig. 151, centre, right). The effects of heat in the immediate neighbourhood of the sinus carry the danger of thrombosis. A technical hint for their avoidance by stitching or clipping on of vein transplants, as practiced by the author, may be permitted (Figs. 152 and 153). The principle of clipping rather than coagulating in the vicinity of the sinus is also expedient in the vicinity of the dural lacunae near the sinus, and prevents extensive thrombosis. An approach from 1 cm^2 surface area must on occasion suffice in order to be able, under microsurgical conditions, to remove space-occupying processes extracerebrally under the veins – e.g., in the region of the parietal lacunae.

E. References

Duvernoy, H. M.: The Superficial Veins of the Human Brain. Veins of the Brain Stem and of the Base of the Brain. Berlin–Heidelberg–New York: Springer. 1975.

Kalkar, J. see Vesalius, A.

Kaplan, H. A.: The transcerebral venous system. An anatomical study. A. M. A. Archives of Neurology **1,** 40/148–44/152 (1959).

Kaplan, H. A., Browder, J.: Importance of veins in partial cerebral lobectomy. J. Neurosurg. **41,** 360–366 (1974).

Kaplan, H. A., Ford, H. D.: The Brain Vascular System. Amsterdam–London–New York: Elsevier Publishing Company. 1966.

Lin, P. M., Mokrohisky, J. F., Stauffer, H. M., et al.: The importance of the deep cerebral veins in cerebral angiography with special emphasis on the orientation of the foramen of monro through visualization of the "venous angle" of the brain. J. Neurosurg. **12,** 256–277 (1955).

Ring, A.: In: The Neglected Cause of Stroke. Occlusion of the Smaller Intracranial Arteries and Their Diagnosis by Cerebral Angiography. St. Louis: Warren H. Green, Inc. 1969.

Stephens, R. B., Stilwell, D. L.: Arteries and Veins of the Human Brain. Springfield, Ill.: Ch. C Thomas. 1969.

Vesalius, A.: De humani corporis fabrica. Basiliae 1543.

Literature for Further Reading

Foix, Ch., Levy, M.: Les ramollissements sylviens. Revue Neurologique **II,** 1, 1–51 (1927).

Yaşargil, M. G., et al.: Arteriovenous malformations of vein of Galen: microsurgical treatment. Surg. Neurol. **6,** 195–200 (1976).

Yaşargil, M. G., et al.: Arteriovenous malformations of the splenium of the corpus callosum: microsurgical treatment. Surg. Neurol. **5,** 5–13 (1976).

F. Illustrations

(Figs. 134–153)

Fig. 134. Orientation in the region of Fissura longitudinalis from frontal to occipital according to the position of Bregma and Lambda, with distance measurements in millimetres (mm). Notice the variable distance (10–30 mm) of the precentral and paracentral regions from Bregma and the relationship between Gyrus praecentralis and Sutura coronalis

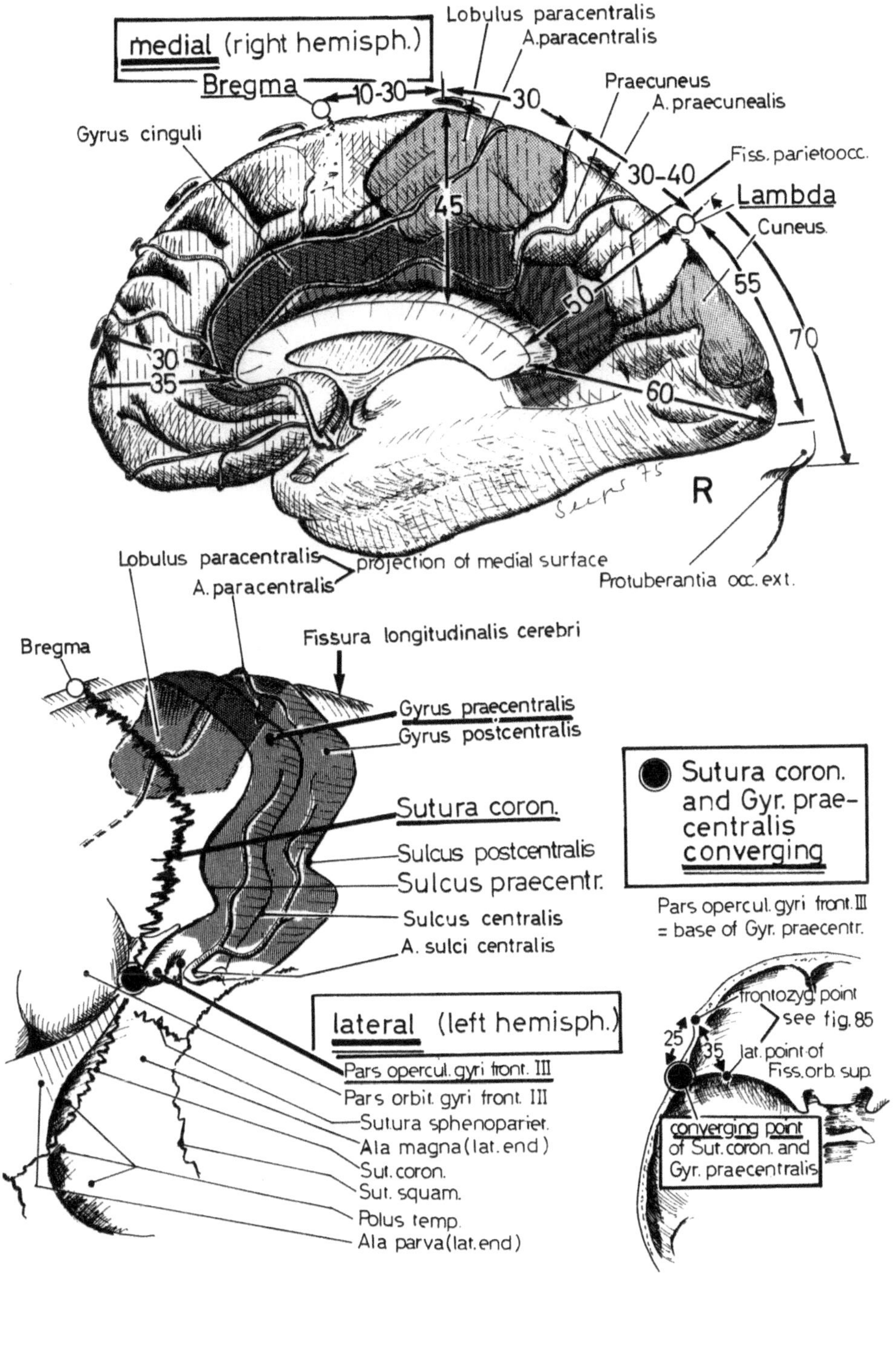
medial (right hemisph.)
Bregma
10-30
30
30-40
45
Lobulus paracentralis
A.paracentralis
Praecuneus
A. praecunealis
Fiss. parietoocc.
Lambda
Cuneus
55
70
50
60
Gyrus cinguli
30
35
R
Lobulus paracentralis
A. paracentralis
projection of medial surface
Protuberantia occ. ext.
Bregma
Fissura longitudinalis cerebri
Gyrus praecentralis
Gyrus postcentralis
Sutura coron.
Sulcus postcentralis
Sulcus praecentr.
Sulcus centralis
A. sulci centralis
Sutura coron. and Gyr. praecentralis converging
Pars opercul. gyri front. III = base of Gyr. praecentr.
lateral (left hemisph.)
Pars opercul. gyri front. III
Pars orbit. gyri front. III
Sutura sphenopariet.
Ala magna (lat. end)
Sut. coron.
Sut. squam.
Polus temp.
Ala parva (lat. end)
frontozyg. point
see fig. 85
25
35
lat. point of Fiss. orb. sup.
converging point of Sut. coron. and Gyr. praecentralis

Fig. 135. Parietal preparation; measurements in millimetres (mm).
Between the roof of the ventricle and the bottom of Fissura lat. (Sylvii) the white matter is only 15–20 mm wide and it contains Corona radiata. Complete hemiplegia and hemihypaesthesia may possibly result from slight lateral deviation in the midline approach (see 'Operative techniques – some aspects', Fig. 143). Note the relationships between gyri (+ arteries) and Ventriculus lat. in the posterior parietal region

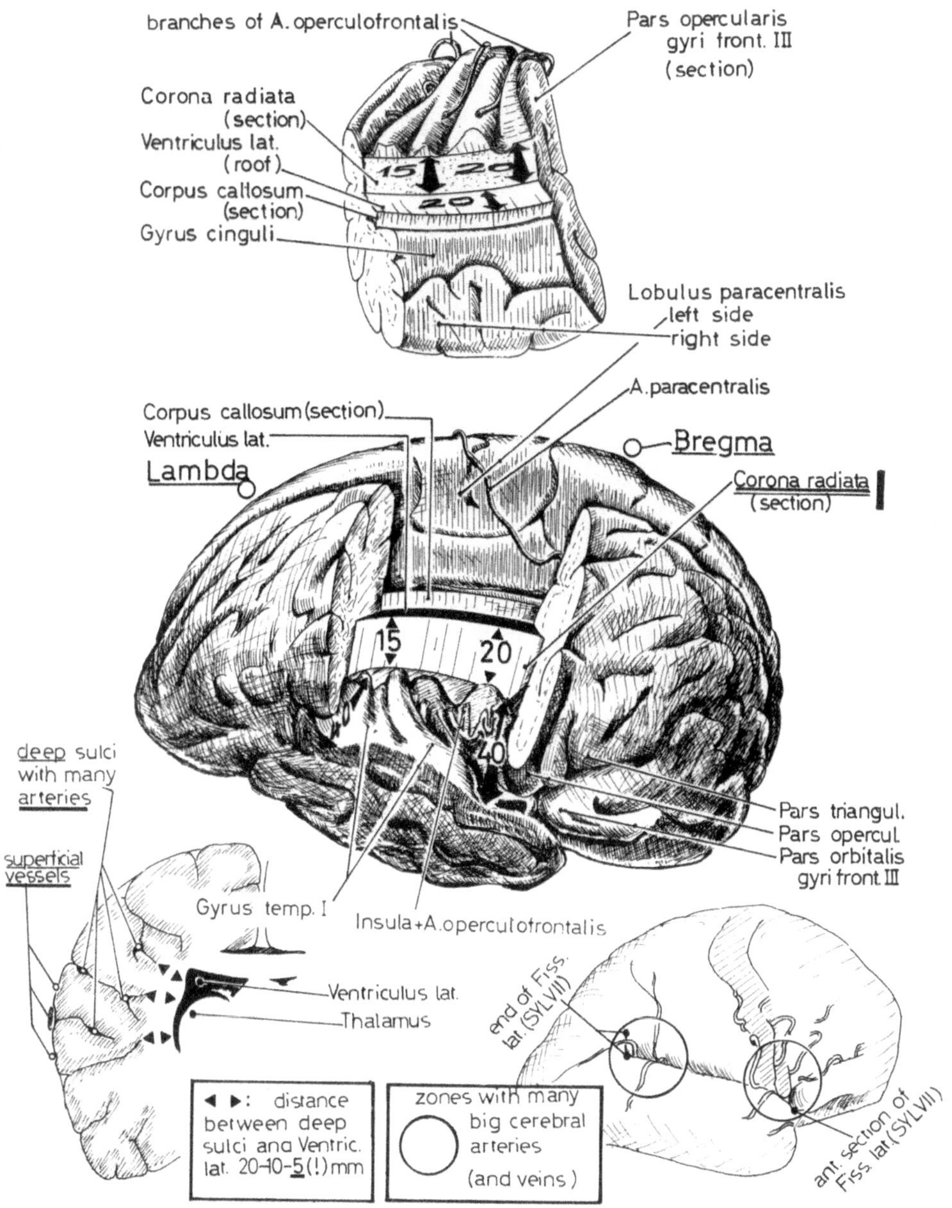
branches of A. operculofrontalis
Pars opercularis gyri front. III (section)
Corona radiata (section)
Ventriculus lat. (roof)
Corpus callosum (section)
Gyrus cinguli
15
20
20
Lobulus paracentralis
left side
right side
A. paracentralis
Corpus callosum (section)
Ventriculus lat.
Lambda
Bregma
Corona radiata (section)
15
20
40
Pars triangul.
Pars opercul.
Pars orbitalis gyri front. III
Gyrus temp. I
Insula+A. operculofrontalis
deep sulci with many arteries
superficial vessels
Ventriculus lat.
Thalamus
◄ ►: distance between deep sulci and Ventric. lat. 20-10-5(!) mm
zones with many big cerebral arteries (and veins)
end of Fiss. lat. (SYLVII)
ant. section of Fiss. lat. (SYLVII)

Fig. 136. Preparation of Fig. 135 from the medial view; even the small section of the lateral ventricle allows easy orientation by means of the landmarks (Stria terminalis, Plexus chorioideus, venous system). Fornix and Septum pellucidum are not sharply demarcated from each other

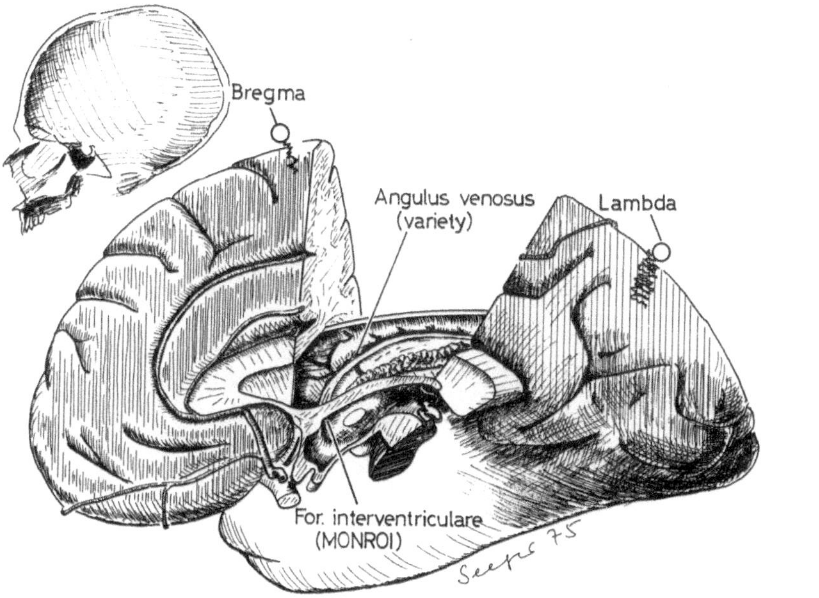
Bregma
Angulus venosus
(variety)
Lambda
For. interventriculare
(MONROI)
Seeger 75

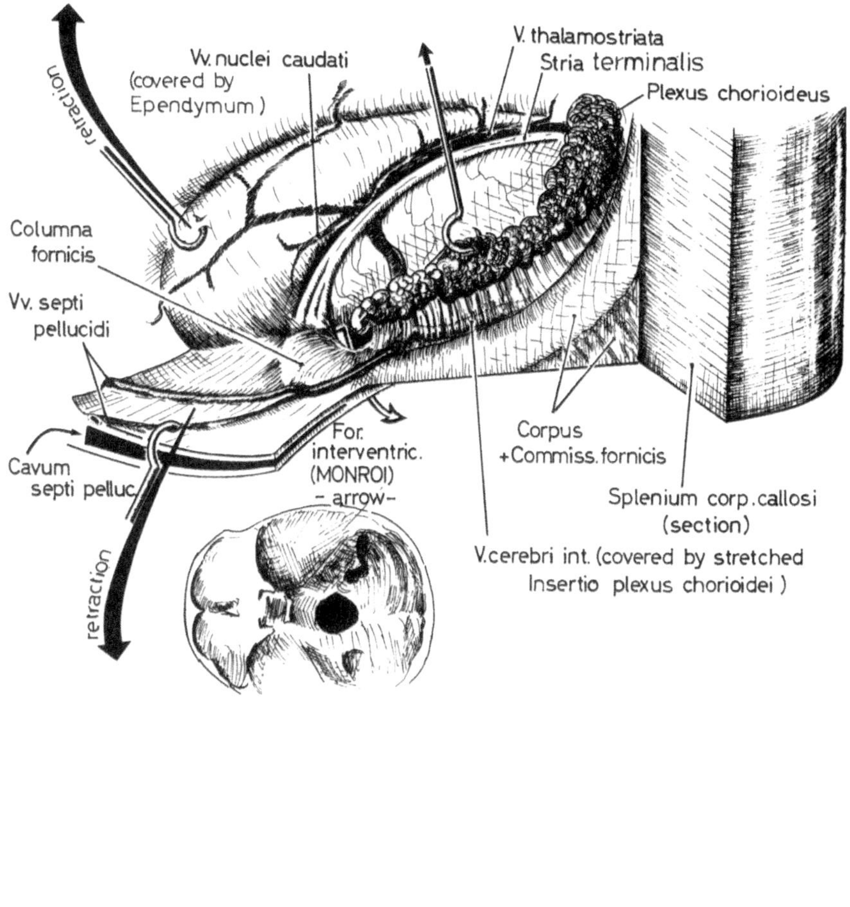
retraction
Vv. nuclei caudati
(covered by
Ependymum)
V. thalamostriata
Stria terminalis
Plexus chorioideus
Columna
fornicis
Vv. septi
pellucidi
Cavum
septi pelluc.
For.
interventric.
(MONROI)
- arrow -
Corpus
+Commiss. fornicis
Splenium corp. callosi
(section)
V. cerebri int. (covered by stretched
Insertio plexus chorioidei)
retraction

Fig. 137. Relationships between parietal lobe and surroundings. Notice the venous course to Sinus sagittalis sup. and its ill-defined lateral margins with transition into Lacunae, which can reach several centimetres laterally

FIG. 137

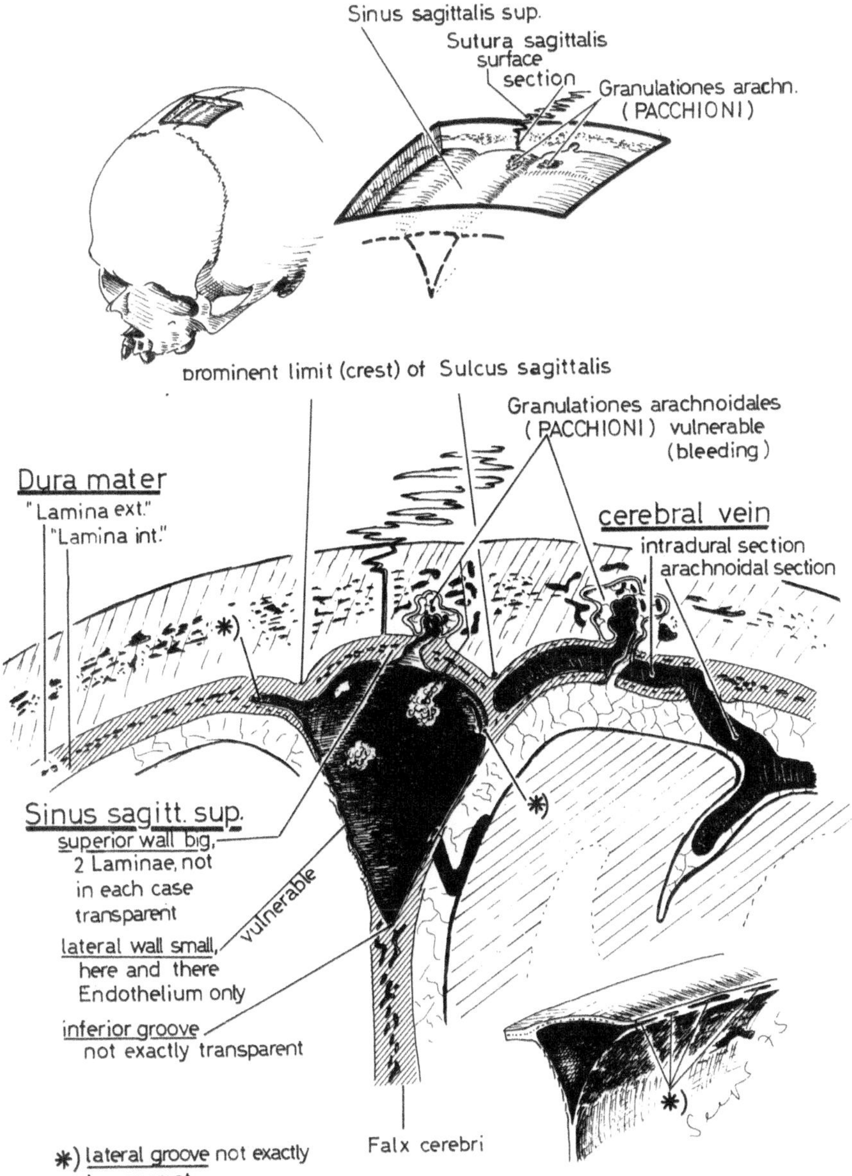

*) lateral groove not exactly transparent,
lateral extension of Sinus variable ⟶ Lacunae

Fig. 138. Example of a collapsed cerebral venous system. Well-known historical oblique view (veins drawn black on the copy). Mainly right-angled junctions of the cerebral veins with Sinus sagittalis sup.; situation unclear in high frontal region (arrow)

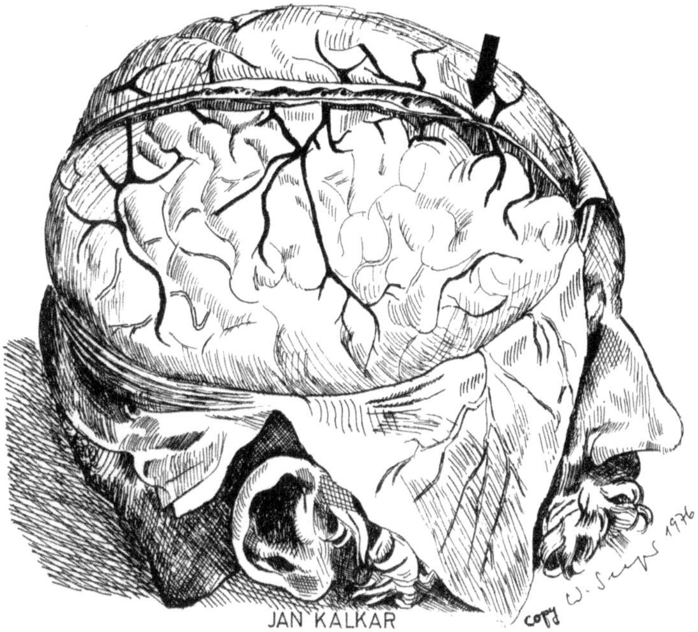

JAN KALKAR
ANDREAS VESALIVS (1543)

Fig. 139. Example of a tensely filled cerebral venous system
A Indian ink copy of an injection preparation by Stephens and Stilwell, 1969. Even with venous course against direction of flow of the sinus (see Fig. 138), junction is rectangular or in direction of flow. Single or multiple septa in Sinus sagittalis sup. are a frequent normal finding
B Junction of left cerebral veins with the right half of a divided sinus; pronounced lateral outcurving of the left part of the sinus (variety, compare also Fig. 138)
C In the vicinity of Lacuna parietalis pronounced branching and lateral widening of the sinus on both sides, instead of a single central lumen

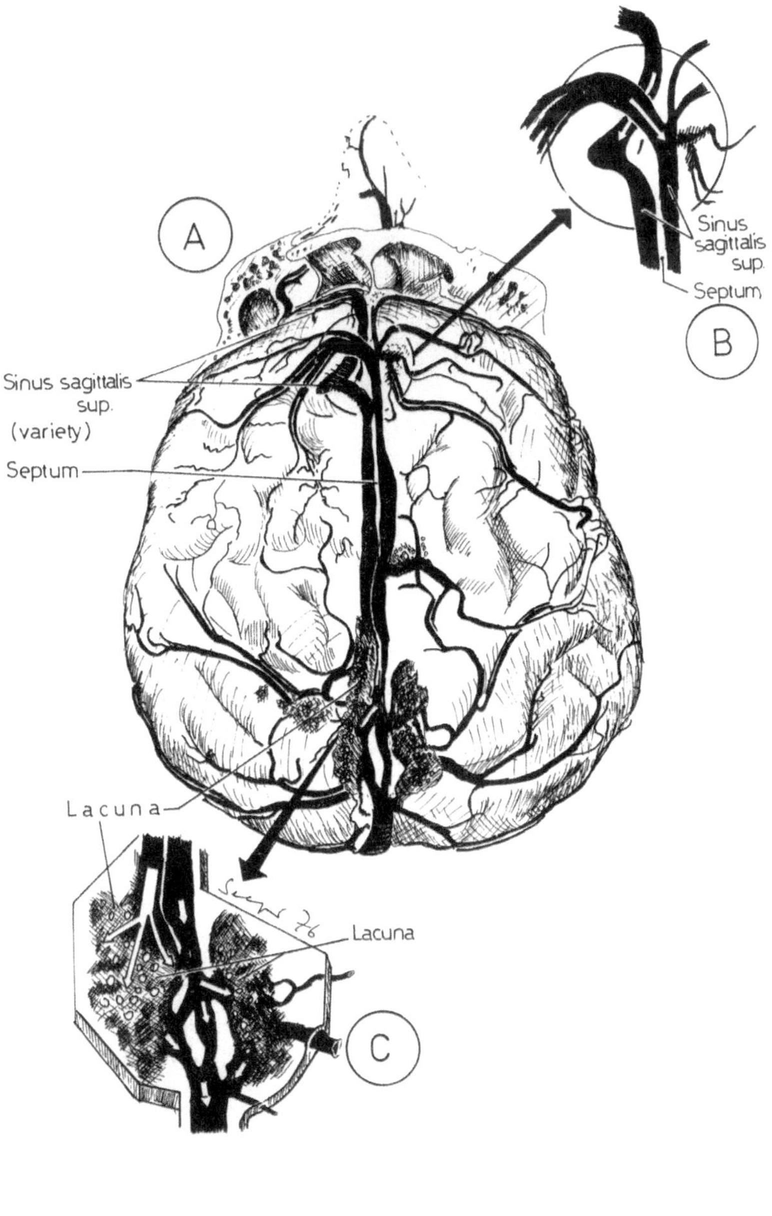
A
Sinus sagittalis
sup.
(variety)
Septum
Sinus
sagittalis
sup.
Septum
B
Lacuna
Lacuna
C

Fig. 140. Preoperative radiological details. Correction of tilting of roentgenogram (*A*, left) and of a lateral projection not exactly corresponding to a-p (*A*, right). Apart from the orbital roof and the petrous bone, Lambda and Bregma are – if recognizable – particularly useful for exact orientation
Projection of deep-seated processes onto the external surface of the skull (shortest distance) *B* and *C*. Notice projective foreshortening at *c*

FIG. 140

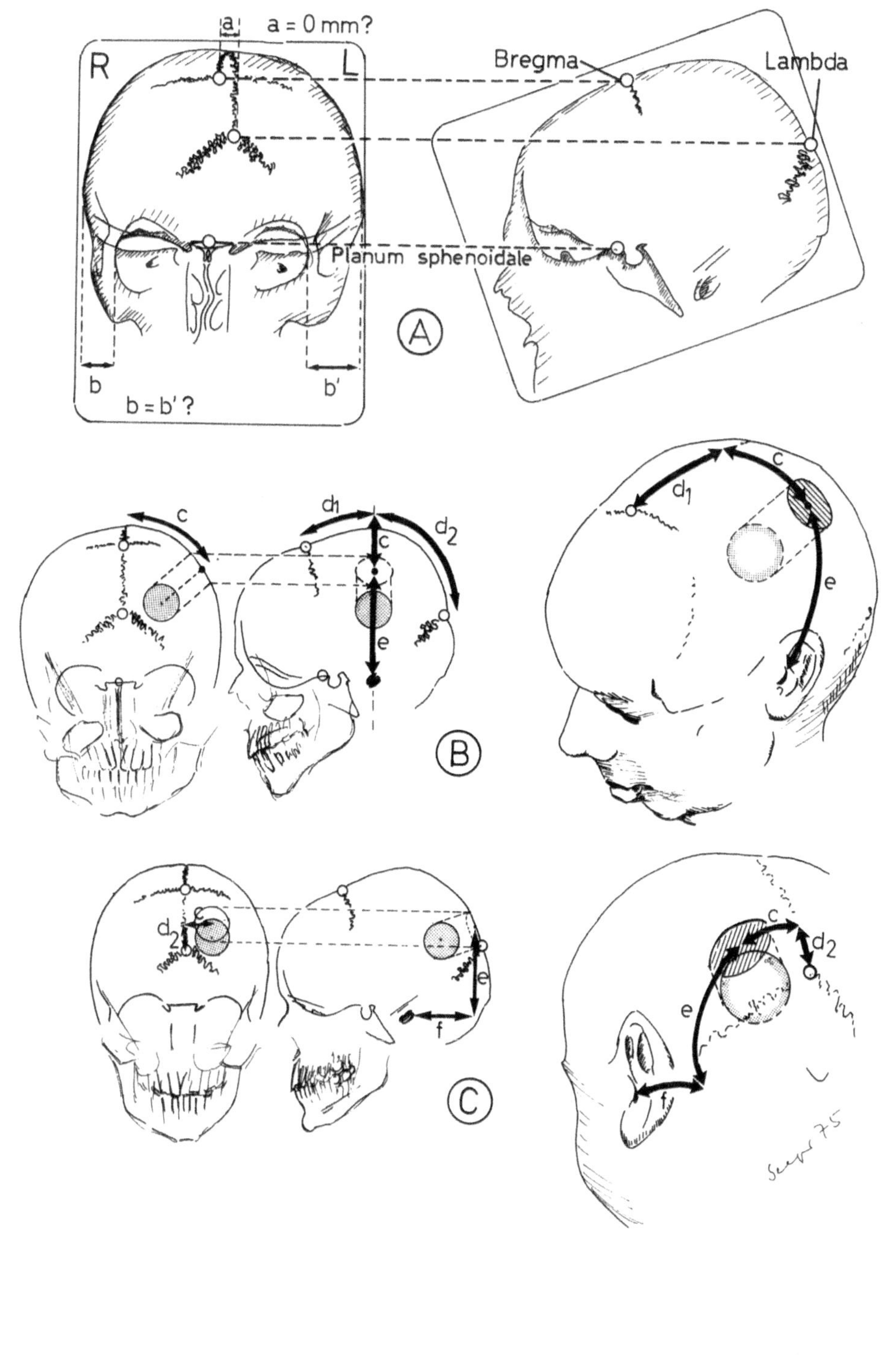
a
a = 0 mm?
R
L
Bregma
Lambda
Planum sphenoidale
b
b'
b = b' ?
A
c
d_1
d_2
e
B
f
C

Fig. 141
A The sinus and example of a cerebral vein. The last stretch (*a–b*) before the junction with Sinus sagitt. sup. is projected onto the sinus in the lateral projection and is not recognizable
B Frontal view of *A*
C View from above
D In the oblique projection, recognizable final stretch of vein before junction. Lacuna parietalis is also more easily recognizable than in lateral projection (*A*)

FIG. 141

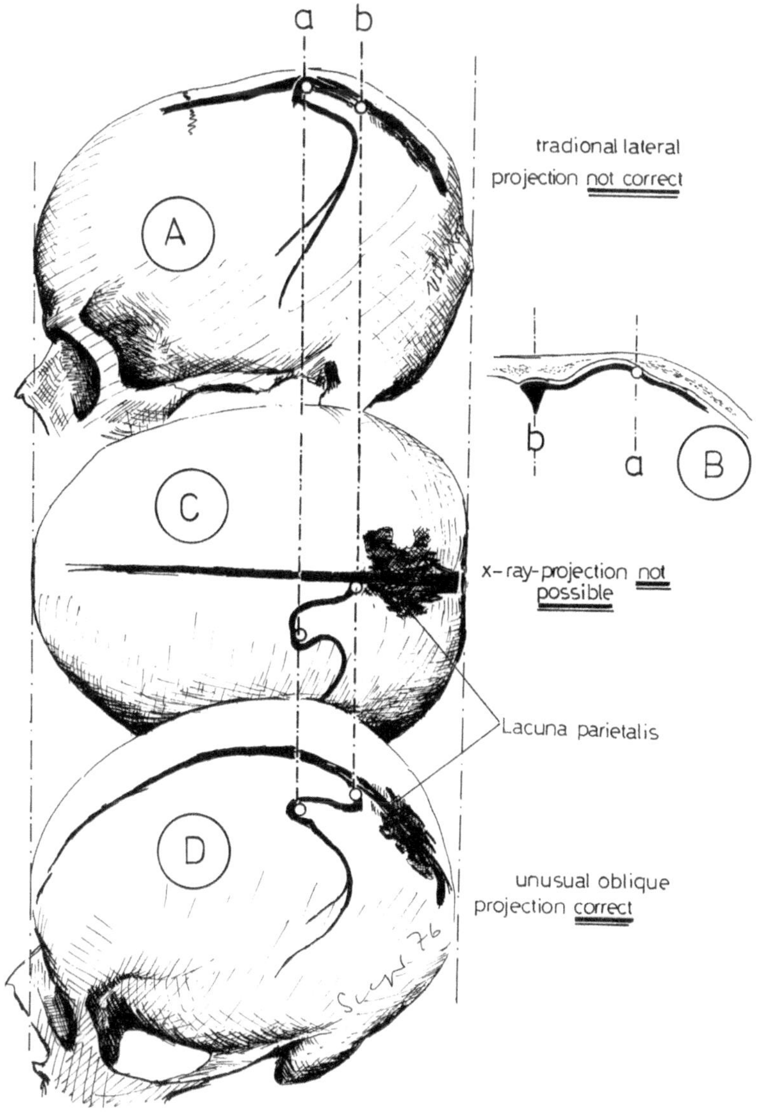
a
b
A
tradional lateral
projection not correct
b
a
B
C
x-ray-projection not possible
Lacuna parietalis
D
unusual oblique
projection correct

Fig. 142. Practical use in a successfully operated AV malformation of Corpus callosum. Only in the oblique projection is the possible approach (large arrow) recognizable

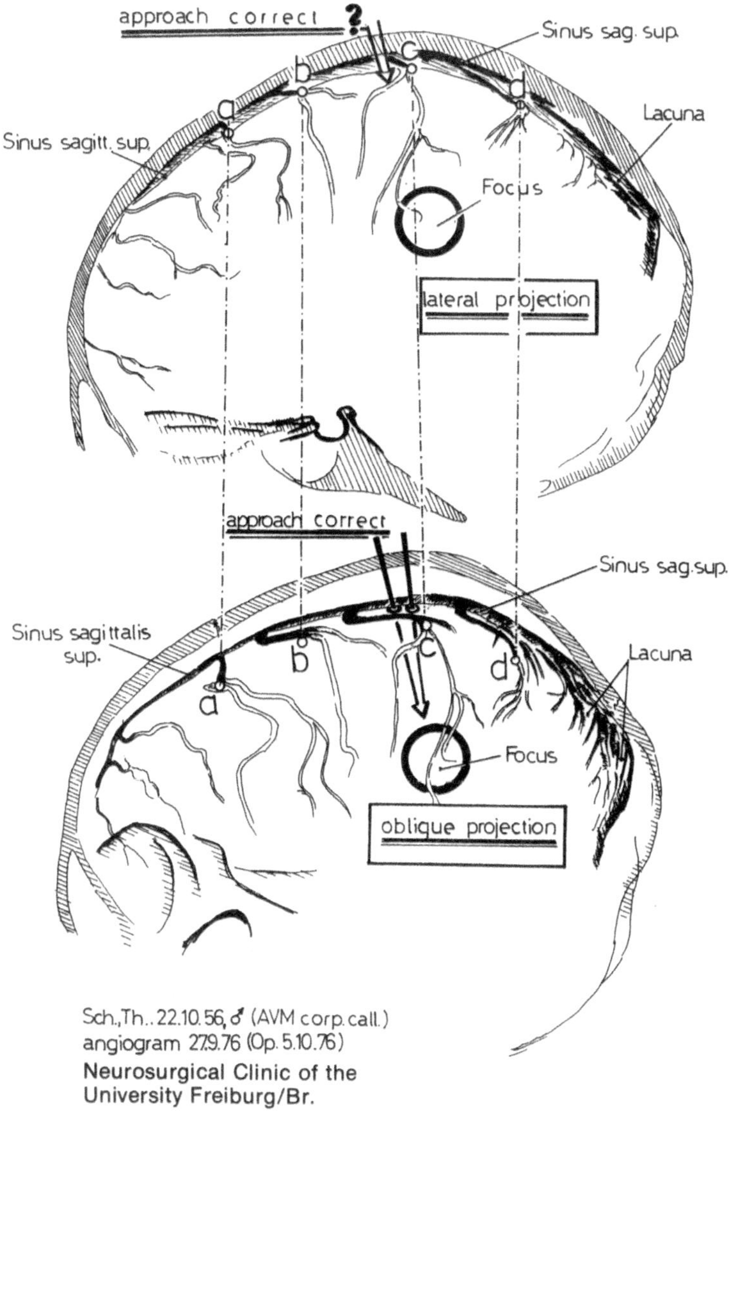

Sch.,Th.. 22.10.56, ♂ (AVM corp. call.)
angiogram 27.9.76 (Op. 5.10.76)
Neurosurgical Clinic of the
University Freiburg/Br.

Fig. 143. Projection of a deep-seated parietal process into the projection fields (*A* above) and frontally in front of the projection fields (*A* below). Measurement of the distance from important arteries of Fissura longitudinalis in various stretches of their course (*B*)

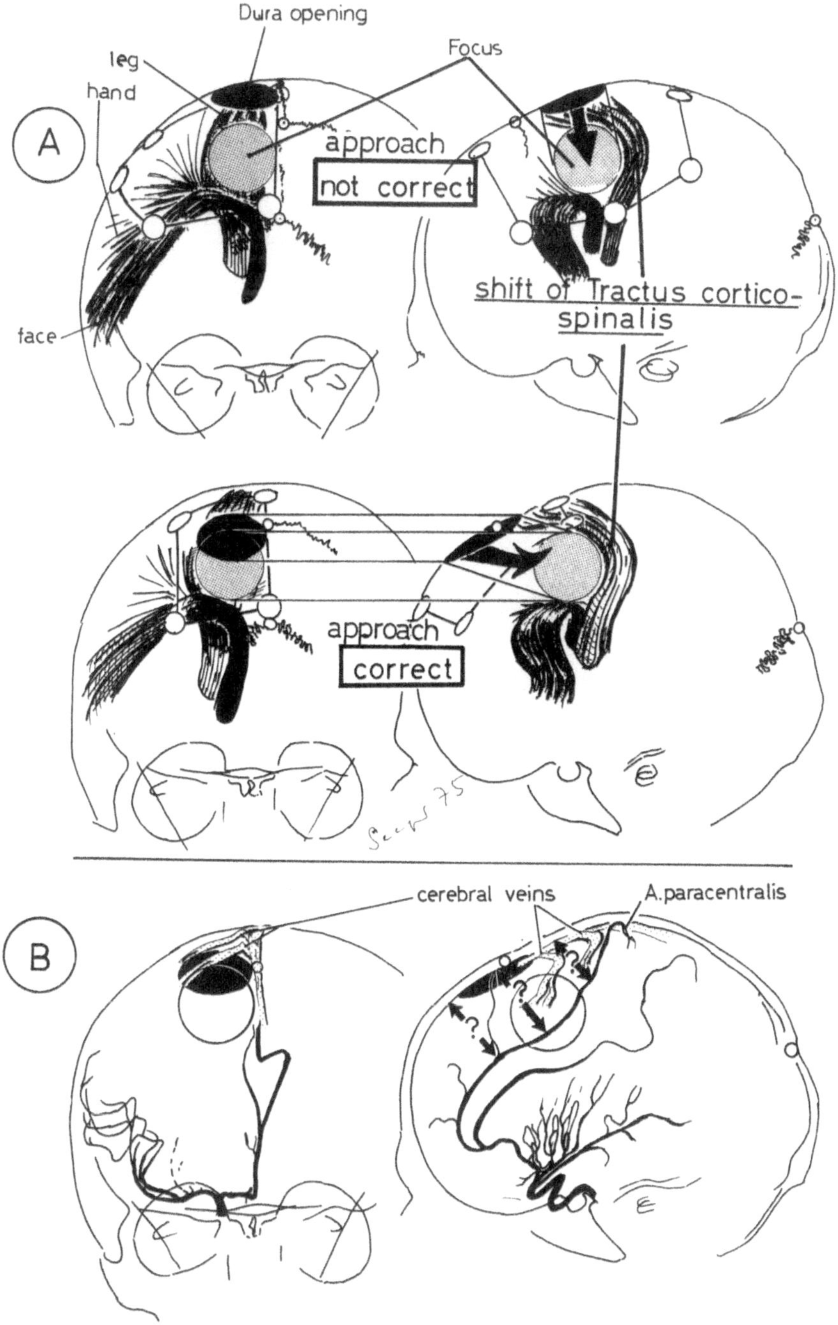
Dura opening
leg
hand
Focus
A
approach
not correct
shift of Tractus cortico-
spinalis
face
approach
correct
B
cerebral veins
A.paracentralis

Fig. 144. Parietooccipital projection of deep-seated parietal processes with bypassing of the motor and sensory fields *A*. Positional relationships of arteries of Fissura longitudinalis to the process (white) and in view *A* determined operative field (black). The projection field (operative approach) was chosen in a region that is free of larger connecting veins
Below: Schematic section *S*: the lower border of the process can be projected onto Sinus rectus, V. cerebri magna (Galeni), and Splenium, which lie medially higher than the parietooccipital white matter

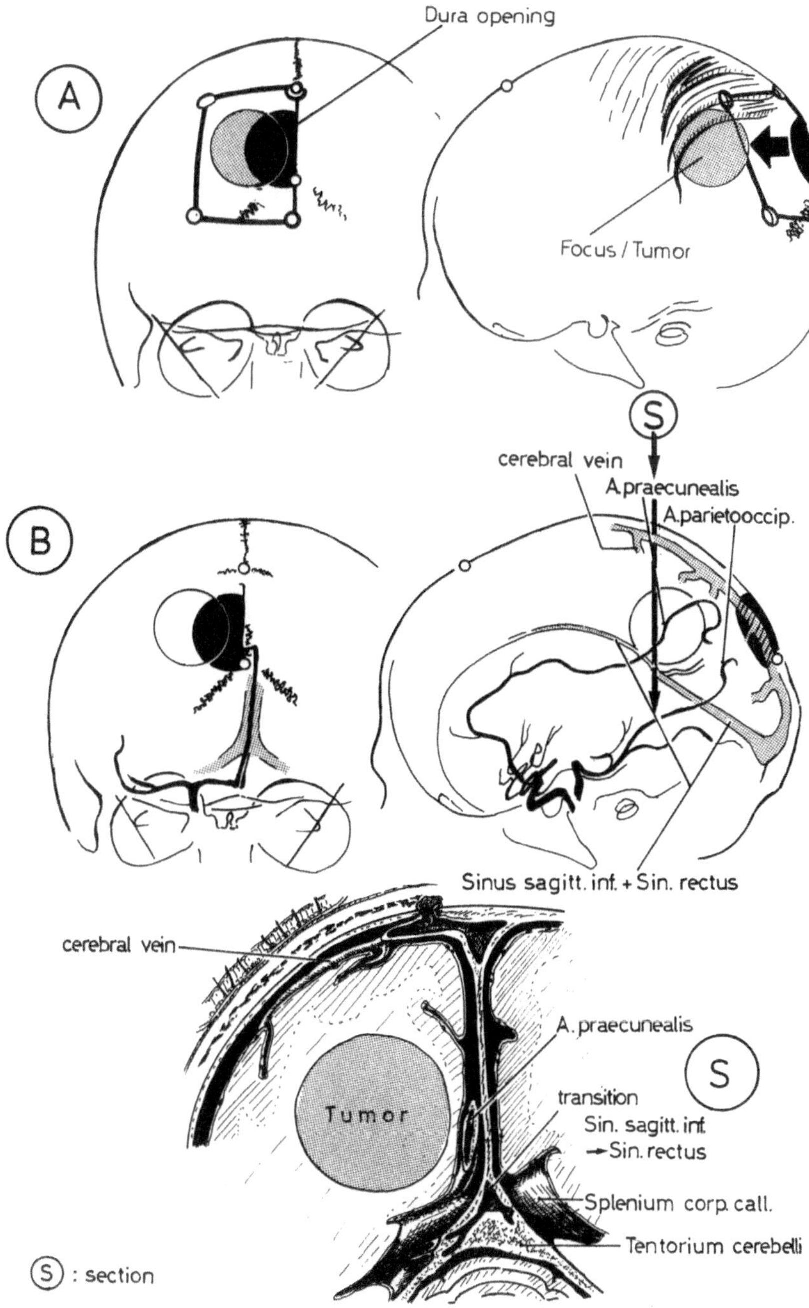
Dura opening
A
Focus / Tumor
S
cerebral vein
A.praecunealis
A.parietooccip.
B
Sinus sagitt. inf. + Sin. rectus
cerebral vein
A. praecunealis
S
transition
Sin. sagitt. inf.
→Sin. rectus
Tumor
Splenium corp. call.
Tentorium cerebelli
S : section

Fig. 145. Variable possibilities for skin incision with and without injury to R. temp. n. facialis

FIG. 145

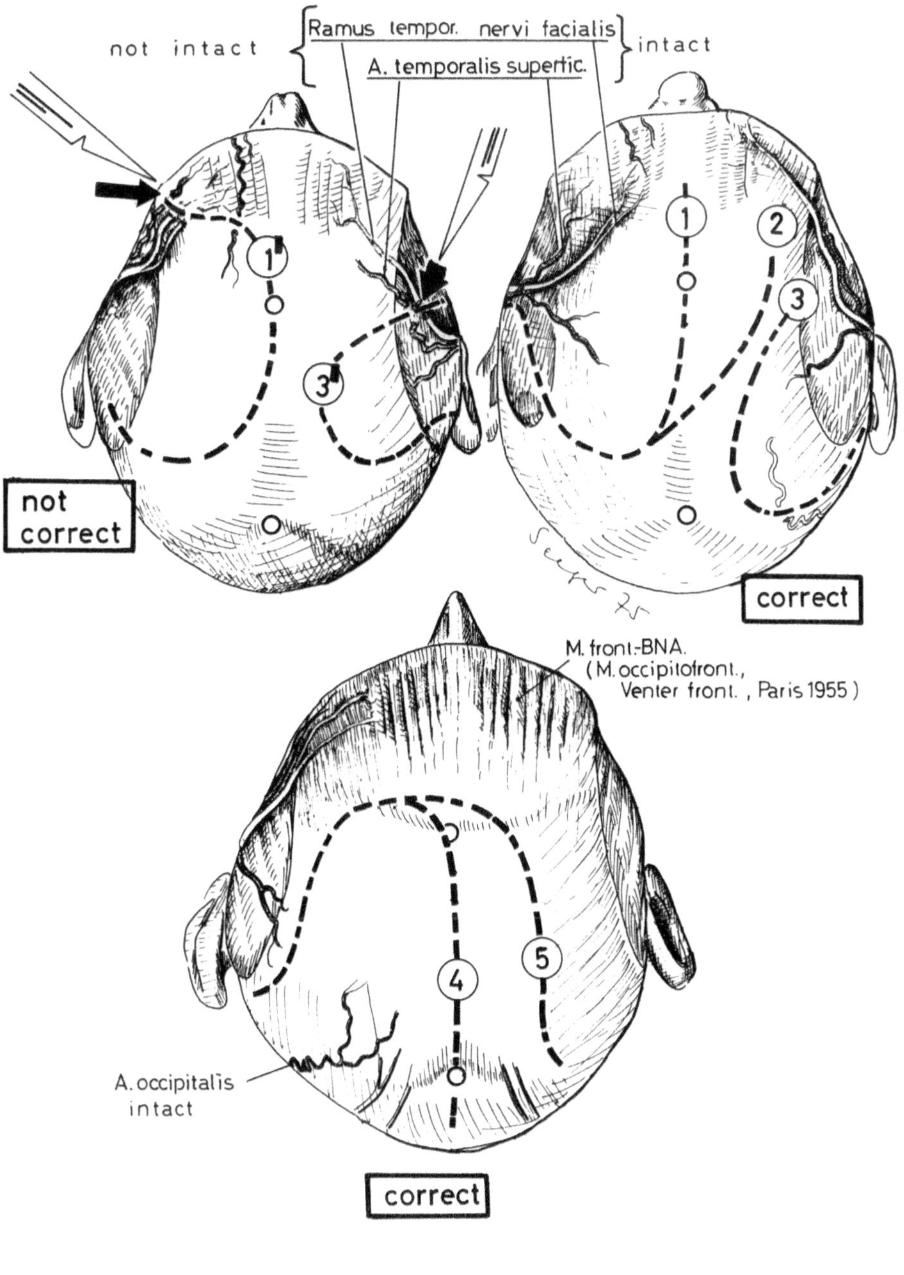
not intact
Ramus tempor. nervi facialis
A. temporalis superfic.
intact
1
3
2
not correct
correct
M. front.-BNA.
(M. occipitofront.,
Venter front., Paris 1955)
4
5
A. occipitalis
intact
correct

Fig. 146. Approach to processes near the midline

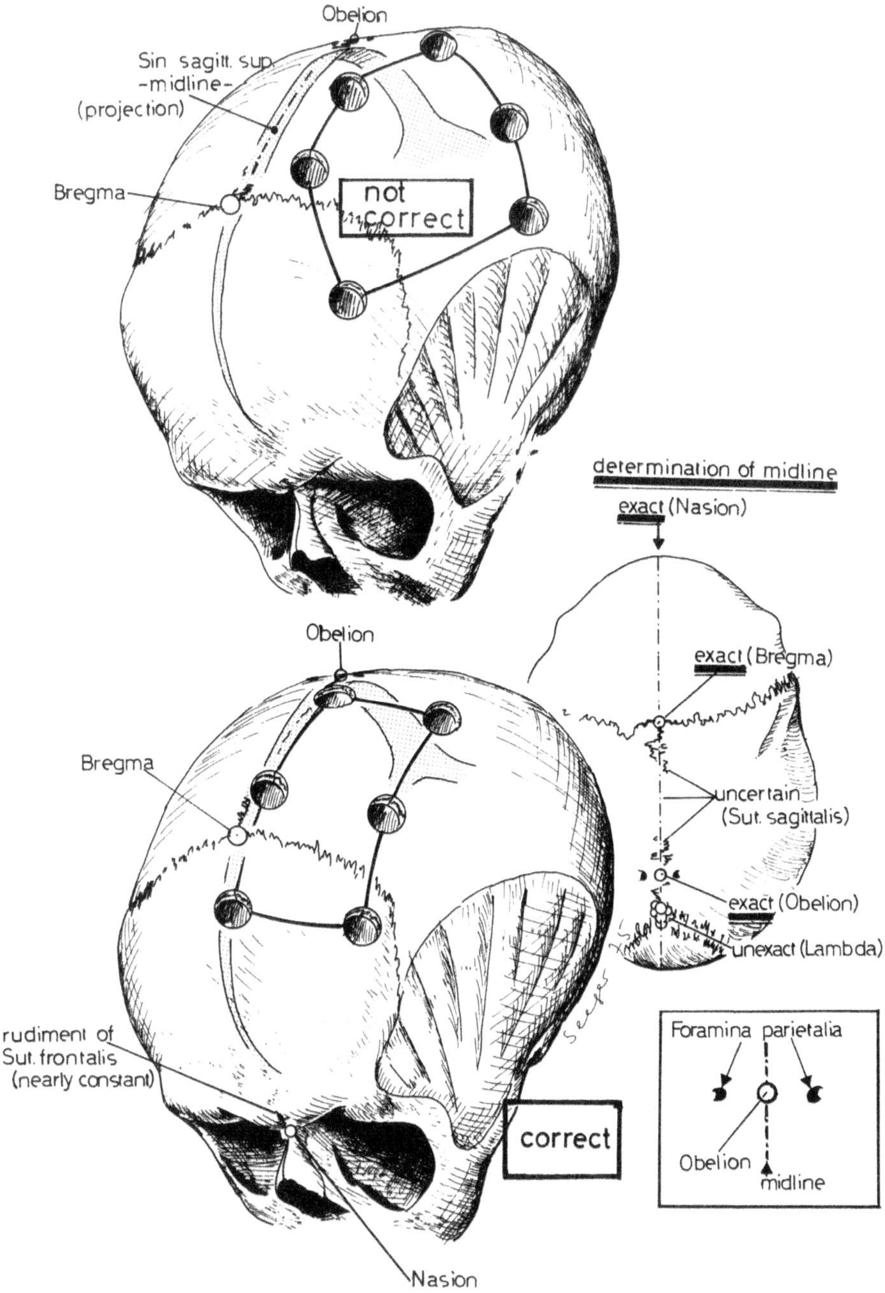
Obelion
Sin. sagitt. sup.
-midline-
(projection)
Bregma
not correct
determination of midline
exact (Nasion)
exact (Bregma)
uncertain (Sut. sagittalis)
exact (Obelion)
unexact (Lambda)
Obelion
Bregma
rudiment of Sut. frontalis (nearly constant)
correct
Nasion
Foramina parietalia
Obelion
midline

Fig. 147. Trepanation for bilateral midline processes. Displacement syndrome, position of the arteries and veins can be measured on the angiogram. Points of reference – Bregma and Lambda (see also Fig. 148)

FIG. 147

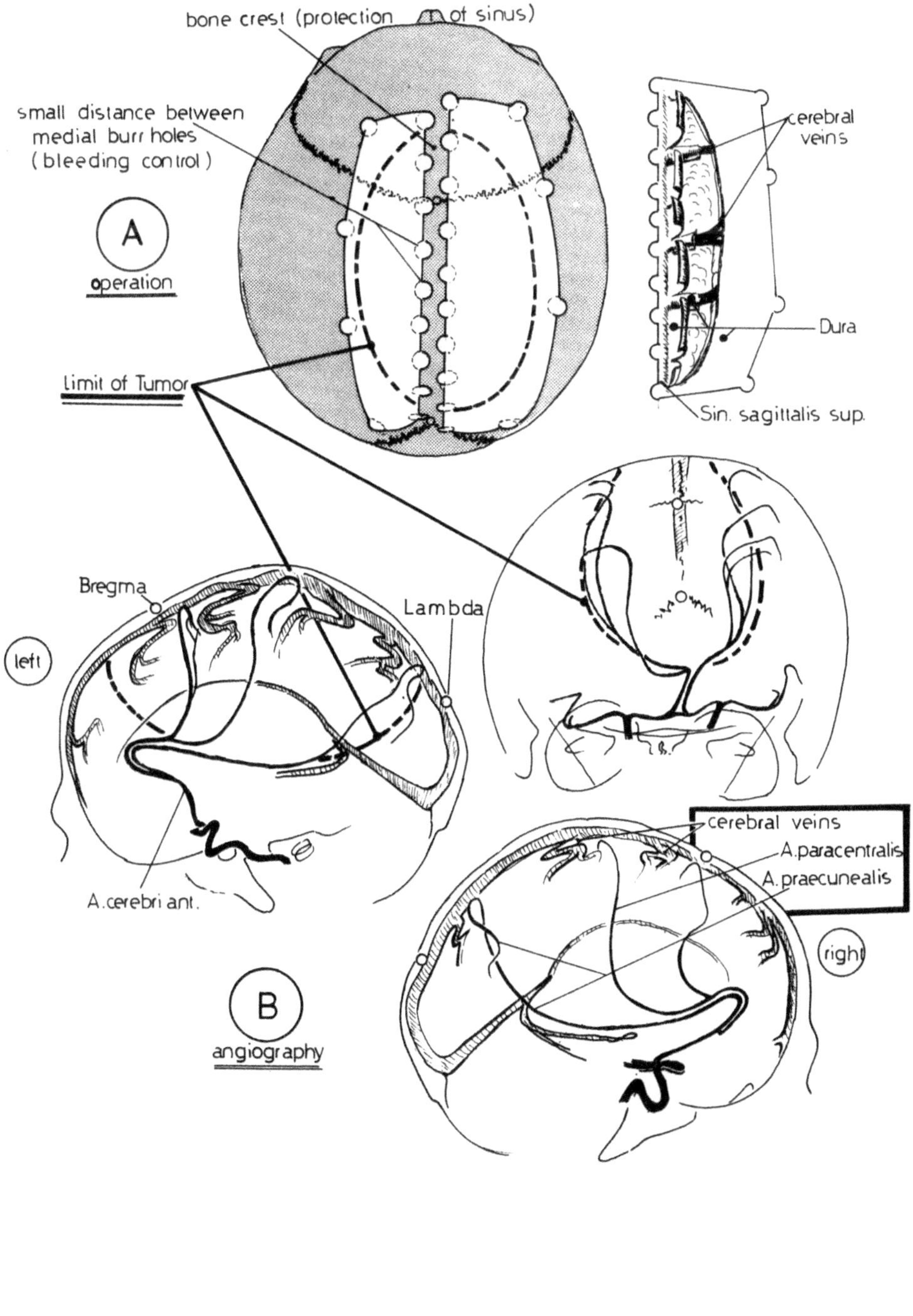
bone crest (protection of sinus)
small distance between medial burr holes (bleeding control)
A
operation
limit of Tumor
cerebral veins
Dura
Sin. sagittalis sup.
Bregma
Lambda
left
A.cerebri ant.
cerebral veins
A.paracentralis
A.praecunealis
right
B
angiography

Fig. 148. Measurements taken for bilateral midline processes: distance from lower border of the falx (Sinus sagittalis inf. distance *b1*), position of Corpus callosum (A. pericallosa, distance *b2*, or *b1* + *b2*)
A right: Partial occlusion of Sinus sagittalis inf.
B Interposition of Gyrus cinguli between tumour and Corpus callosum with site of tumour initially superficial
C Direct contact of primarily deep-seated tumour to A. pericallosa and Corpus callosum

FIG. 148

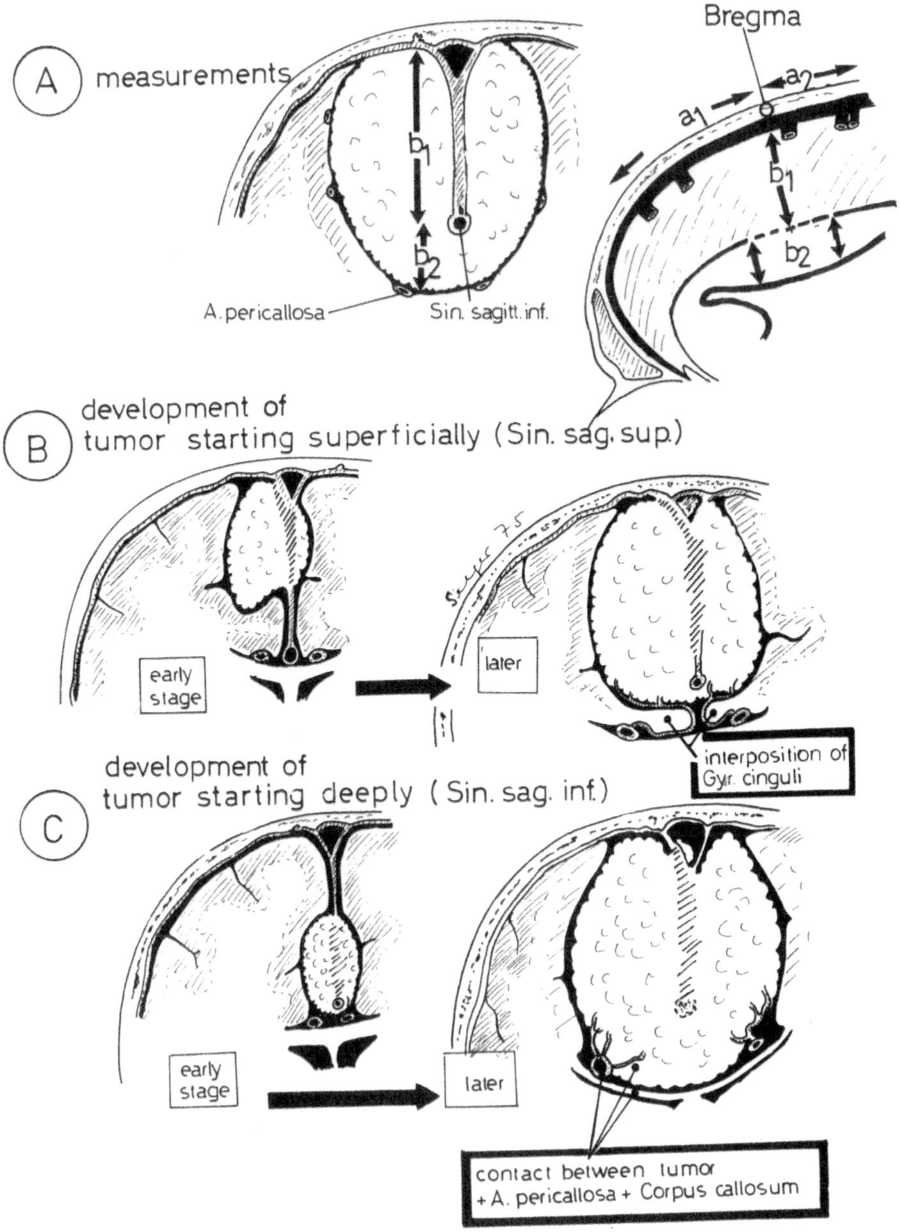
A
measurements
Bregma
a1
a2
b1
b2
A. pericallosa
Sin. sagitt. inf.
development of
B
tumor starting superficially (Sin. sag. sup.)
early stage
later
interposition of Gyr. cinguli
development of
tumor starting deeply (Sin. sag. inf.)
C
early stage
later
contact between tumor + A. pericallosa + Corpus callosum

Fig. 149. See Fig. 150

FIG. 149

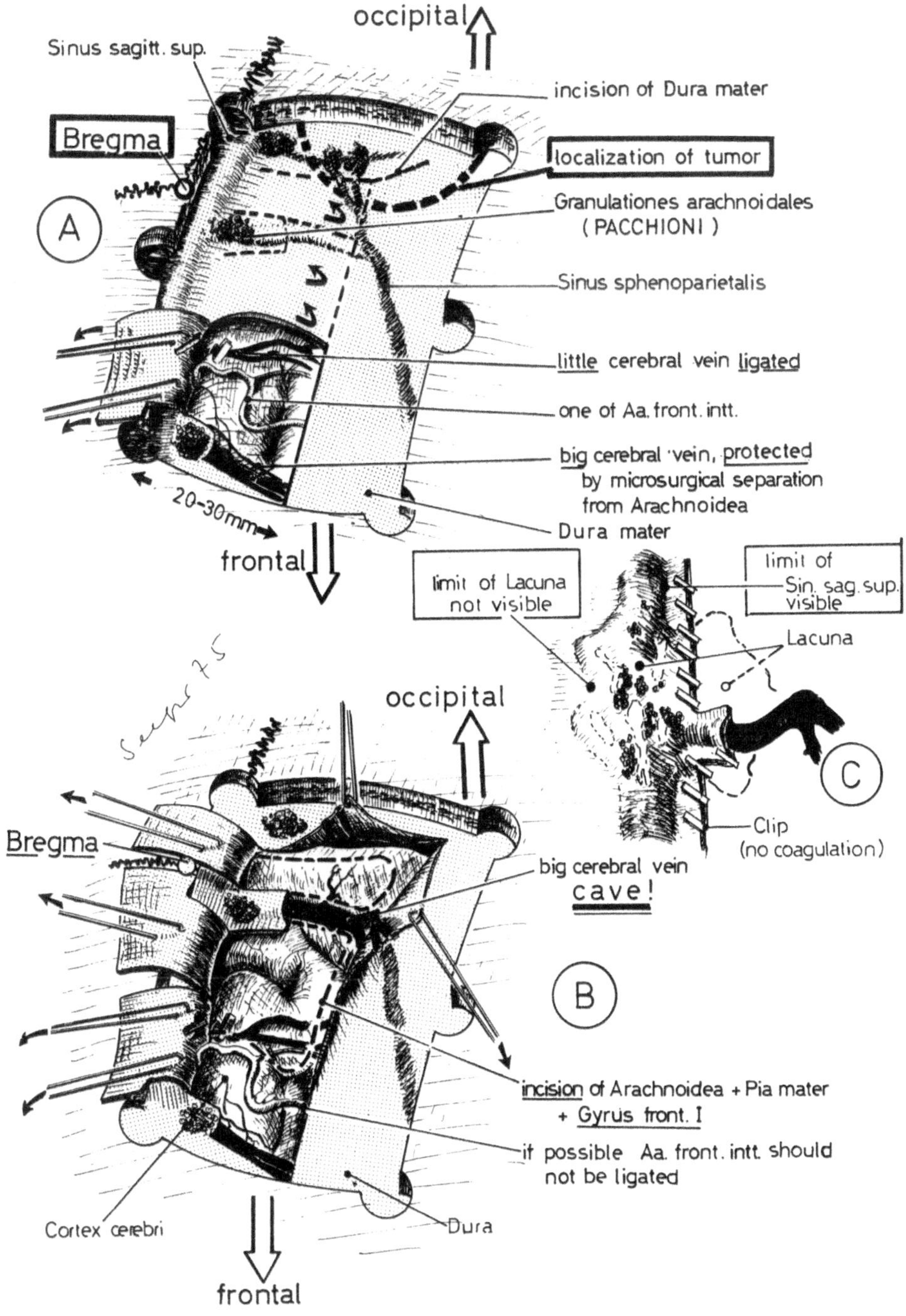

occipital
Sinus sagitt. sup.
incision of Dura mater
Bregma
localization of tumor
A
Granulationes arachnoidales (PACCHIONI)
Sinus sphenoparietalis
little cerebral vein ligated
one of Aa. front. intt.
big cerebral vein, protected by microsurgical separation from Arachnoidea
20-30mm
Dura mater
frontal
limit of Lacuna not visible
limit of Sin. sag. sup. visible
Lacuna
C
Clip (no coagulation)
occipital
Bregma
big cerebral vein cave!
B
incision of Arachnoidea + Pia mater + Gyrus front. I
if possible Aa. front. intt. should not be ligated
Cortex cerebri
Dura
frontal

Fig. 150. Approach to structures near the midline with conservation of important vessels. Subpial approach for protection of the arteries (*C*). Diminution of tumour viewed from frontal direction (*D*)
Below right: Direction of viewing at the surface of the skull and brain in Figs. 149 and 150

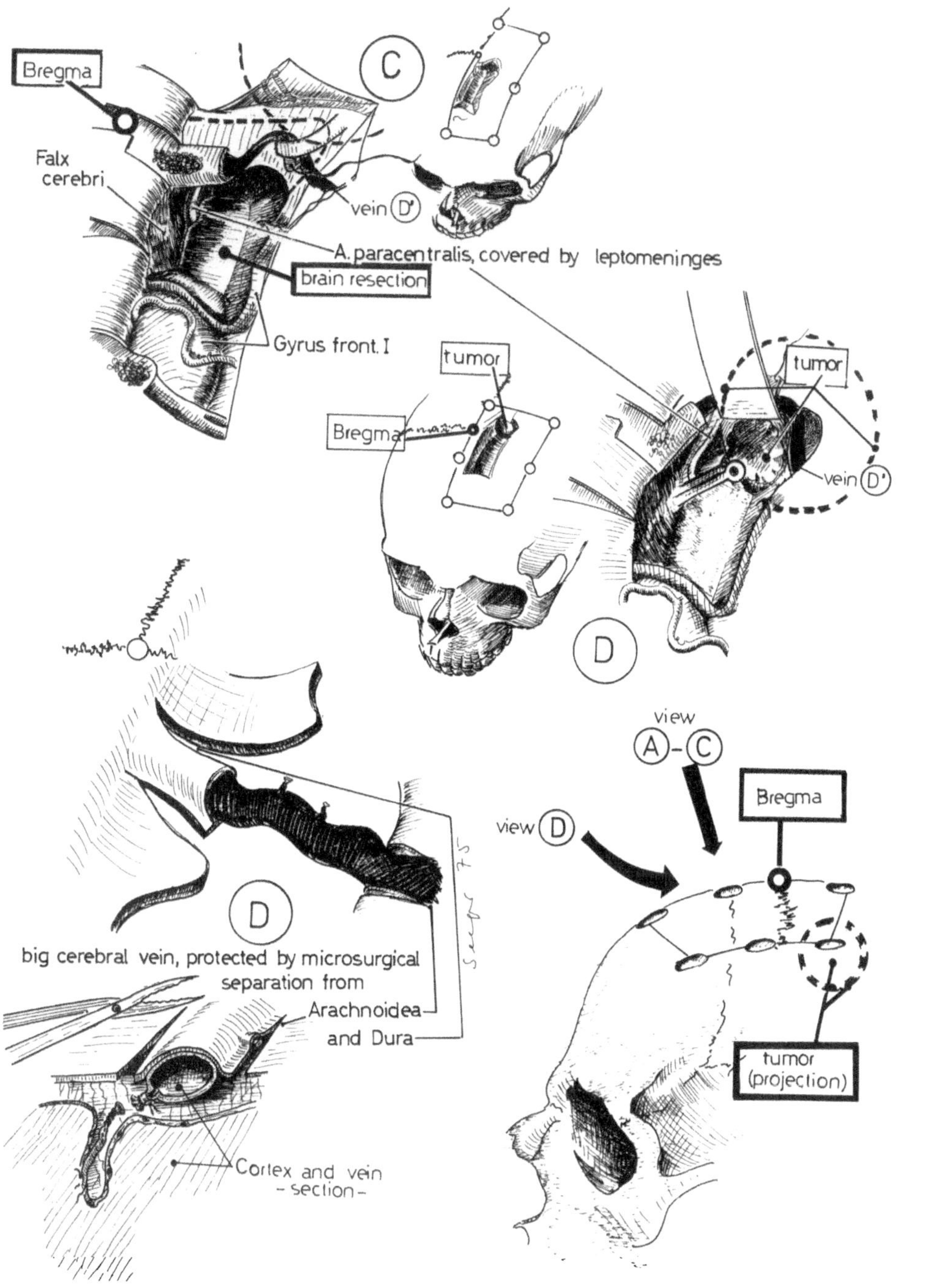

Bregma
C
Falx cerebri
vein D'
A. paracentralis, covered by leptomeninges
brain resection
Gyrus front. I
tumor
Bregma
tumor
vein D'
D
view
A - C
Bregma
view D
D
big cerebral vein, protected by microsurgical separation from
Arachnoidea
and Dura
tumor (projection)
Cortex and vein - section -

Fig. 151. Danger of injury to vessels due to trepanation performed too far laterally *A*, and trepanation reaching too far medially *B*

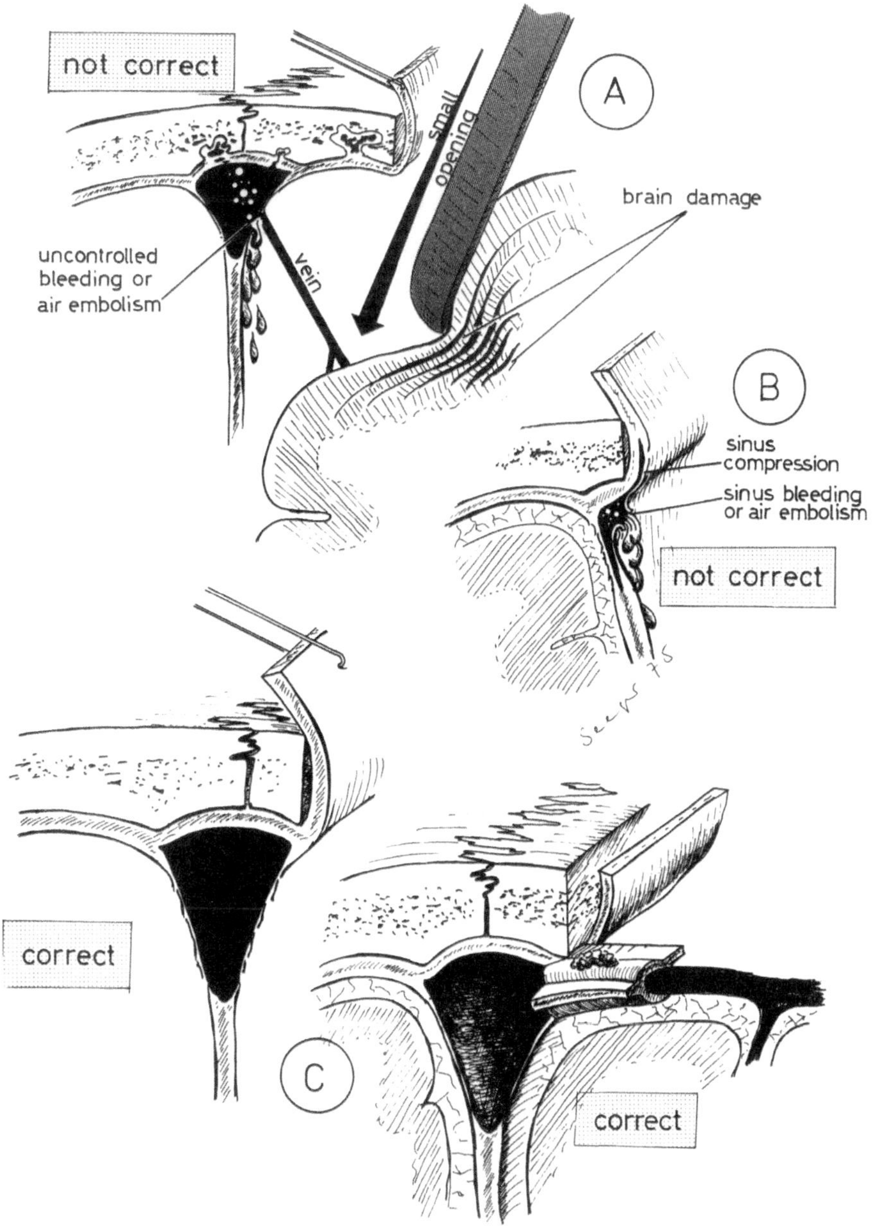
not correct
A
small opening
brain damage
uncontrolled bleeding or air embolism
vein
B
sinus compression
sinus bleeding or air embolism
not correct
correct
C
correct

Fig. 152 and 153. Avoidance of venous thrombosis in Sinus sagittalis sup.

Fig. 152

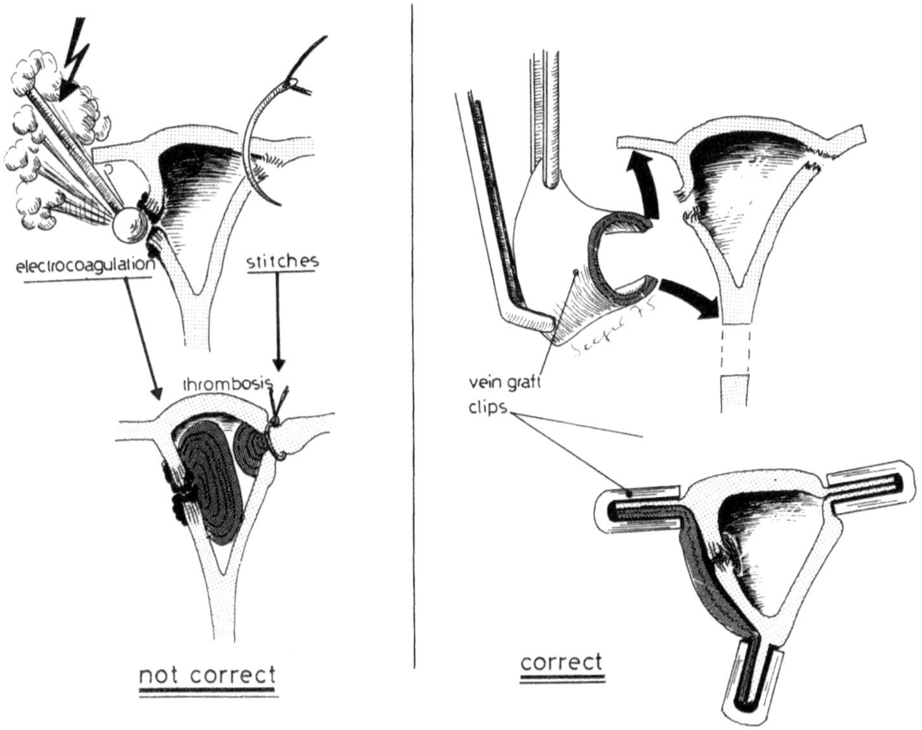
electrocoagulation
stitches
thrombosis
not correct
vein graft
clips
correct

FIG. 153

Fig. 153

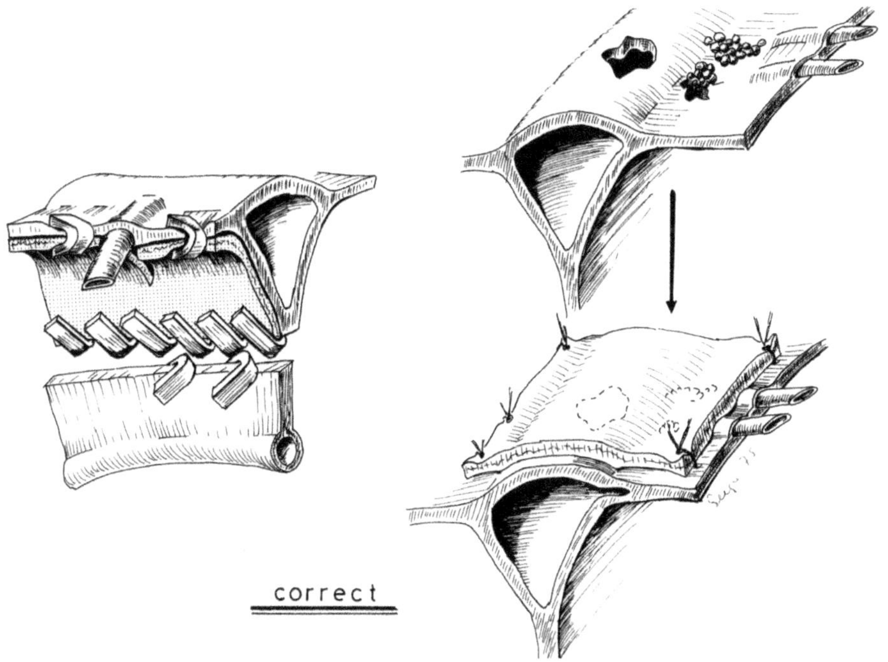

correct

Chapter 5
Occipital Region and Lamina quadrigemina

A. Surface of Occipital Lobe

The shape of the occipital lobe cannot be outlined from the surface of the skull. Its irregularities are compensated for by bony irregularities, so that between Lambda and Protuberantia occipitalis ext. – distance approx. 70 mm (Figs. 154 and 155) – there is fairly even external vaulting of the bone. Below this the dural relief shows the tapering bulge of the occipital pole. Over it the bone is considerably thinned out. In the midline in the vicinity of Protuberantia occipitalis ext. and int. the bone is particulary strongly developed. Asymmetries of both occipital poles and corresponding deviation of Sinus sagittalis sup. are typical asymmetries of this cerebral region. Vermis cerebelli is usually displaced contralaterally to the displacement of the occipital poles, with corresponding asymmetries of the falx, tentorium, and the large blood vessels (Fig. 156). The pole encroaches in a hooked shape into a hollow in the posterior tentorial region, and is convex on its undersurface, whereas the anterior portions of the occipital lobe base rise concavely in a forward and medial direction, corresponding to the shape of Tentorium and the slightly convex form of the underlying Lobulus quadrangularis of Cerebellum. The lateral surface shows generally an almost even curvature. The transition between the level medial surface and the base occurs gradually (Fig. 156). Fissura calcarina begins medially in the central polar region and lies in the transitional curvature between medial plane and base, rising forward. Despite all variations there is always a sharp bend forward and basally at its meeting with Sulcus cinguli. It may completely divide Isthmus gyri cinguli and end in Cisterna ambiens (in the example of Fig. 155).

As is well known, the visual pathway ends in the occipital Cortex (Area striata, Fig. 157) and reaches from the posterior border of Gyrus parahippocampalis to the superior precuneus region (see also Chapter 6).

Surface Arteries:
The border area of A. cerebri ant. (A. praecunealis) and post. (A. parietooccipitalis) may vary considerably in its position in the anterior or posterior precuneus or cuneus region (Ring, 1969). The deeply indented Fissura calcarina which pushes Calcar avis forward into the lumen of the posterior horn and forms the medial surface of the (in cross-section, triangular) posterior horn (see Fig. 156) often reveals deep loops of A. calcarina, which may lie near the ventricular system (see Chapter 1, Fig. 22). Usually it lies more superficially than is shown in Fig. 156.
A. angularis originating from A. cerebri media (see Chapter 1) supplies occipital pole from a lateral direction.

Surface Veins:
Drainage takes place mainly into the superior sagittal sinus occasionally over veins of large calibre which may also serve extensive areas of the neighbouring parietal and temporooccipital cortex. Veins between the under surface of the occipital lobe and tentorium require particularly careful preparation. At Sinus transversus the venous drainage between confluens sinuum and the entry point of V. Labbé to Sinus transversus is rarely a factor of importance so that the basal approach here is not hindered. Not until the medial occipital veins may there be hindrance to the further approach to Splenium corporis callosi, V. cerebri magna (Galeni), and Cisterna ambiens. The exit of the medial occipital veins from Fissura collateralis can be seen in Fig. 158. They may form connections anteriorly with V. basalis (Rosenthal), V. cerebri magna (Galeni) or to Lacunae of Tentorium, or the connections may be completely absent. Almost the whole tentorium is permeated by venous lacunae which form branching arborescent connections with the neighbouring sinus. The particularly well-developed connection to Sinus rectus, which in 15% of cases is bi- or tripar-

tite, have recently been investigated (Browder et al., 1976).

B. Deep Brain Structures

Fissura longitudinalis and "surface" of Tentorium: The width of the falx in the occipital region corresponds to the distance between the occipital pole and Splenium corporis callosi, since at most a few millimetres' space exist between the posterior end of Corpus callosum and the junction of Falx and Tentorium at the entry point of V. cerebri magna (Galeni) into Sinus transversus (Fig. 154). Although the width of the falx in the frontal region is very variable, occipitally it varies little in accordance with its close relationship to Corpus callosum and the vessels in its vicinity. The distance of Splenium from the occipital pole measures approx. 60 mm. Laterally in this frontal plane of Splenium the Cella media is reached; after a depth of 60 mm, Pulvinar thalami lying somewhat in front of the plane of Splenium may be reached (Fig. 154 *B*). When puncturing from a dorsolateral direction at the level of Lambda the Corpus callosum is to be expected at a depth of 50 mm (Fig. 155, above). The border between the surfaces of Falx and Tentorium is so ill-defined that only the discoloration due to Sinus rectus enables it to be recognized from the dorsolateral view (Fig. 155). The border to the upper edge of the petrous bone can be identified at anatomical preparation or operation by its hard consistency. The upper edge of the petrous bone is marked by Sinus petrosus sup. Since the dura is not always transparent and the calibre of Sinus petrosus is liable to vary in size, the upper edge of the petrous bone must occasionally be localized by instrumental palpation (tentorium soft, surface of petrous bone hard; see Fig. 155). In Fig. 155 the width of the falx is given as 60 mm – i.e., narrower than the distance laterally between the edge of Tentorium and the protrusion of Dura and Squama occipitalis caused by the occipital pole. This corresponds to the projection of Protuberantia occipitalis int. or the two ridges of Sulcus longitudinalis sup. into the interior of the skull, whereas the occipital pole bulges backwards.

Border area between Cisterna ambiens and ventricular atrium:

Whereas in Fig. 154 the posterior horn was reached at a depth of 45 mm, the plane of incision in Fig. 158 lies immediately in front of Pulvinar thalami at 65 mm. A thin slice of Hippocampus is still connected medially with Splenium radiation and laterobasally with Isthmus gyri cinguli. At *B* a triangle can be seen representing the posterior horn section. Despite the large-surfaced slice of Gyrus parahippocampalis, the Pulvinar thalami is only a few millimetres away. Between this slice and Pulvinar thalami lies the posterior part of Fissura transversa cerebri at the transition to Cisterna quadrigemina. This section is shown enlarged in Fig. 159. Cerebrum and Cerebellum are slightly pulled apart in order to show Lamina quadrigemina which is otherwise hidden between Splenium and Culmen (cf. Fig. 158). The structures shown here are difficult to demonstrate at operation because of superimposition by Plexus chor., vessels, and in the cisternal region by arachnoidal trabeculae. Attention should, therefore, be paid to the reference structures which are more easily recognizable at operation: Stria terminalis, V. thalamostriata, Cauda nuclei caudati. Plexus chorioideus, which is most strongly developed in the ventricular atrium, can easily be luxated, in which case injuries to its vessels must be avoided (see Chapter 6). At the same time the point of attachment of Plexus chorioideus to the floor of the ventricle marks medially the edge of Fornix and laterally the border of Pars affixa thalami, which becomes narrower posteriorly until the insertion of Plexus chorioideus reaches Stria terminalis. Basal to Plexus chor. in the occipital horn the protrusion of Hippocampus is flattened out in the presence of ventricular dilatation. Laterally it forms a sulcus (section in Fig. 159, left). Posteriorly it merges without a recognizable border line into Fornix and Corpus callosum.

Arteries and veins: From the section preparation *A* in Fig. 159 and Fig. 160 a slice has been cut out in Fig. 160, below. The quadrigeminal region and Pulvinar thalami can now be well seen. The presentation of the arteries (Fig. 161, above left) shows lateral branches of A. chorioidea post. lying over the thalamus. These penetrate the insertion of Plexus chor. and supply not only Plexus chor. but very often encroach beyond Plexus chor. into the border area between Thalamus and Caudatum (Lamina affixa thalami). After resection of Plexus chorioideus, encephalomalacia in the region of the basal ganglia is to be expected. In Fig. 161 these arteries are demonstrated in isolation. Only under the microscope can they be recognized in a broad sheet of connective tissue, together with the veins, which are demonstrated in Figs. 160, 161, 163, and 166. On the operating table the arteries and veins in their loose bed of connective tissue can be more easily differentiated under the microscope, owing to the differences in colour and transparency of the structures, than is possible with collapsed vessels. One of the many possible venous courses is illustrated in Fig. 160 above. These have been described in recent years, particularly by Huang and Wolf (1965) and by Brown et al. (1975). Detailed neuroradiological data are given particularly by Potts et al. (1974). Hammock et al. (1971) demonstrated recently that after ligation. of V. cerebri magna (Galeni) in 16 rhesus monkeys, a hydrocephalus was not found, in contrast to earlier observations in man, originating with Dandy (1919). In the assessment of such findings it must be considered that the accompanying veins, the cerebellar veins (V. supraculminata, V. praecentralis cerebellaris), and not infrequently V. mesencephalica lateralis as well, flow into either V. cerebri magna (Galeni) itself or into the often missing V. basalis (Rosenthal). Operative ligations of some of these small veins are possibly of more significance than ligation of the main venous trunk, V. cerebri magna (Galeni) itself, particularly if it is ligated immediately at its entry into Sinus rectus. Potent collaterals may develop over V. basalis (Rosenthal) to the group of Sylvian veins, or over the above-named cerebellar veins to the undersurface of Tentorium (Lacunae of Sinus rectus) or Sinus transversus. According to the writer's own observations on injection preparations the elimination of single, smaller veins appears to be perhaps more significant. In every case, therefore, an analysis of the venous connections must be made both angiographically and at operation, before an elimination of veins during exposure of the dorsal brainstem region is possible. The symmetrically structured veins near the midline are almost constantly present but even two Vv. pericallosae postt., as well as the veins of Culmen and Lobulus centralis, may be completely absent or replaced by asymmetrically developed irregular venous structures. In Figs. 162 and 165 an operative approach from the supratentorial direction to the quadrigeminal region has been simulated in an anatomical preparation. Fig. 162 above *A* shows the preparation from the basal direction. In the centre *B* the occipital lobe has been drawn aside and Corpus callosum can be seen lying close to Tentorium. It can also be seen from section *C* that Lamina quadrigemina can only be demonstrated by resection of Tentorium, since it lies predominantly infratentorially. Even after tentorial resection (see Fig. 163) the approach is hampered by occipitomedial veins. After these have been interrupted the lower part of Lamina quadrigemina is still concealed by Culmen. Because of these difficulties, Yaşargil prefers the infratentorial approach, as described by Fedor Krause (1913 and 1926) and taken up again by Zapletal (1956). Since, however, supratentorial processes near Lamina quadrigemina, – e.g., meningeomas in the rostral region of Sinus rectus or venous aneurysms in the vicinity of V. cerebri magna (Galeni) – would in some circumstances also necessitate preparation of this region from the supratentorial direction, and since a demonstration of the structures without considerable perspective distortion is only possible from that direction, the supratentorial approach was chosen in the anatomical preparation.

Special problems of operative technique are dealt with at the end of this chapter. If Cerebellum is pushed aside and Tentorium lifted from the infratentorial direction, the same site is visible with distortion.

Fig. 164 gives a schematic enlarged view of Fissura transversa cerebri visible after Corpus callosum has been raised and the quadrigeminal region pushed aside (the pineal has been removed). The preparation comes from an old person with correspondingly pronounced widening of Commissura fornicis resulting from cerebral atrophy with dilatation of the ventricles. This view is not normally possible in the brains of younger persons. In the presence of space-occupying processes, on the other hand, the flattening out caused by the tumour also makes this view possible. In such cases the whole mat of vessels, made up mainly of the veins described in the previous illustrations and Aa. chorioideae posteriores, is wide-meshed.

Fissura transversa cerebri and Cisterna quadrigemina merge laterally into Cisterna ambiens. Here the more instructive representation is not from the dorsal, but from the medial and anterior direction, as can be seen in Fig. 165.

In the illustrations of this preparation typical vessel courses have been entered (Fig. 166). Since in the literature arteries and veins are rarely shown together in detail, and also their combined radiological visualization is not usually possible, injection preparations have been used. These show better than combinations of angiograms the positional relationships between the more basally lying A. cerebri post. V. basalis (Rosenthal) lying above it, with their branches.

C. Preoperative Radiology – Some Aspects

The determination of asymmetries of Sinus sagittalis sup. and Sinus transversus (Fig. 167 *A*) is important. Asymmetries of the skull are often not noticeable in the roentgenogram, so these must be looked for on the clean-shaven head. Asymmetries of the sinus region, on the other hand, may be present even if the external appearance of the head is symmetrical.
For details of the deeper vessels the reader is referred to Chapter 3, "Temporal Lobe". The angiographic interpretation of the vessels courses can be difficult. In Fig. 114 a variant of A. chorioidea ant. is shown. This was discovered in the preparation but would have been difficult to interpret angiographically due to the superimposition of other arterial vessels, particularly A. cerebri post. of the opposite side. As is well known, A. quadrigemina, A. thalamogeniculata, and the other branches supplying the quadrigeminal region are most easily demonstrable in children. The use of enlargement techniques with tomograms will enable this region and in particular the area of Trigonum lemnisci to be better explored in the future. Dyed injection preparations by the author show that this is the only part of the brainstem in which the perforating arteries may form many anastomoses. Since the trunk of A. cerebri post. and A. quadrigemina, V. thalamogeniculata, as well as the medial branch of A. chorioidea posterior group, and also A. cerebelli superior, may send branches into the matted layer of arteries of Trigonum lemnisci, the possibility of a collateral circulation arising here after elimination of one or more branches of the above-named arteries is more likely than in the case of the other perforating arteries which only rarely anastomose before entering the brain substance. In principle, no anastomosing takes place in the cerebral parenchyma.

D. Operative Techniques – Some Aspects

In opening the skull the frequently seen asymmetries of the occipital region are of importance. If, however, the darkcoloured and somewhat protruding lateral region of Sinus sagittalis superior and the upper edge of Sinus transversus have been identified, disorientation inside the brain, as shown in Fig. 168 (*A* and *B*), is not possible. In elderly patients, when the dura adheres to the skull the trepanation should initially be made at some distance from the sinus. Then after angiographic orientation the trepanation should be enlarged by drilling towards the edge of the sinus (Fig. 167 *B*).
Resections of the occipital lobe are associated with visualfield defects because the optic radiation enfolds the whole temporal horn and the occipital horn and from here spreads out broadly to reach Area striata (Fig. 157 and Fig. 204 of Chapter 6: "Supratentorial Structures near the Ventricles").
As is well known, Area striata reaches from the posterior part of Gyrus parahippocampalis to Praecuneus into the longitudinal fissure, and laterally lies 2.5-3 cm away from the midline (see Fig. 204, Chapter 6). In occipital lobe resections orientation on Falx and Tentorium is possible, with the distance measurements given in Figs. 154 and 155. The measurements of the posterior horn tip are not given because of their high degree of variability. The ventricular triangle and Thalamus, on the other hand, vary little in their localization (Fig. 169). If one loses the way in the occipital lobe as a result of asymmetrical conditions (Fig. 168), the ventricular system may seem to lie at greater depth (*A* in Fig. 168), or may not be reached at all (*B* in Fig. 168). In both cases destruction of Corona radiata of the internal capsule with Hemiplegia and Hemihypaesthesia is to be expected, particularly if the approach is made too high and deep into the white matter. Otherwise, resection of the occipital lobe is a simple matter if orientation is taken from the dural duplications. Cisterna quadrigemina and ambiens are covered at the edge of Tentorium and Falx with a tough arachnoidal layer. After opening this laterally, attention should be paid to the danger of injury to N. trochlearis, as in temporal exposure. The large venous trunks lie near the midline. Coming from the lateral direction, partly above and partly below the veins, lie the branches of A. chorioidea posterior group. Because of its proximity to the ventricular system this group is dealt with in Chapter 6.
In the supratentorial approach to the quadrigeminal region, first described by Dandy in 1921, it is necessary to clip the medial occipital veins. Since the quadrigeminal region lies mainly under the tentorium, Irsigler, like Poppen, recommends splitting the tentorium in order to reach Lamina quadrigemina. The longitudinal splitting of Splenium

corporis callosi specified by many authors is problematical, since under normal conditions with its numerous vessels Tela chorioidea lies above the quadrigeminal region (see Chapter 6, Figs. 182 and 183) hindering the approach. Only if space-occupying processes push the vascular system apart is the approach simpler. The same is true of the transventricular approach, described by von Wagenen in 1931, which necessitates incision of Fornix and Corpus callosum with splitting of the medial wall of the posterior horn.

Under microsurgical conditions such destructions of parts of the limbic system, Corpus callosum, or the veins of the quadrigeminal area are avoidable.

There are two possibilities:

1) the supratentorial, lateral approach to the quadrigeminal region, which does not provide a reliable view over the contralateral side. From the posterior, temporal-basal direction over Tentorium, splitting of Tentorium enables Crus cerebri, Trigonum lemnisci, and lateral quadrigeminal region to be clearly exposed (Fig. 170 was prepared from an operative case of the author – AV malformation of Brachium pontis covered by Lobulus quadrangularis). It shows the (normal) site without the eliminated angioma (no additional neurological deficits occurred postoperatively). This approach is very useful for all processes in the vicinity of Crus cerebri – e.g. aneurysms of A. cerebri post. or tentorial meningeomas. If Tentorium is split widely it is possible to expose not only Lobulus quadrangularis cerebelli but also in particular the quadrigeminal region from the lateral direction. Cisterna is larger than would be expected from formalin preparations, in which all the vessels and arachnoidal meshes are adherent and more difficult to separate than at the site of operation.

2) the infratentorial approach, described by Fedor Krause in 1913 and 1926, taken up again by Zapletal in 1965, and modified in recent years by Yaşargil (see Chapter 7).

E. References

Braun, J. P., et al.: The importance of normal venous landmarks in the topography of the mesencephalon, pons and cerebellum. Neuroradiology **10,** 43–46 (1975).

Browder, J., Kaplan, H., Krieger, A. J.: Anatomical features of the straight sinus and its tributaries. J. Neurosurg. **44,** (1976).

Dandy, W. E. (1919) s. Irsigler, F. J.

Dandy, W. E.: Orbital Tumor: Results Following the Transcranial Operative Attack. New York: O. Piest. 1941.

Dandy, W. E.: Operation for removal of pineal tumors. Surg. etc. **33,** 113 (1921).

Hammock, M. K., et al.: Vein of Galen ligation in the primate angiographic gross, and light microscopic evaluation. J. Neurosurg. **34,** 77–83 (1971).

Huang, Y. P., Wolf, B. S.: The veins of the posterior fossa-superior or Galenic draining group. Amer. J. Roentgenol. **95,** 808–821 (1965).

Irsigler, F. J.: Allgemeine Operationslehre. In: Handbuch der Neurochirurgie, herausgeg. von Olivecrona, H., Tönnis, W. Berlin–Göttingen–Heidelberg: Springer. 1960.

Krause, F., Schum, H.: Die spezielle Chirurgie der Gehirnkrankheiten. Stuttgart: F. Enke. 1932.

Newton, Th., Potts, D. G.: Radiology of the Skull and Brain Angiography. St. Louis: The C. V. Mosby Company. 1974.

Voigt, K., Yaşargil, M. G.: Cerebral cavernous haemangiomas or cavernomas. Neurochirurgia **19,** 59–68 (1976).

Van Wagenen, W. P.: Surg. etc. **53,** 216 (1931) zitiert nach Irsigler, F. J.

Zapletal, B.: Zbl. Neurochir. **16,** 64, 154 (1956).

Literature for Further Reading

Ferner, H., Kautzky, R.: Angewandte Anatomie des Gehirns und seiner Hüllen. In: Handbuch der Neurochirurgie, Bd. 1, Teil 1. Berlin–Göttingen–Heidelberg: Springer. 1959.

Pernkopf, E.: Topographische Anatomie des Menschen, Bd. IV: Topographische und stratigraphische Anatomie des Kopfes. München–Berlin–Wien: Urban & Schwarzenberg. 1957.

Zuleger, S., Staubesand, J.: Schnittbilder des Zentralnervensystems. München–Wien–Baltimore: Urban & Schwarzenberg. 1976.

F. Illustrations

(Figs. 154 to 170)

Fig. 154.
A Width of different regions of Falx
B Distance of Polus occipitalis from medial and lateral reference structures of Cerebrum
Measurements in millimetres (mm)

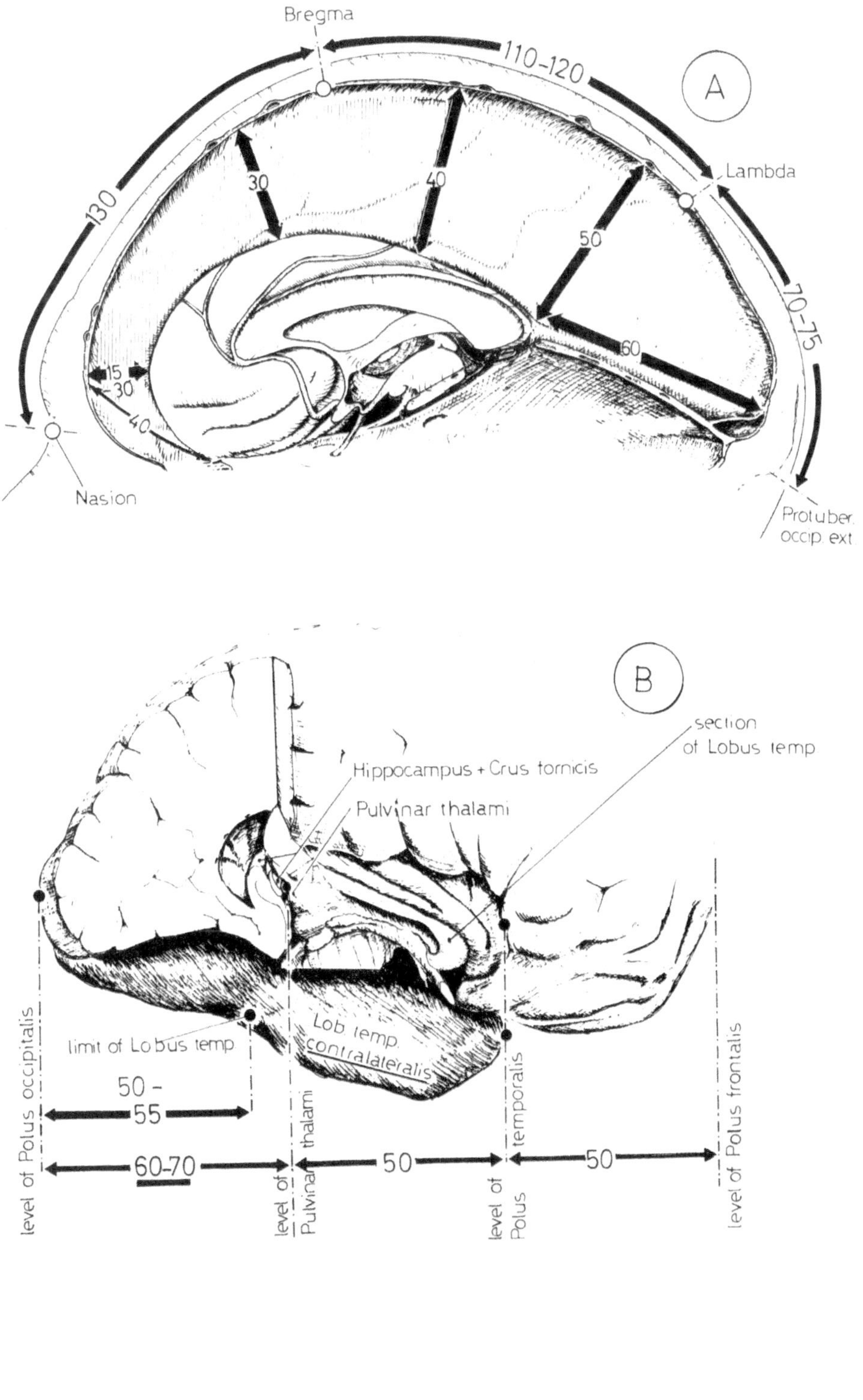
Bregma
110-120
A
130
30
40
Lambda
50
70-75
60
15
30
40
Nasion
Protuber. occip. ext.
B
section of Lobus temp.
Hippocampus + Crus fornicis
Pulvinar thalami
limit of Lobus temp
Lob. temp. contralateralis
50 - 55
60-70
50
50
level of Polus occipitalis
level of Pulvinar thalami
level of Polus temporalis
level of Polus frontalis

Fig. 155. Width of Falx and Tentorium. Measurements in millimetres (mm). Reference structure between Falx and Tentorium: Sinus rectus. Reference structure between Tentorium and middle cranial fossa: Sinus petrosus superior (if not transparent, recognizable by the difference in consistency between Tentorium and Eminentia arcuata)

FIG. 155

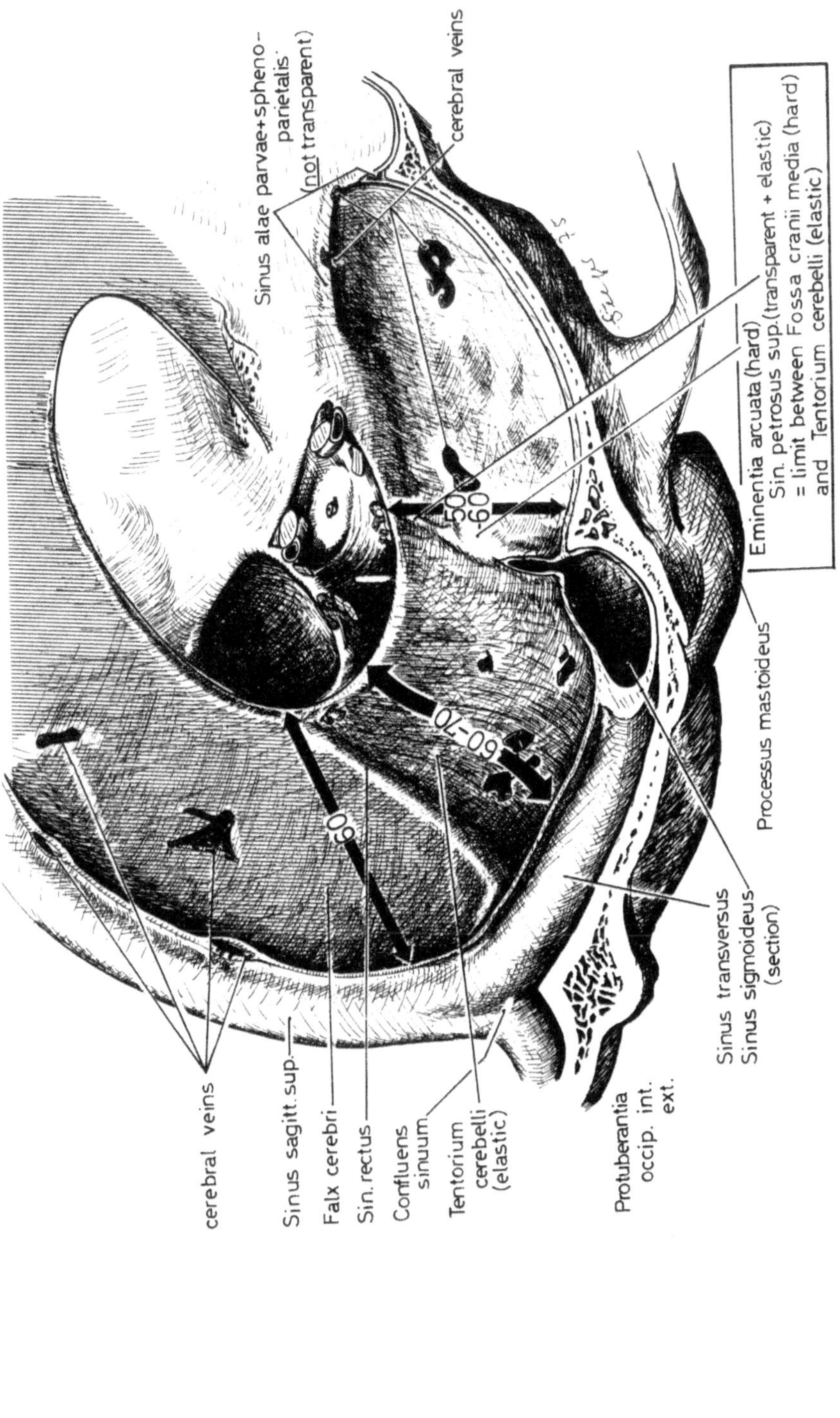
Sinus alae parvae+spheno-parietalis (not transparent)
cerebral veins
Eminentia arcuata (hard)
Sin. petrosus sup. (transparent + elastic)
= limit between Fossa cranii media (hard)
and Tentorium cerebelli (elastic)
50
60
60–70
60
Processus mastoideus
Sinus transversus
Sinus sigmoideus
(section)
Protuberantia
occip. int.
ext.
Tentorium
cerebelli
(elastic)
Confluens
sinuum
Sin. rectus
Falx cerebri
Sinus sagitt. sup.
cerebral veins

Fig. 156.
A Frontal section 45 mm from occipital pole. Characteristic asymmetry of the occipital poles, Confluens sinuum and the cerebellar hemispheres
B Sectioned area enlarged. Incision of triangular tip of Cornu post., the roof of which is formed by the fibres radiating from Corpus callosum (Tapetum). Deep fissures push the pallium down to form contours around the ventricular system

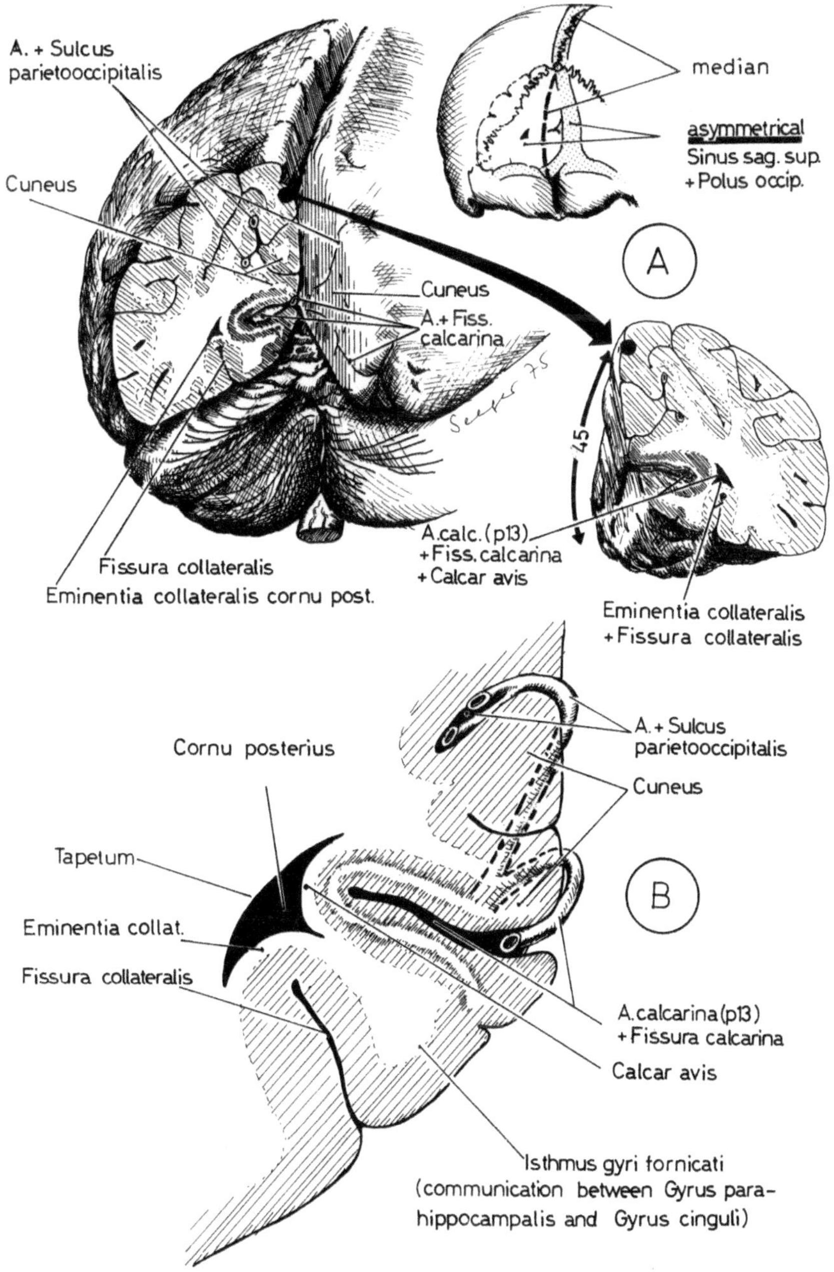
A. + Sulcus parietooccipitalis
Cuneus
median
asymmetrical
Sinus sag. sup. + Polus occip.
A
Cuneus
A.+ Fiss. calcarina
45
A.calc. (p13) + Fiss. calcarina + Calcar avis
Fissura collateralis
Eminentia collateralis cornu post.
Eminentia collateralis + Fissura collateralis
A. + Sulcus parietooccipitalis
Cornu posterius
Cuneus
Tapetum
B
Eminentia collat.
Fissura collateralis
A. calcarina (p13) + Fissura calcarina
Calcar avis
Isthmus gyri fornicati (communication between Gyrus parahippocampalis and Gyrus cinguli)

Fig. 157. Schematic representation of the visual pathway, according to Elze (1932) and Pfeiffer (1925), modified considerably

FIG. 157

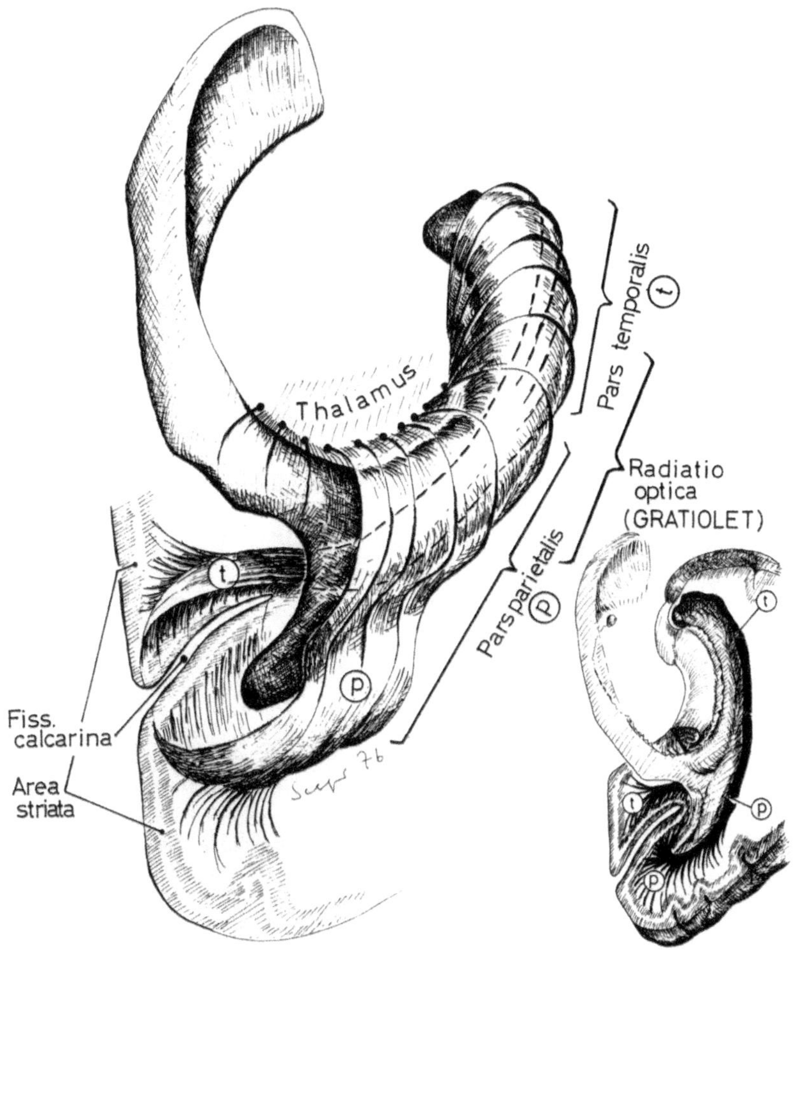
Thalamus
Pars temporalis
t
Radiatio
optica
(GRATIOLET)
Pars parietalis
p
t
p
Fiss.
calcarina
Area
striata
t
p
t
p

Fig. 158. Frontal section 70 mm from Polus occipit. Pulvinar thalami is still covered by a thin layer of the tangentially incised Hippocampus and Gyrus parahippocampalis. Isthmus gyri cinguli is very variable and may be divided by Fissura calcarina. Fanning out of Tapetum radiation, along the under side of which Gyrus dentatus/fasciolaris and Hippocampus lie

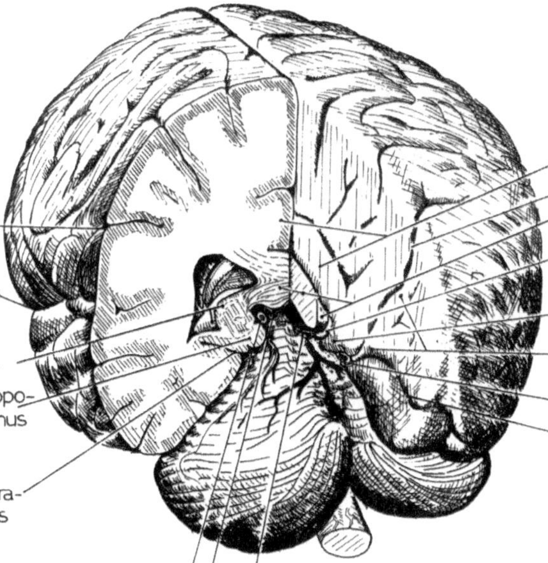
Gyrus cinguli
Fiss. parietooccip.
Splenium corp. call.
Gyrus dentatus /Gyrus fasciolaris
Isthmus gyri cinguli
Cuneus
W. occpitales mediales
Fissura calcarina
Fiss. lat. (SYLVII)
Hippocampus
Gyrus parahippocampalis/Isthmus gyri cinguli
Fissura collateralis
V.cerebri magna (GALENI)
V. basalis (ROSENTHALI)
A. cerebri post. (p1)

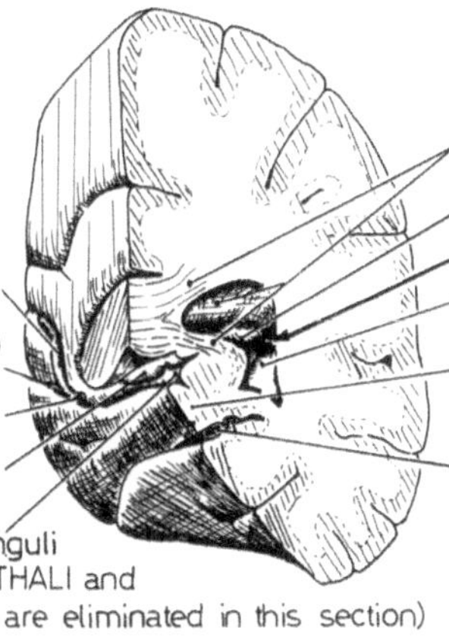
Splenium, 3divisions of Radiatio corporis callosi
Tapetum
Calcar avis
top of Cornu post.(section) ▷
Eminentia collateralis
Gyrus occipitotempor.med.
Fiss. collat.+Vv. occip. med.
A. parietoocipit. (p12)
A. calcarina (p13)
A.cerebri post. (p1)
Gyrus dentatus /Gyr. fasciolaris
Isthmus gyri cinguli
(V. bas. ROSENTHALI and
A.cerebri post. are eliminated in this section)

Fig. 159. Enlarged sectioned area of Fig. 158. Leptomeninges and vessels left out. Cerebellum (Culmen) has been retracted caudally in order to bring the quadrigeminal region into view

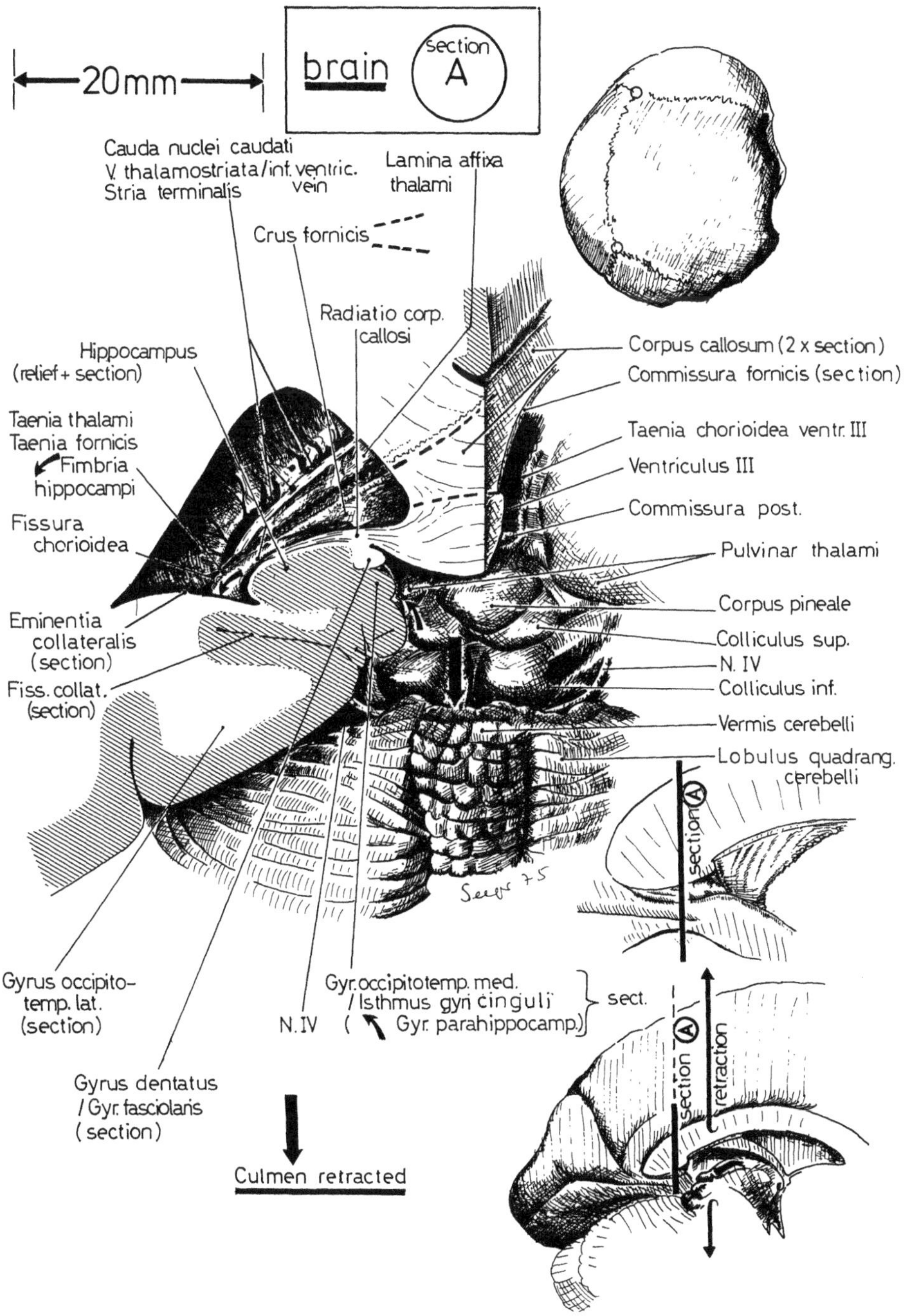
20mm
brain
section A
Cauda nuclei caudati
V. thalamostriata / inf. ventric. vein
Stria terminalis
Lamina affixa thalami
Crus fornicis
Radiatio corp. callosi
Hippocampus (relief + section)
Taenia thalami
Taenia fornicis
Fimbria hippocampi
Fissura chorioidea
Eminentia collateralis (section)
Fiss. collat. (section)
Corpus callosum (2 x section)
Commissura fornicis (section)
Taenia chorioidea ventr. III
Ventriculus III
Commissura post.
Pulvinar thalami
Corpus pineale
Colliculus sup.
N. IV
Colliculus inf.
Vermis cerebelli
Lobulus quadrang. cerebelli
section A
Gyrus occipito-temp. lat. (section)
N. IV
Gyr. occipitotemp. med. / Isthmus gyri cinguli (Gyr. parahippocamp.)
sect.
section A
retraction
Gyrus dentatus / Gyr. fasciolaris (section)
Culmen retracted

Fig. 160.
Section *A* Section plane of Fig. 159 with vessels drawn in
Section *B* Removal of a slice of brain (B'). Leptomeninges and vessels not shown. Here too Culmen is retracted downwards in order to show Lamina quadrigemina

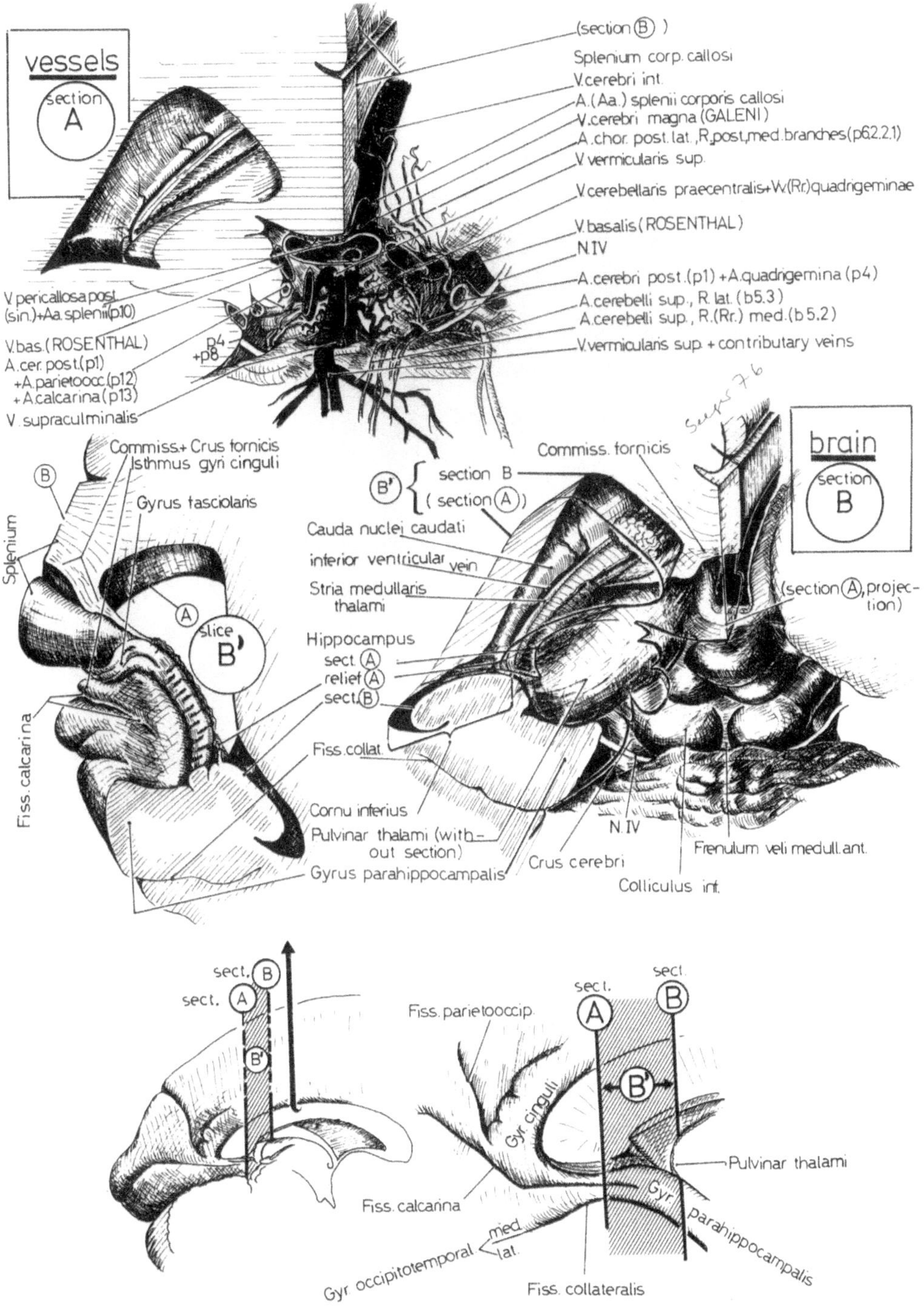
vessels
section A
(section B)
Splenium corp. callosi
V.cerebri int.
A.(Aa.) splenii corporis callosi
V.cerebri magna (GALENI)
A.chor. post. lat., R.post, med. branches (p6.2.2.1)
V.vermicularis sup.
V.cerebellaris praecentralis+Vv.(Rr.)quadrigeminae
V.basalis (ROSENTHAL)
N.IV
A.cerebri post.(p1) + A.quadrigemina (p4)
A.cerebelli sup., R. lat. (b5.3)
A.cerebelli sup., R.(Rr.) med.(b5.2)
V.vermicularis sup. + contributary veins
V.pericallosa post. (sin.)+Aa.splenii(p10)
V.bas.(ROSENTHAL)
A.cer. post.(p1)
+A.parietoocc.(p12)
+A.calcarina (p13)
p4
+p8
V. supraculminalis
Commiss.+ Crus fornicis
Isthmus gyri cinguli
B
Gyrus fasciolaris
Splenium
A
slice B'
Fiss. calcarina
B' { section B
(section A)
Cauda nuclei caudati
inferior ventricular vein
Stria medullaris thalami
Hippocampus
sect. A
relief A
sect. B
Fiss. collat.
Cornu inferius
Pulvinar thalami (without section)
Gyrus parahippocampalis
Commiss. fornicis
brain
section B
(section A, projection)
N.IV
Crus cerebri
Frenulum veli medull. ant.
Colliculus inf.
sect. B
sect. A
B'
sect. A
sect. B
Fiss. parietooccip.
Gyr. cinguli
B'
Pulvinar thalami
Fiss. calcarina
Gyr. parahippocampalis
med.
lat.
Gyr. occipitotemporal
Fiss. collateralis

Fig. 161. Section *B* of Fig. 160 with vessels drawn in

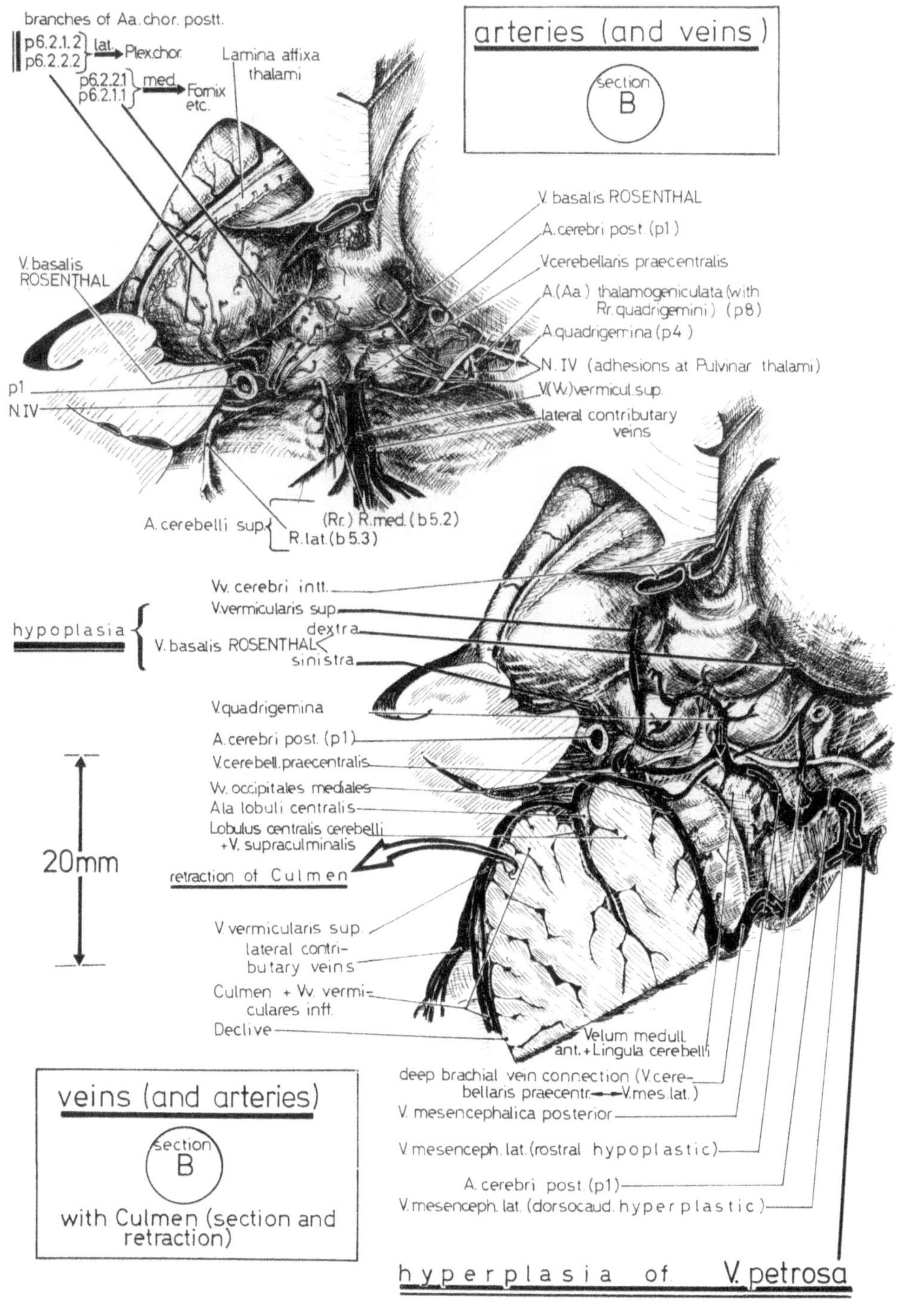

branches of Aa. chor. postt.
p6.2.1.2 p6.2.2.2 lat. Plex. chor.
p6.2.2.1 p6.2.1.1 med. Fornix etc.
Lamina affixa thalami
arteries (and veins)
section B
V. basalis ROSENTHAL
A. cerebri post. (p1)
V. cerebellaris praecentralis
A. (Aa.) thalamogeniculata (with Rr. quadrigemini) (p8)
A. quadrigemina (p4)
N. IV (adhesions at Pulvinar thalami)
V. (Vv.) vermicul. sup.
lateral contributary veins
V. basalis ROSENTHAL
p1
N. IV
A. cerebelli sup.
(Rr.) R. med. (b5.2)
R. lat. (b5.3)
Vv. cerebri intt.
V. vermicularis sup.
hypoplasia
V. basalis ROSENTHAL dextra sinistra
V. quadrigemina
A. cerebri post. (p1)
V. cerebell. praecentralis
Vv. occipitales mediales
Ala lobuli centralis
Lobulus centralis cerebelli + V. supraculminalis
retraction of Culmen
20mm
V. vermicularis sup.
lateral contributary veins
Culmen + Vv. vermiculares inft.
Declive
Velum medull. ant. + Lingula cerebelli
deep brachial vein connection (V. cerebellaris praecentr. ↔ V. mes. lat.)
V. mesencephalica posterior
V. mesenceph. lat. (rostral hypoplastic)
A. cerebri post. (p1)
V. mesenceph. lat. (dorsocaud. hyperplastic)
veins (and arteries)
section B
with Culmen (section and retraction)
hyperplasia of V. petrosa

Fig. 162
A Basal view (midbrain section) with nomenclature of structures
B Occipital view with dural duplications preserved after retraction of Polus occ. For nomenclature see *A*
C Enlarged detail from *B*, for nomenclature see *A*. Leptomeninges and vessels not shown

FIG. 162

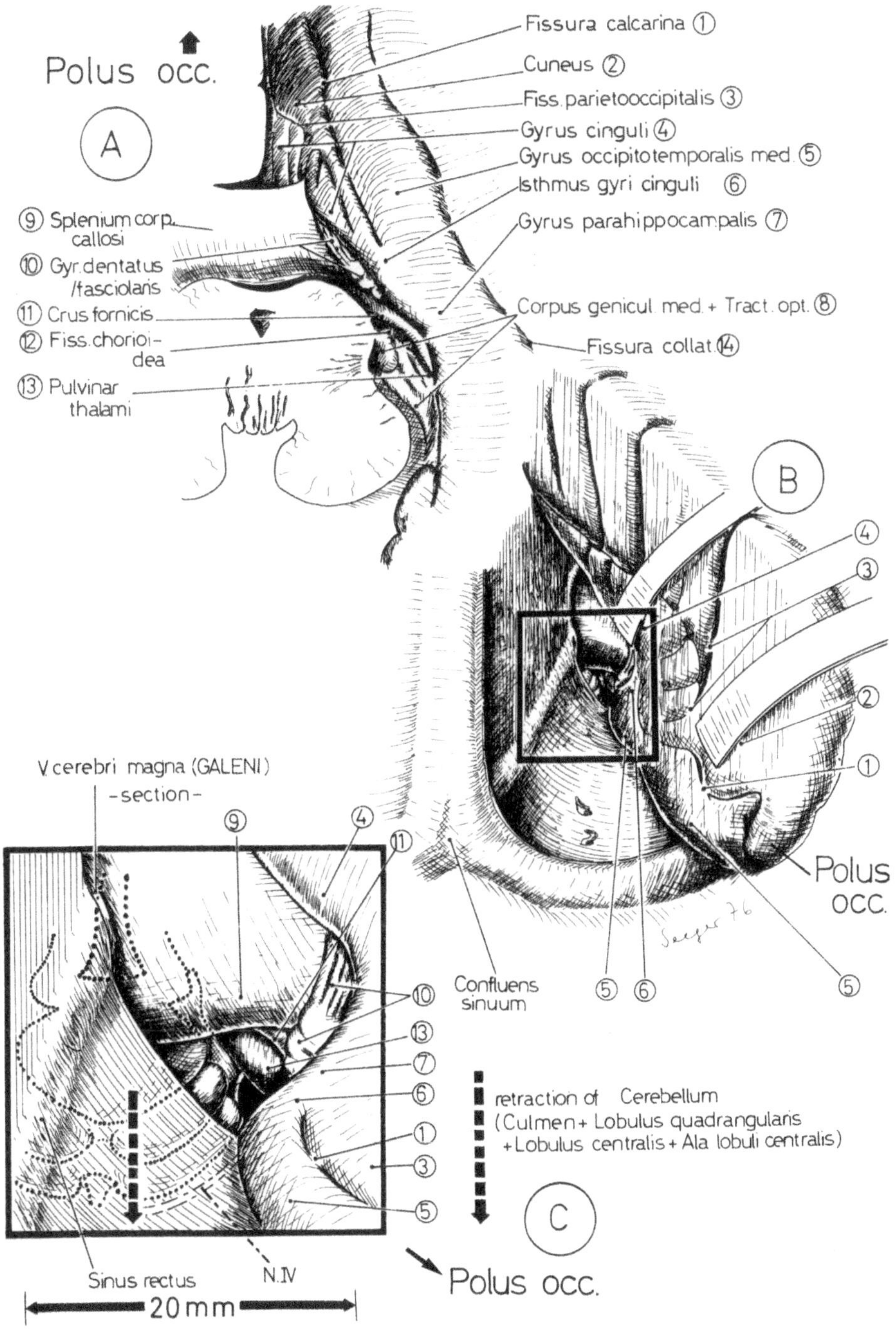
Polus occ.
A
Fissura calcarina ①
Cuneus ②
Fiss. parietooccipitalis ③
Gyrus cinguli ④
Gyrus occipitotemporalis med. ⑤
Isthmus gyri cinguli ⑥
Gyrus parahippocampalis ⑦
Corpus genicul. med. + Tract. opt. ⑧
Fissura collat. ⑭
⑨ Splenium corp. callosi
⑩ Gyr. dentatus /fasciolaris
⑪ Crus fornicis
⑫ Fiss. chorioi-dea
⑬ Pulvinar thalami
B
Polus occ.
Confluens sinuum
V cerebri magna (GALENI) -section-
Sinus rectus
N.IV
20 mm
retraction of Cerebellum (Culmen + Lobulus quadrangularis + Lobulus centralis + Ala lobuli centralis)
C
Polus occ.

Fig. 163. Preparation of Fig. 162 with tentorial resection and vessels drawn in.

D Connections between medial occipital region and V. magna (Galeni). Cerebellum and quadrigeminal veins removed in order to show Corpus pineale

E Cerebellum and quadrigeminal veins drawn in, occipital veins A. cerebri post. and V. basalis (Rosenthal) removed in order to show Pulvinar thalami

F More extensive tentorial resection. Almost all vessels shown must be preserved at operative interventions

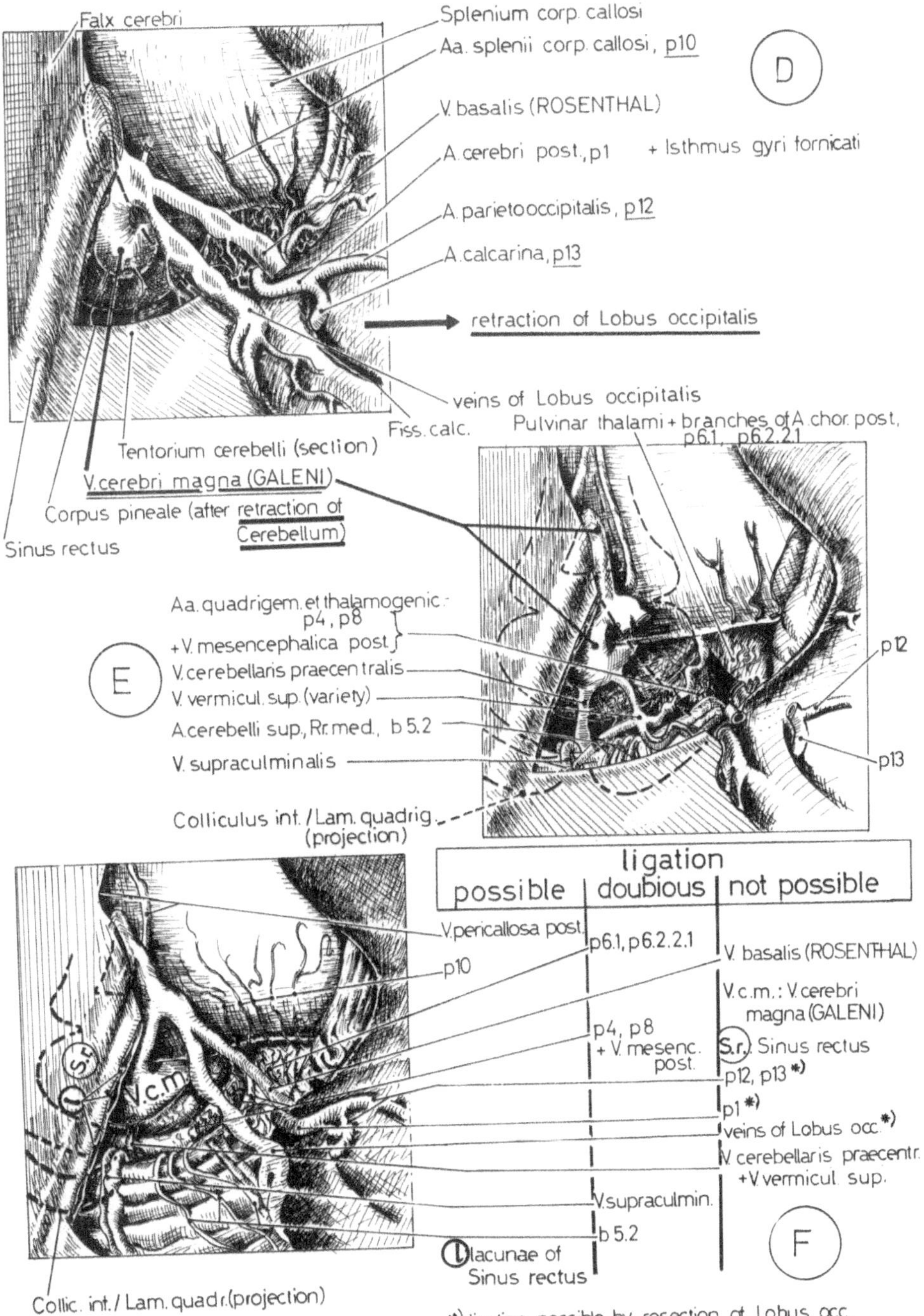

*) ligation possible by resection of Lobus occ.

Fig. 164. View of Fissura transversa cerebri from behind in senile atrophic brain with extremely widened Commissura fornicis (vessels, leptomeninges, and Corpus pineale not shown)

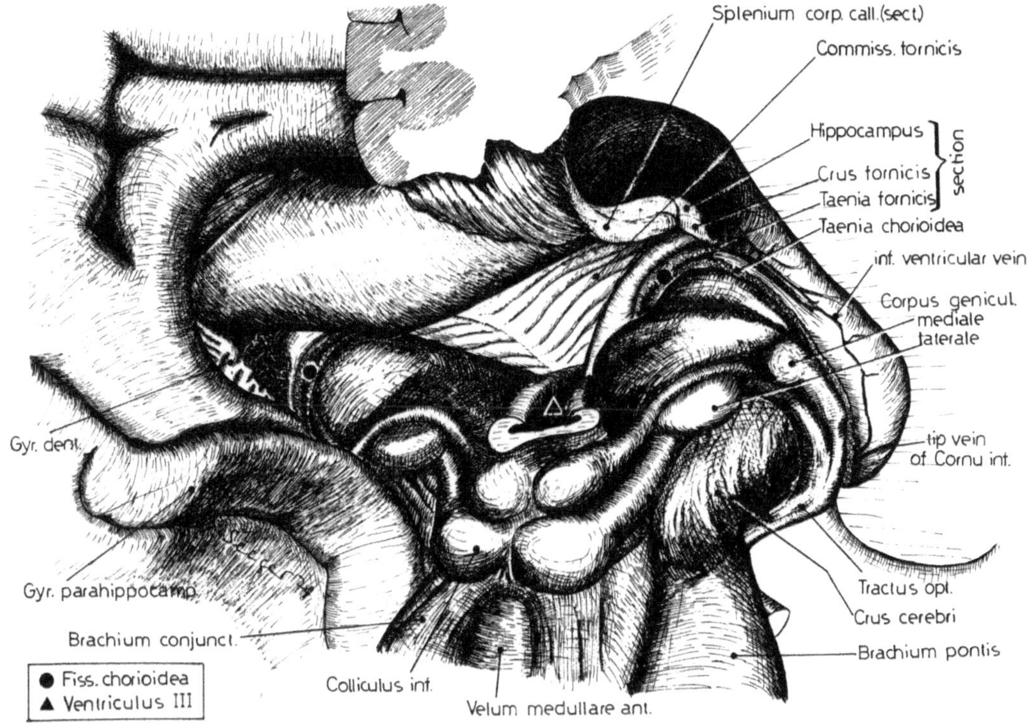
Splenium corp. call. (sect.)
Commiss. tornicis
Hippocampus
Crus tornicis
Taenia fornicis
section
Taenia chorioidea
inf. ventricular vein
Corpus genicul.
mediale
laterale
tip vein
of Cornu int.
Tractus opt.
Crus cerebri
Brachium pontis
Gyr. dent.
Gyr. parahippocamp.
Brachium conjunct.
Colliculus int.
Velum medullare ant.
● Fiss. chorioidea
▲ Ventriculus III

Fig. 165. General view of Fig. 166. For nomenclature see Fig. 162. The same structures which are shown there from the occipital direction can be seen here from the medial anterior view. Corpus callosum and Fornix are divided a few millimetres contralaterally to the midline. Pallium has been removed laterally in the parietotemporooccipital vicinity of Fissura lat. (Sylvii), (drawn from a preparation of Dr. H. Eggert, Neurosurgical Clinic of the University Freiburg i. Br.)

FIG. 165

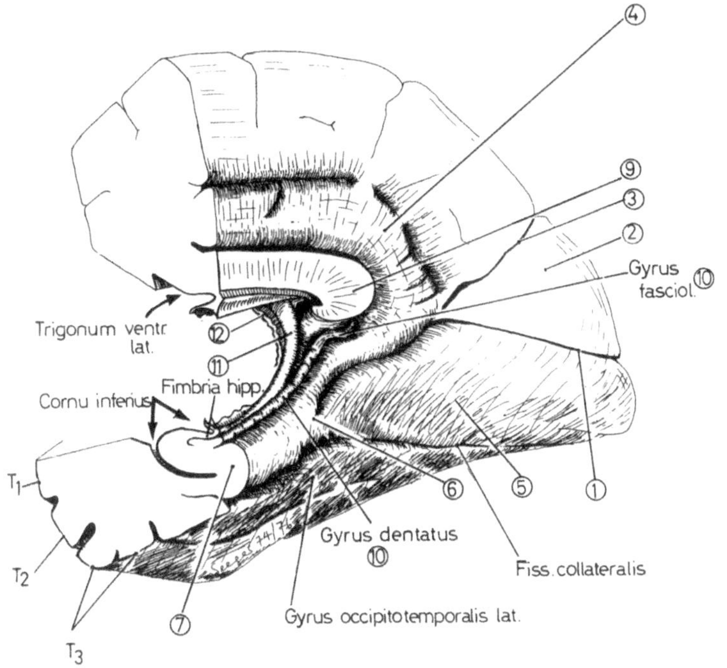

④
⑨
③
②
Gyrus fasciol. ⑩
Trigonum ventr. lat.
⑫
⑪
Fimbria hipp.
Cornu inferius
T_1
T_2
T_3
⑦
⑥
⑤
①
Gyrus dentatus ⑩
Fiss. collateralis
Gyrus occipitotemporalis lat.

Fig. 166. Enlarged details from Fig. 165. Leptomeninges, parts of Falx and Tentorium have been left out, and vessels drawn in

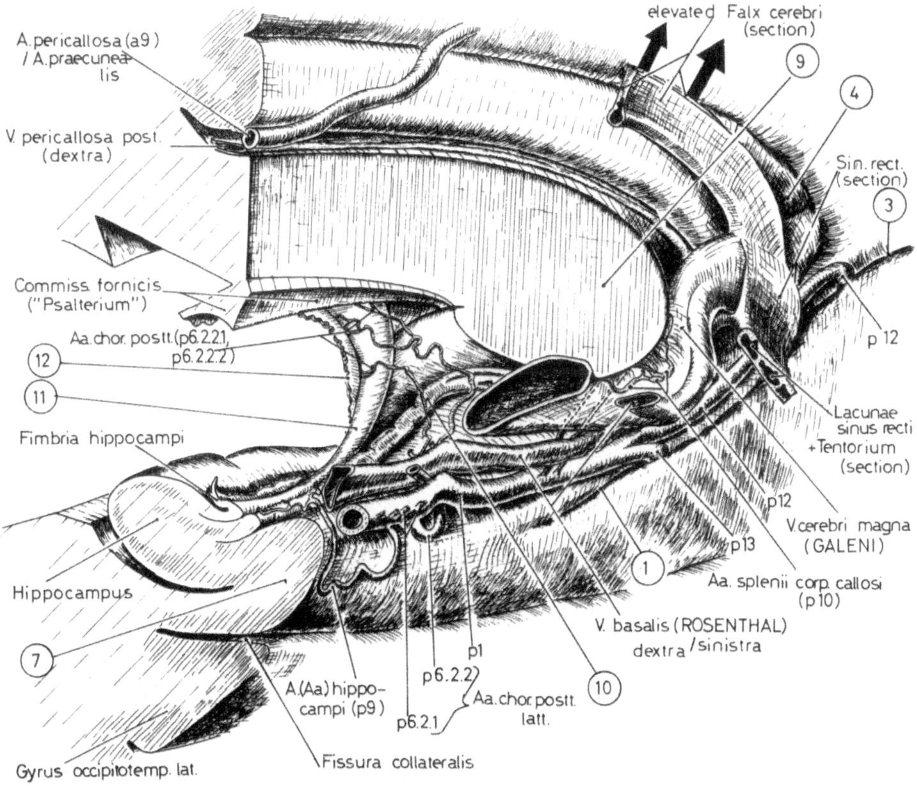
elevated Falx cerebri (section)
A. pericallosa (a9) / A. praecunealis
V. pericallosa post. (dextra)
9
4
Sin. rect. (section)
3
Commiss. fornicis ("Psalterium")
Aa. chor. postt. (p6.2.2.1, p6.2.2.2)
p 12
12
11
Lacunae sinus recti + Tentorium (section)
Fimbria hippocampi
p12
V. cerebri magna (GALENI)
p13
Hippocampus
1
Aa. splenii corp. callosi (p 10)
V. basalis (ROSENTHAL) dextra / sinistra
7
p1
p6.2.2
10
A.(Aa) hippocampi (p9)
Aa. chor. postt. latt.
p6.2.1
Gyrus occipitotemp. lat.
Fissura collateralis

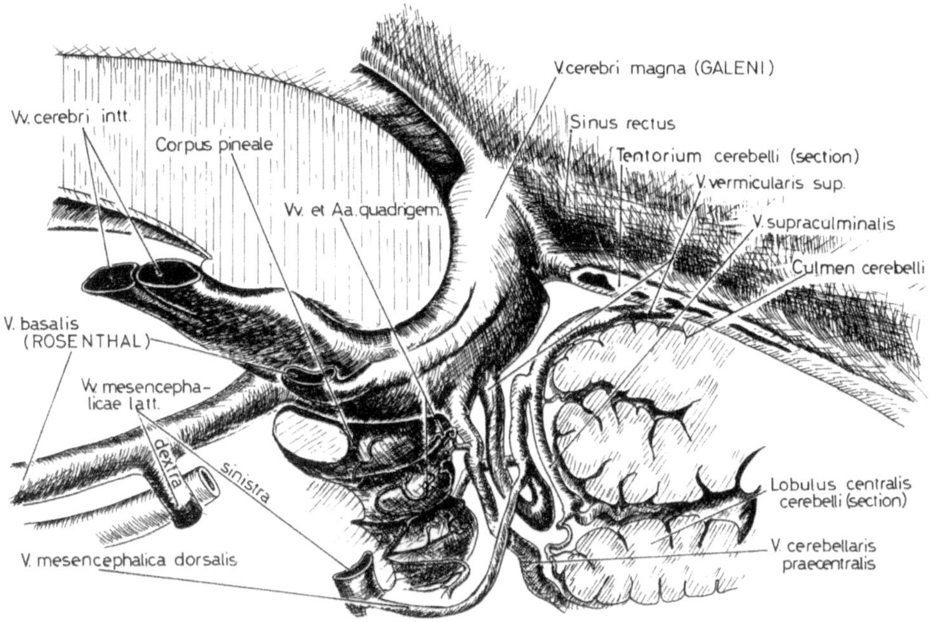
V. cerebri magna (GALENI)
Sinus rectus
Vv. cerebri intt.
Corpus pineale
Tentorium cerebelli (section)
V. vermicularis sup.
Vv. et Aa. quadrigem.
V. supraculminalis
Culmen cerebelli
V. basalis (ROSENTHAL)
Vv. mesencephalicae latt.
dextra
sinistra
Lobulus centralis cerebelli (section)
V. cerebellaris praecentralis
V. mesencephalica dorsalis

Fig. 167. Asymmetry of the skull and course of the sinus
A Preoperative recognition
B Demonstration of edges of the sinus at operation
C Anatomical preparation

FIG. 167

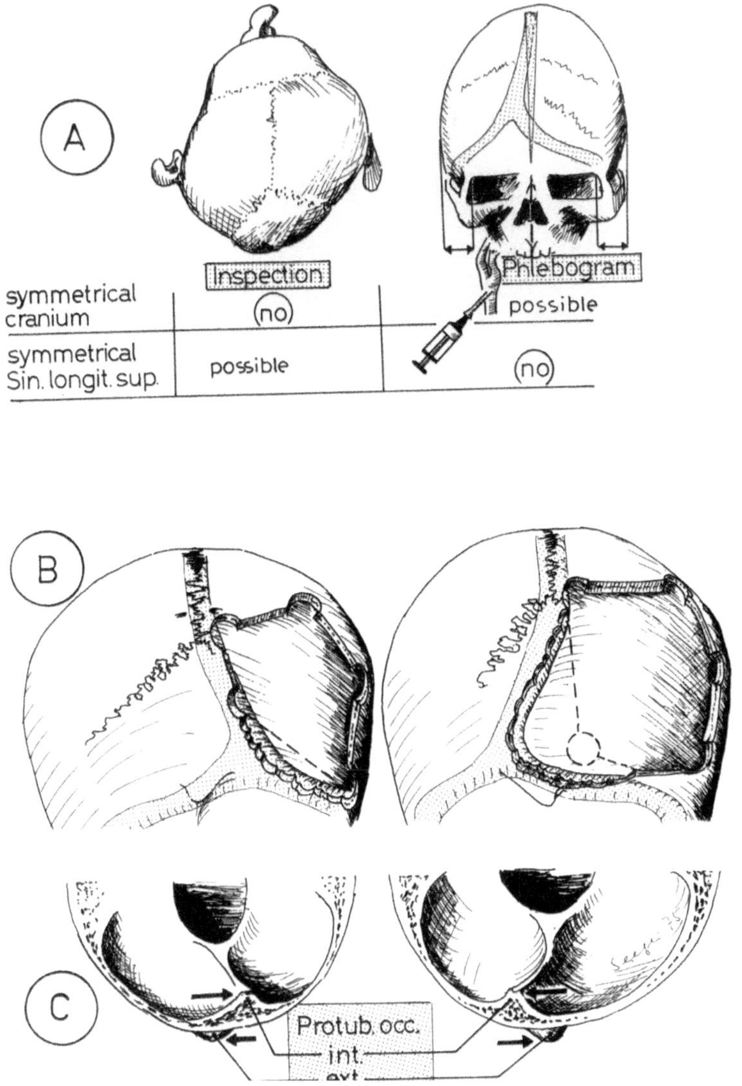
A
Inspection
Phlebogram
symmetrical cranium
no
possible
symmetrical Sin. longit. sup.
possible
no
B
C
Protub. occ.
int.
ext.

Fig. 168
A Difficulties of orientation due to contralateral deviation of Sinus sagittalis superior
B Difficulties of orientation due to homolateral deviation of Sinus sagittalis superior
C Correct procedure for Sinus deviation

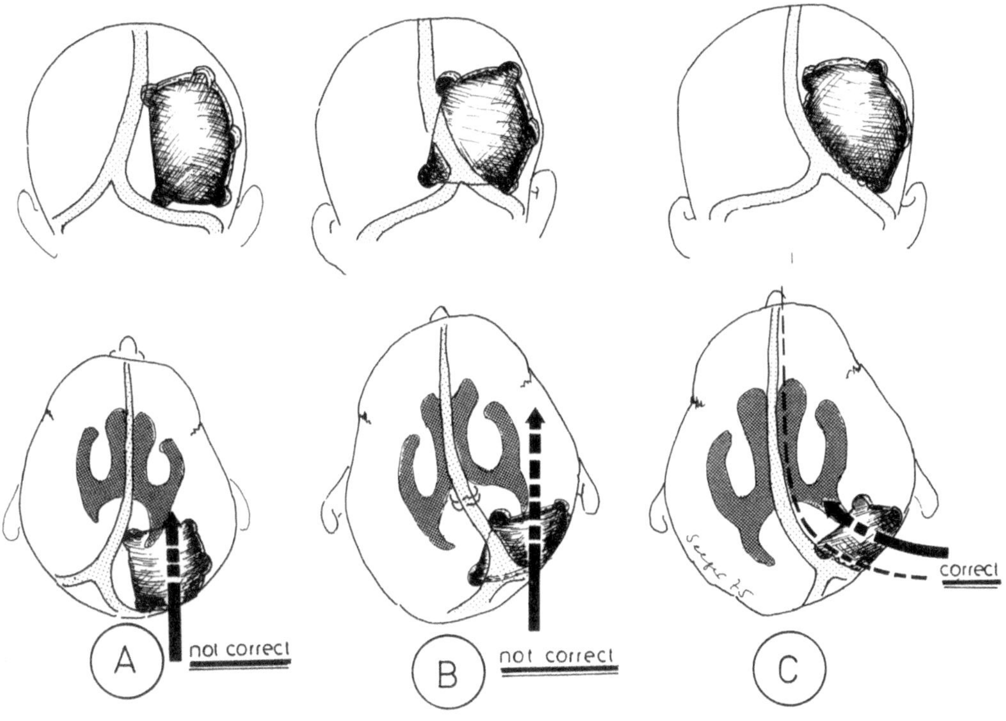
not correct
not correct
correct
A
B
C

Fig. 169. Positional relationships of deeper veins of the occipital region to surrounding brain structures. Measurements in millimetres (mm)

A General lateral view

B Frontal section (*S*)

C Enlarged detail from *A*

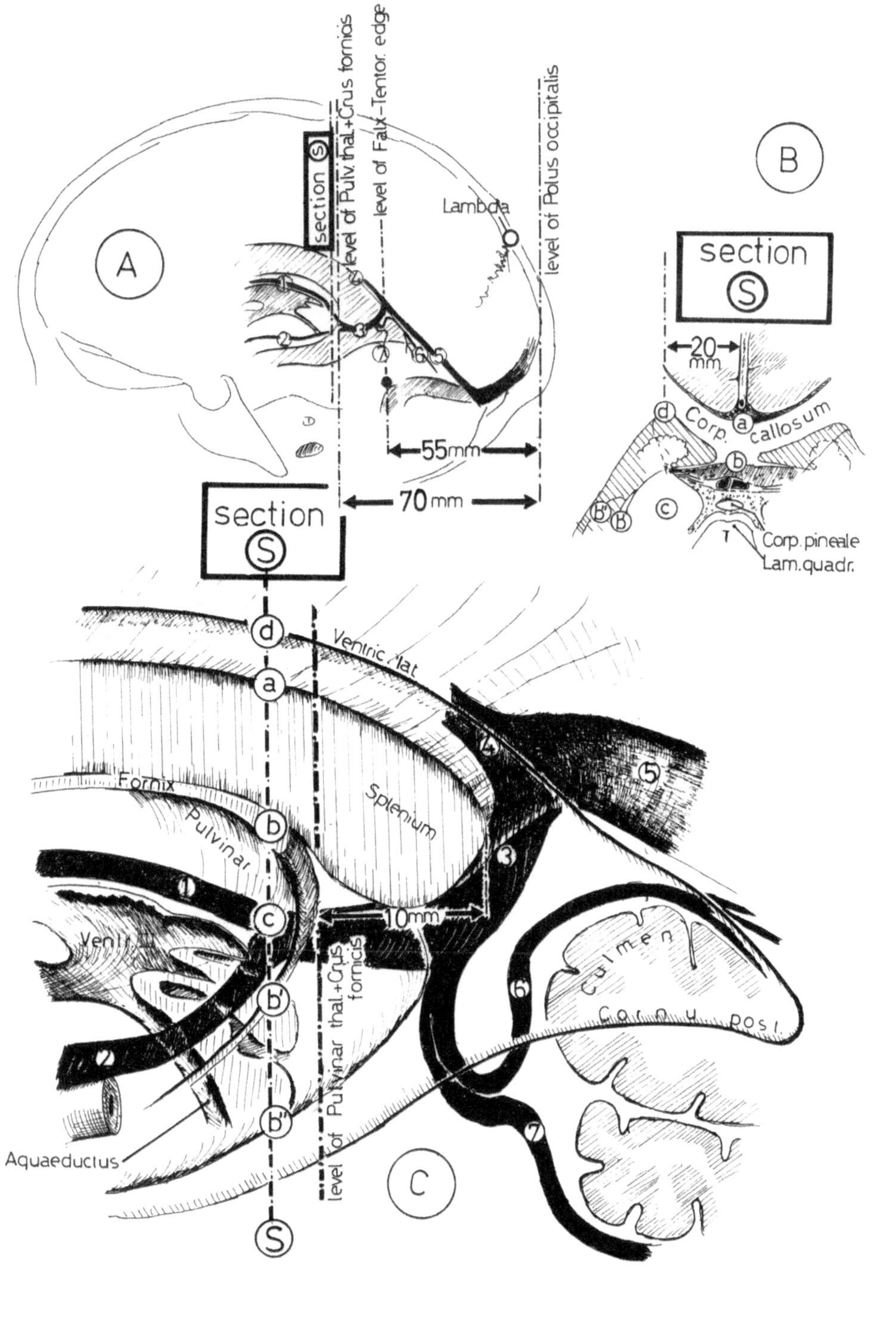
A
B
C
section S
level of Pulv. thal.+Crus fornicis
level of Falx-Tentor. edge
level of Polus occipitalis
Lambda
55mm
70 mm
20 mm
Corp. callosum
Corp. pineale
Lam. quadr.
Ventric. lat.
Fornix
Pulvinar
Splenium
10mm
Ventr.
level of Pulvinar thal.+Crus fornicis
Culmen
Cornu post.
Aquaeductus

Fig. 170. Operation site composed of several views with the surgical microscope
Circle: One of the microscopic views in the middle range of magnification. Occasion was the preparation of an AV malformation of Brachium pontis, overlapped by Lobulus quadrangularis

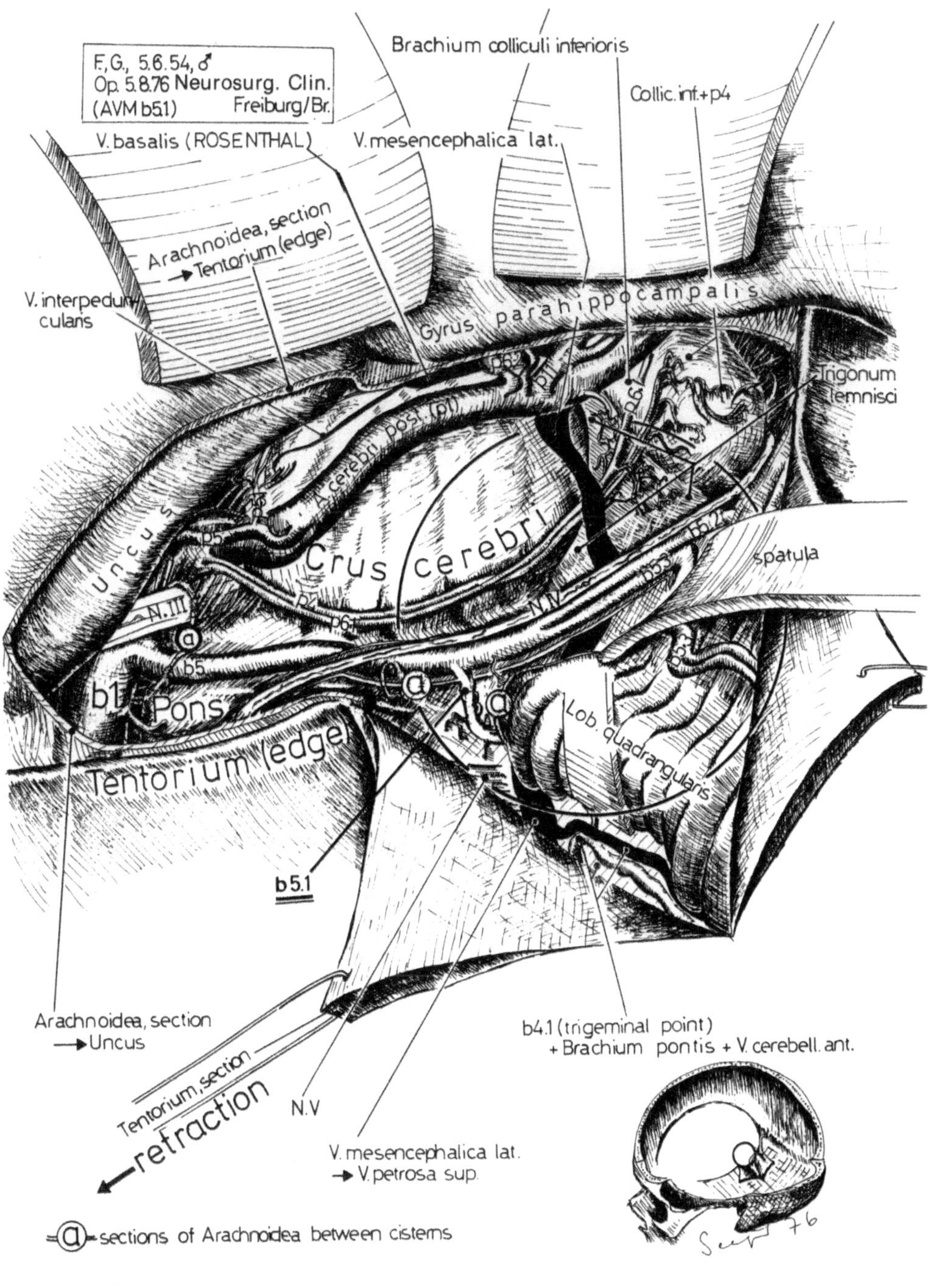
F.,G., 5.6.54, ♂
Op. 5.8.76 Neurosurg. Clin.
(AVM b5.1) Freiburg/Br.
Brachium colliculi inferioris
Collic. inf.+p4
V. basalis (ROSENTHAL)
V. mesencephalica lat.
Arachnoidea, section
→ Tentorium (edge)
V. interpeduncularis
Gyrus parahippocampalis
Trigonum lemnisci
Uncus
Crus cerebri
spatula
N.III
N.V
b1
Pons
Tentorium (edge)
Lob. quadrangularis
b5.1
Arachnoidea, section
→ Uncus
b4.1 (trigeminal point)
+ Brachium pontis + V. cerebell. ant.
Tentorium, section
retraction
N.V
V. mesencephalica lat.
→ V. petrosa sup.
(a) sections of Arachnoidea between cisterns

Chapter 6
Supratentorial Structures Near the Ventricles

A. Schematic Representation of Structural Composition

A knowledge of the relationships between Plexus chorioideus, Fornix, and Thalamus is the basis of an understanding of the structural composition of the ventricular system. After Plexus chorioideus is removed, Taenia fornicis can be seen to arise at Fornix, and Taenia chorioidea at Thalamus. A thin residual part of Pallium, which is attached to Stria medullaris and secondarily welded to the surface of Thalamus, is designated Lamina affixa. Taenia chorioidea passes round the thalamus as far as the roof of Cornu inf. After removal of Plexus chorioid. a gaping hole (= Fiss. chorioidea) is left between Taenia fornicis and Taenia chor., which now connects the lateral ventricle with the extracerebral space: under the lateral ventricle Fissura transversa cerebri, and medial to Cornu inf. the Cisterna ambiens.

The artificially formed Fissura chorioidea is illustrated schematically in Fig. 171. It marks the course of Plexus chor. Fig. 171 shows a model of the course of Fissura chorioidea: Caudatum and Lamina affixa are demonstrable separately from Fornix-Hippocampus-complex (*A* in Fig. 171). In *B* of Fig. 171 the two structures are dovetailed together and it can be seen that the darkly shaded floor of Cornu ant. and Atrium pass into the roof of Cornu inf. The medially lying, lightly sketched Fornix and Fimbria hippocampi pass into the floor of Cornu inf. Further neighbouring structures have been included in Fig. 172 in order to make the subsequent illustrations intelligible. Figs. 173 to 176 show the relationships of Fornix to its surroundings with progressive resection of Corpus callosum. In Figs. 177 to 180 an attempt has been made, by means of stepwise resection of Corpus callosum and Fornix, to elucidate schematically the attachment sites of Plexus chorioideus to Fornix and Pars affixa.

B. Discussion of (Anatomical) Preparations

On the outer surface of the brain the veins usually lie close to the surface, whereas the arteries pass freely in the cisternal space. After opening Fissura chorioidea (Fig. 181) the picture is reversed: Vv. cerebri intt. and V. cerebri magna (Galeni) run medially in the C. S. F. space of Fissura transversa. The branches of A. chorioidea post. lie close to the surface of the thalamus. The lateral branches of Aa. chorioideae postt. may take a particularly regular course (*p6.2.2.2*), apart from exceptions (Fig. 182, left half of picture).
The anterior part of the floor of the lateral ventricle shows V. thalamostriata. The typical acute-angled form of its Angulus venosus can only be seen on lateral X-ray projection. In reality it is a wide arch of V. thalamostriata which extends along the margin of Caudatum and usually under Stria medullaris in a medial direction. In the area of Caudatum, V., thalamostriata may still lie rostrally to Foramen interventriculare (Monroi) in lateral projection (see Fig. 182, left half of anatomical preparation). It may also pass as the so-called V. lateralis directa far behind Foramen interventriculare (Monroi) across and over the thalamus (see Fig. 182, right half of preparation, see also Newton and Potts, 1974). Thus its value as a neuroradiological criterium for the assessment of mass displacement is poor. After crossing under Plexus chorioideus, V. thalamostriata passes into V. cerebri int. which runs in the extracerebral space (Fissura transversa cerebri). There it takes up V. septi pellucidi outside the ventricular system (Fig. 182). Here too exceptions are possible whereby V. septi pellucidi enters intraventricularly (Fig. 185). Intraventricularly the veins run subependymally, and extraventricularly in the C. S. F.-filled arachnoidal trabecular system of Fissura transversa cerebri.
The medial ventricle wall shows V. septi pellucidi with crossover of the fornix (Fig. 181). The pos-

terior septal veins which pass between Septum pellucidum and Crus fornicis subependymally are particularly variable. The third group of medial ventricular veins, the medial atrial veins, pass from the fibres of Corpus callosum in the ventricular triangle to Crus fornicis and Hippocampus (Figs. 181, 182 and 184). In contrast to the other two groups of veins, they enter V. basalis (Rosenthal), and not V. cerebri interna.

The lateral ventricle wall exhibits V. thalamostriata anteriorly. Usually V. thalamostriata terminates before the ventricular triangle (Figs. 181 and 182). At the level of Pulvinar thalami and the roof of Cornu inf. beside Stria medullaris and Cauda nuclei caudati runs the inferior ventricular vein, which can easily be damaged in the effort to free Plexus chorioideus. It may occur as a continuation of V. thalamostriata. The veins passing over Corpus nuclei caudati, the lateral atrial veins, may also run into an inferior ventricular vein, which does not follow the course of Stria terminalis. It then passes directly over Pulvinar thalami to V. basalis (Rosenthal) (Fig. 182, left half of picture). The typical course is illustrated in Fig. 184. These veins are thus unsuitable as reference structures at radiological examination or intraventricular operations. Since they drain approximately 1 cm of brain substance under the surface of the ventricular system, their preservation is necessary in view of the importance of the brain structures drained. Further details of variability and fine arborization can be obtained from Newton and Potts (1974) and from Hölzel (1977). Only in cases of ventricular enlargement is the relief of Caudatum, Stria medullaris, and Lamina affixa thalami up to the insertion of Plexus chorioideus flat and difficult to recognize. Due to the vaulting of the thalamus, Foramen interventriculare (Monroi) cannot be seen into from the occipital direction; this is possible only from the frontal or parietal direction.

The lateral tip-vein should be mentioned as the last lateral vein coming from the roof of the ventricle. It can very easily be damaged during isolation of the temporal lobe. Like the inferior ventricular vein, it enters V. basalis (Rosenthal) at the level of Cornu inferius. The relationships between Cornu inf. and V. basalis (Rosenthal), which lies in Cisterna ambiens, can be seen after splitting Fissura chorioidea and removing Plexus chorioideus (Fig. 184).

If Plexus chorioideus of the lateral ventricle is removed, and the posterior end of Corpus callosum including the fornix cut and opened up, the whole Fissura transversa cerebri lies exposed (see Figs. 182 and 183). Between the fornix and thalamus there is a loose arachnoidal trabecular system, interlaced with small branches of A. chorioidea post., and veins, running to Fornix and Corpus callosum. Tela chorioidea ventriculi tertii is a tough, vascular arachnoidal sheet which not only adjoins the roof of the 3rd ventricle (Fig. 183) but also covers the extraventricular free part of Thalamus. In a posterior direction Tela chorioidea ventriculi III merges into the, also dense, tightly knit arachnoidal network of Cisterna quadrigemina. The rule applies here that the veins supplying the quadrigeminal region lie medially, and the arteries laterally (*A* in Fig. 183). They become visible at anatomical or neurosurgical preparation if Culmen of Cerebellum is somewhat retracted. At the same time the neighbouring medial veins of Cerebellum become visible. The most important lateral vein which should be preserved at operation is V. basalis (Rosenthal), which is usually spanned by arteries. Thus in the region of Cisterna ambiens the principle is maintained that cerebral veins keep close to the surface and arteries run freely in the cisternal space.

Fig. 185 shows the close relationships between Foramen interventriculare (Monroi), the anterior portion of Plexus chorioideus, and Fissura transversa cerebri (Tela chorioidea ventriculi tertii). In the preparation of Fig. 185 note the intraventricular entry of V. septi pellucidi after it has initially passed under or through Plexus chor. to reach the extracerebral space of Fissura transversa. When tumours in the 3rd ventricle are prepared through Foramen interventriculare (Monroi) attention must be paid to the positional relationships between Columna fornicis, the most anterior portion of the thalamus, V. thalamostriata, V. septi pellucidi, and Plexus chorioideus. Therefore in Figs. 186 and 187 these positional relationships between Commissura ant., Columnae fornicis, and Lamina terminalis are shown.

Fig. 188 is a schematic reproduction of a preparation from an elderly person with atrophic enlargement of the ventricular system. The otherwise cramped space of the 3rd ventricle does not normally allow an oblique view of these structures. Similarly in enlargement of the 3rd tumours or hydrocephalus ventricle is to be expected.

The structural composition of the brain in the vicinity of the wall of the 3rd ventricle is difficult to understand because of its deep position between the basal ganglia and the long tracts. The preparations reproduced in Figs. 189 to 196 are intended to clarify this complicated spatial structural composition. Details of the nuclear regions and the white matter have been given in serial sections with staining of the matter by Zuleger and Staubesand (1976).

C. Preoperative Radiology – Some Aspects

In ventriculography the relief of the wall structures is of particular interest. Ventriculograms with positivecontrast media give a plastic impression of the structures near the ventricles, of a kind which was formerly only possible with cast preparations. A cast by Retzius published in 1900 (quoted according to Corales and Torrealba, 1976), is reproduced in Figs. 197 and 198. The designations chosen by Retzius are not all contained in the Basle or the Paris nomenclature. The structural peculiarities in the immediate neighbourhood of Sulcus hypothalamicus up to Recessus opticus are, however, of increasing clinical significance at the present time.

D. Operative Techniques – Some Aspects

The distance measurements at the floor of the lateral ventricle from the dorsal direction are given in Fig. 199. Ventricular puncture requires an exact knowledge of the positional relationships between the external surface of the skull and the ventricular system.

Details of the surface relief of the skull are inadequately described in the anatomical literature. In clinical work, too, they are neglected, as can be seen from the modern schematized illustrations of the skull. The varying irregularities of the convexity of the skull stand out under the skin of the shaved head. The course of the sutures in visible externally. The anatomical research of earlier authors also served artistic expression (Fig. 200). They exhibit exaggerations of structural irregularities which can facilitate the localization of the skull sutures for the clinician (Fig. 201).

Distance measurements of topographic orientation points on the surface of the head (skull) are given in Fig. 202 for orientation before carrying out ventricular puncture. With regard to the localization of Foramen interventriculare (Monroi), the reader is referred to Rothman et al. (1976). The data given by Robertson and Denton (1973) were tested on a skull preparation into which an almost congruent formalinfixed brain had been inserted (in collaboration with Gilsbach and Friedrich). Section preparations were made according to the directions of the punctures. Figs. 203 and 204 are taken from these preparations and demonstrate the possibilities of injury to important cerebral structures resulting from faulty attempts at puncturing.

In the vicinity of the foramen of Monro, particular attention should be paid to the medial position of Genu capsulae internae (Fig. 205). Immediately laterally to the foramen of Monro and Massa intermedia lie tracts which serve the upper extremities. This relationship is also important at operations in the region of the 3rd ventricle.

Details of brain structure in the vicinity of the ventricles are given in the voluminous literature on stereotactic brain surgery. (For a general survey see Schaltenbrand, 1959; for Thalamus see van Buren, 1972).

E. References

Van Buren, J. M., Boske, R. C.: Variations and Connections of the Human Thalamus. Berlin–Heidelberg–New York: Springer. 1972.
Corales, M., Torrealba, G.: The third ventricle. Normal anatomy and changes in some pathological conditions. Neuroradiology **11**, 271–277 (1976).
Hölzel, G.: Dissertation Freiburg 1978.
Kalkar, J., s. Vesalius, A.
Newton, Th., Potts, D. G.: Radiology of the Skull and Brain Angiography. St. Louis: The C. V. Mosby Company. 1974.
Retzius, C., s. Corales, M., Torrealba, G.
Robertson, J. T., Denton, J. C.: Neurological Surgery, **I**, p. 229–234, ed. by Youmans, J. R. Philadelphia–London–Toronto: Saunders Company. 1973.
Rothman, S. L. G., Allen, W. E., III, Simeone, J. F.: The medial posterior choroidal artery as an indicator of masses at the foramen of Monroi. Neuroradiology **11**, 123–12 (1976).
Schaltenbrand, G., Bailey, P.: Introduction to Stereotaxis With an Atlas of the Human Brain. Stuttgart: G. Thieme. 1959.
Vesalius, A.: De corporis humani fabrica. Baseliensis 1543.
Leonardo da Vinci s. Braunfeld-Esche, S.: Leonardo da Vinci. Das anatomische Werk. 6. Aufl. Wiesbaden–Berlin: E Vollmer. 1955.
Zuleger, S., Staubesand, J.: Schnittbilder des Zentralnervensystems. München–Wien–Baltimore: Urban & Schwarzenberg. 1976.

Literature for Further Reading

Agnoli, A., et al.: Diagnostische Möglichkeiten der positiven Ventrikulographie. Acta Neurochir. (Wien) **31**, 227–24 (1975).

Dürer, A.: Alberti Dureri, clarissimi pictoris et geometrae de symmetria partium in rectis formis humanorum corporum. Nürnberg: Libri in Latinum conversi. 1532.

Giannotta, S. L., et al.: Epidermoid cyst of the third ventricle. Surg. Neurol. **5**, 164–166 (1976).

Kahle, W., Leonhardt, H., Platzer, W.: Nervensystem und Sinnesorgane. dtv-Atlas der Anatomie, Bd. 3. Stuttgart: G. Thieme. 1976.

Krogness, K. G.: Normal position of the aqueduct of Sylvius. J. Neurosurg. **42**, 499–502 (1975).

F. Illustrations
(Figs. 171 to 205)

Figs. 171. Fissura chorioidea, model of structural composition
A Neighbouring structures taken apart
B Neighbouring structures put together

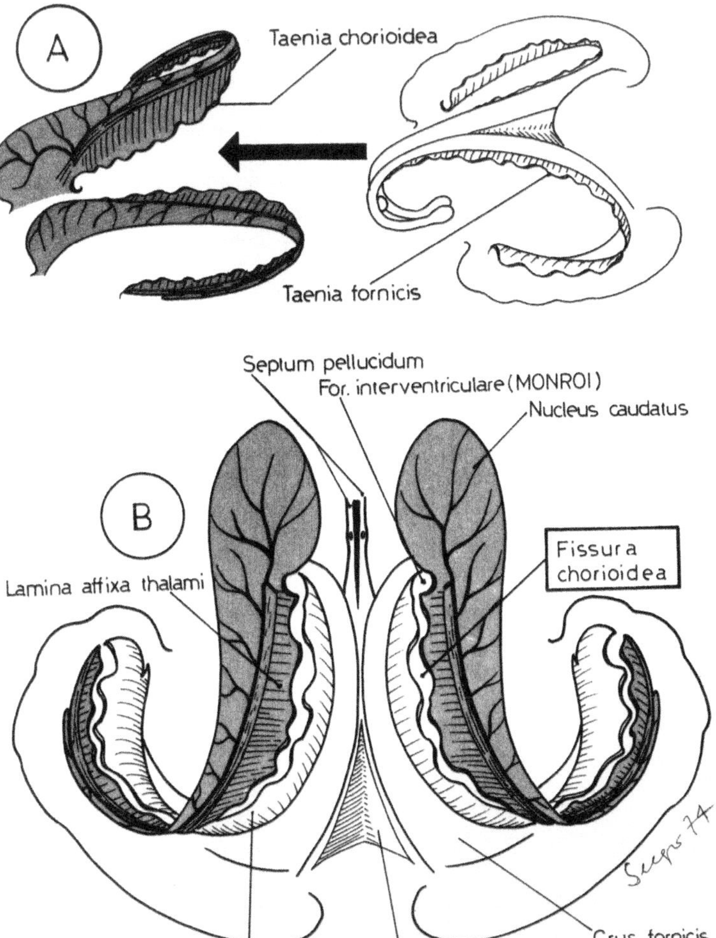
A
Taenia chorioidea
Taenia fornicis
Septum pellucidum
For. interventriculare (MONROI)
Nucleus caudatus
B
Fissura chorioidea
Lamina affixa thalami
Crus fornicis
Commissura fornicis
Pulvinar thalami

Fig. 172. Neighbourhood of ventricular system. Nomenclature applies also to Figs. 173 to 180

1 a Rostrum corporis callosi
1 b Genu corporis callosi
1 c Truncus corporis callosi
1 d Splenium corporis callosi
1 e Splenium corporis callosi
2 Commissura ant.
3 Lamina terminalis
4 a Corpus mamillare
4 b Columna fornicis (Pars tecta)
4 c Columna fornicis (Pars libera)
4 d Corpus fornicis
4 e Corpus fornicis/Commissura fornicis
4 f Crus fornicis
4 g Taenia fornicis et Fimbria hippocampi
4 h Insertion of Septum pellucidum at Corpus callosum
4 i Septum pellucidum, Cavum septi pellucidi
4 k Hippocampus
5 Foramen interventriculare (Monroi)
6 a Caput nuclei caudati
6 b Corpus nuclei caudati
6 c Cauda nuclei caudati
7 a Pulvinar thalami
7 b Corpus geniculatum mediale, Corpus geniculatum laterale
8 a Colliculus superior, Brachium colliculi superioris
8 b Colliculus inferior, Brachium colliculi inferioris
9 Velum medullare ant., Brachium conjunctivum
10 Brachium pontis
11 a Ventriculus III
11 b Ventriculus IV
12 Fissura transversa cerebri (pulled apart by lifting Corpus callosum and Fornix, arrow)
13 Corpus pineale

FIG. 172

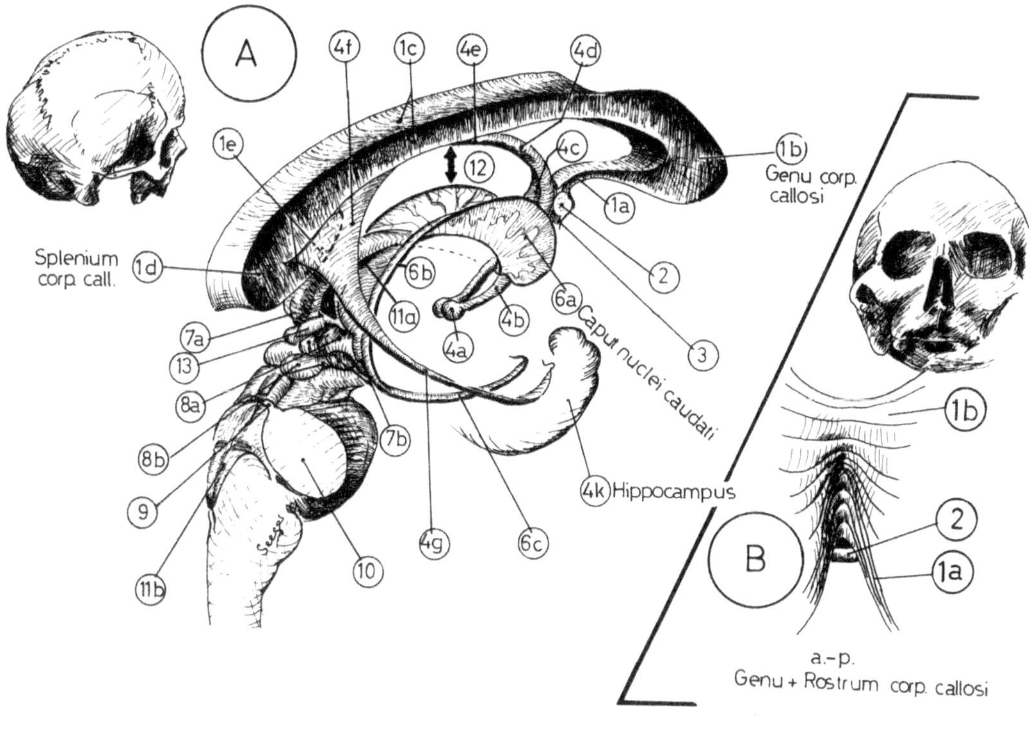
A
4f
1c
4e
4d
1e
12
4c
1b
Genu corp. callosi
1a
2
Splenium corp. call.
1d
6b
6a
11a
4b
4a
3
Caput nuclei caudati
7a
13
8a
7b
8b
9
4k Hippocampus
11b
10
4g
6c
B
1b
2
1a
a.-p.
Genu + Rostrum corp. callosi

Fig. 173. Schematic drawing of Corpus callosum, Fornix, and anterior diencephalic structures, simplified (Genu-Rostrum-block shown transverse instead of forceps-like)*. Lateral (et anterior et basal) view. Pars tecta fornicis left in situ after removal of remaining parts of the 3rd ventricle wall
For nomenclature see Fig. 172

* In the meantime a similar schematic presentation appeared by Kahle, W., M. Leonhard, and W. Platzer (1976).

Fig. 174. Structures of Fig. 173 seen from oblique basal direction, simplified (Genu-Rostrum-radiation, and Lamina terminalis drawn transversely instead of forceps-like)
For nomenclature see Fig. 172

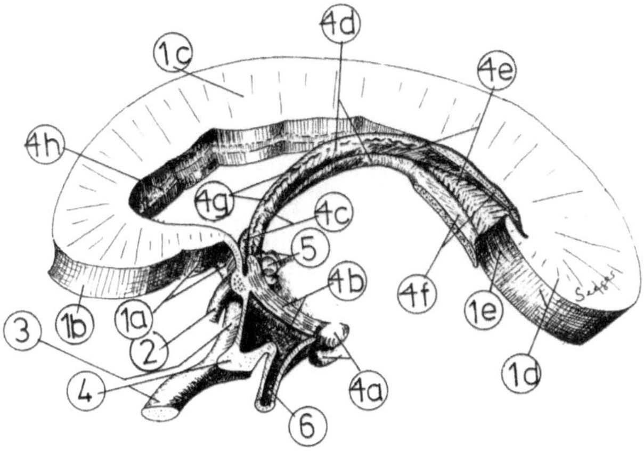
1c
4d
4e
4h
4g
4c
5
4b
4f
1e
1b
1a
2
3
4
4a
6
1d

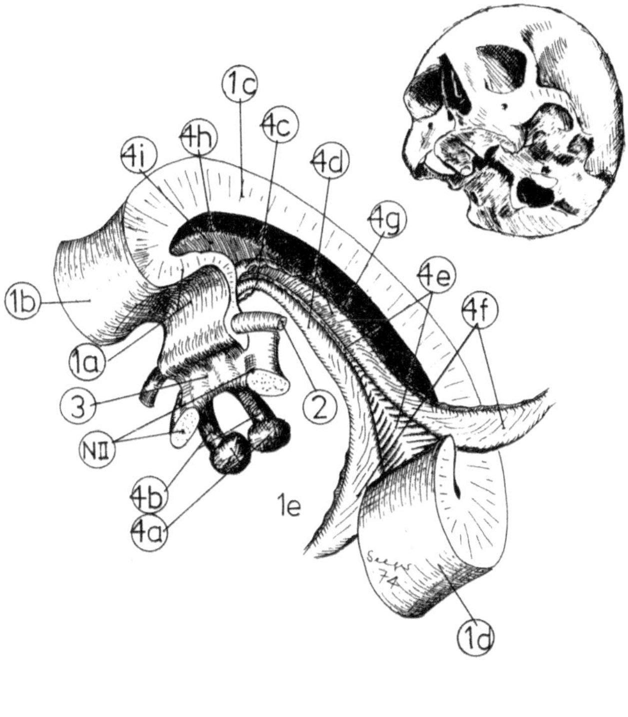
1c
4h
4c
4i
4d
4g
4e
4f
1b
1a
2
3
NII
4b
4a
1e
1d

Fig. 175. Structures of Figs. 173 and 174. Rostrum and Genu corporis callosi removed
For nomenclature see Fig. 172

Fig. 176. Structures of Fig. 175, with further anterior parts of Corpus callosum removed
For nomenclature see Fig. 172

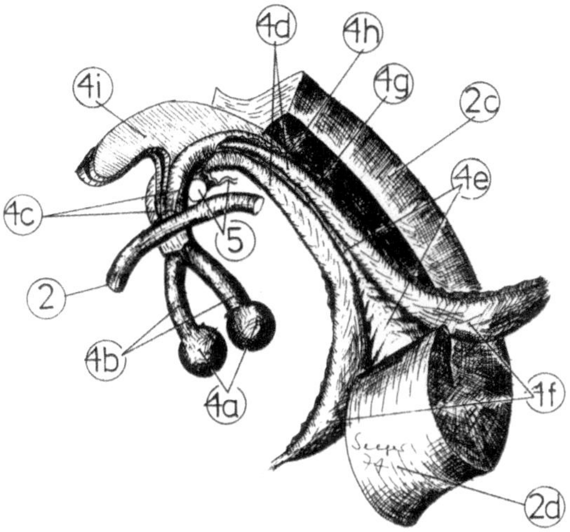
4d
4h
4i
4g
2c
4e
4c
5
2
4b
4a
4f
Seeger 74
2d

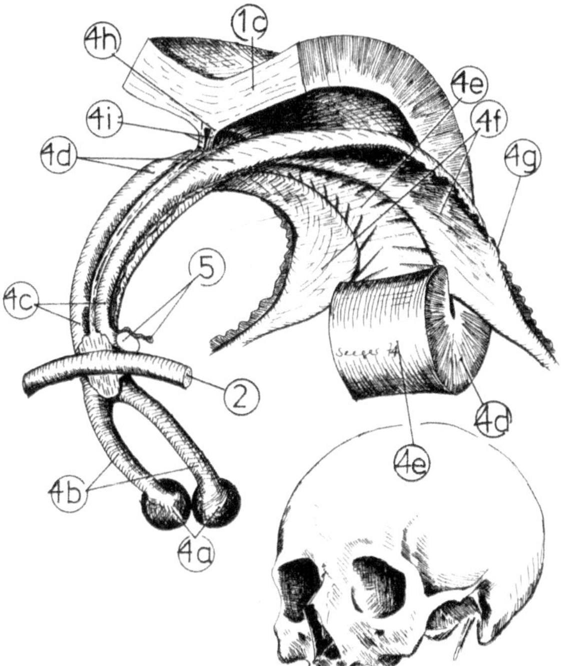
4h
1c
4e
4i
4f
4d
4g
5
4c
2
4d
4e
4b
4a

Fig. 177. Schematic drawing of right lateral ventricle from above. Parts of Corpus callosum and Fornix removed. Relationships between Fornix (*4c, d, f, g*) and Commissura fornicis (*4e*) to Corpus callosum (Septum pellucidum resected). Insertion of resected Plexus chorioideus at Fornix (Taenia fornicis) and at Lamina affixa (Taenia chorioidea). Splenium corporis callosi rolled up (*1d-e*)
For nomenclature see Fig. 172

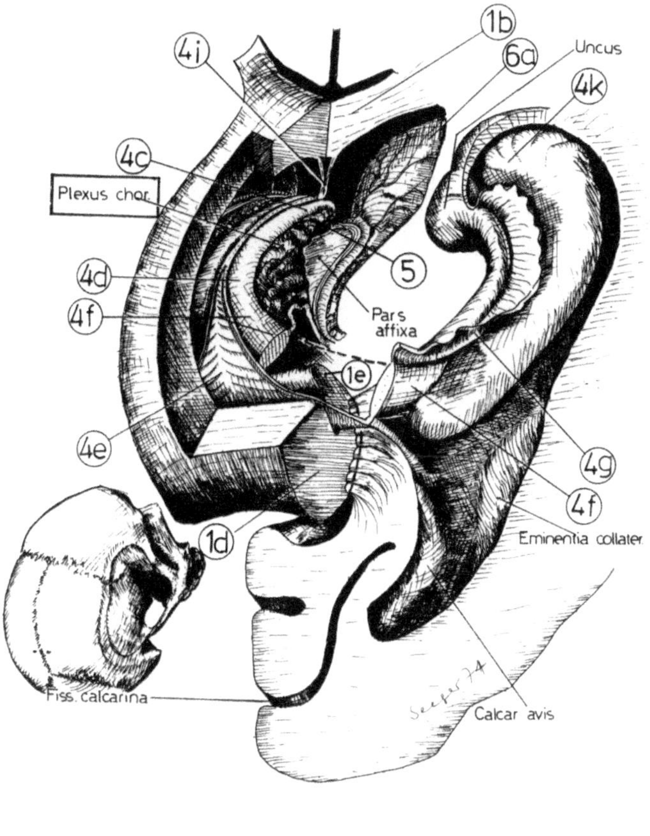
1b
4i
6a
Uncus
4k
4c
Plexus chor.
5
4d
Pars
affixa
4f
1e
4e
4g
4f
1d
Eminentia collater.
Fiss. calcarina
Calcar avis
Seeger 74

Fig. 178. Detail of schematically drawn preparation of Fig. 177. Further parts of Corpus callosum removed. View into both lateral ventricles. Relationships between Plexus chorioideus, Fornix (4d), and Lamina affixa
For nomenclature see Fig. 172

Fig. 179. Exhibit of Fig. 178 after removal of further portions of Fornix, in order to show the relationships between Plexus chorioideus, Fornix, and Thalamus
For nomenclature see Fig. 172

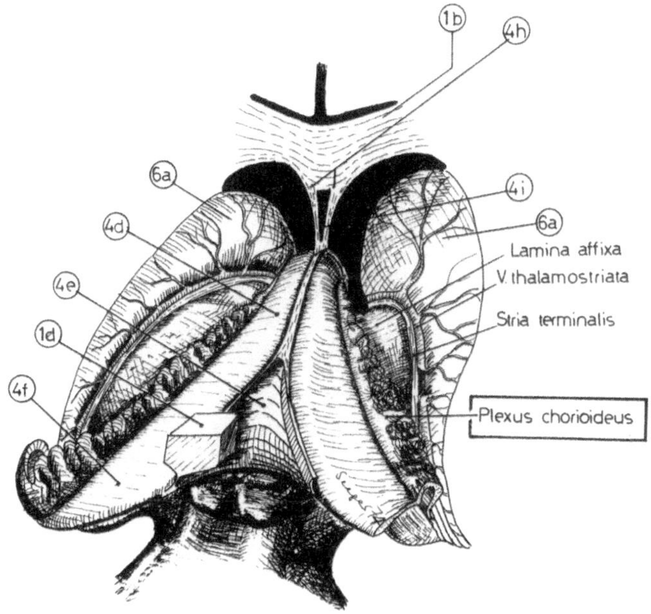
1b
4h
6a
4i
6a
4d
Lamina affixa
V. thalamostriata
4e
Stria terminalis
1d
4f
Plexus chorioideus

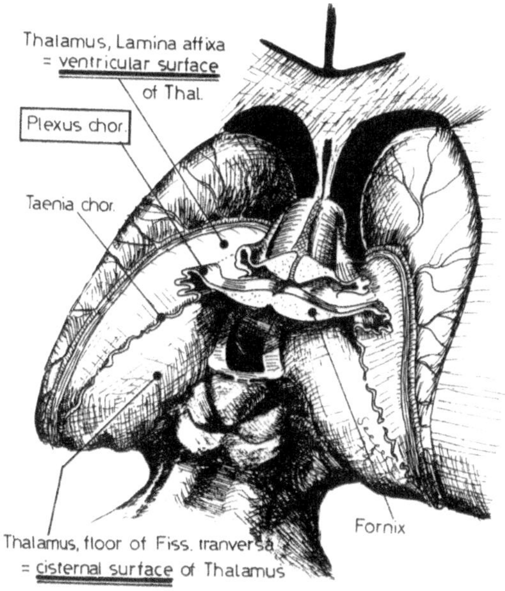
Thalamus, Lamina affixa
= ventricular surface
of Thal.
Plexus chor.
Taenia chor.
Fornix
Thalamus, floor of Fiss. tranversa
= cisternal surface of Thalamus

Fig. 180. Exhibit of Fig. 179, posterior parts of Fornix and Plexus chorioideus completely removed. Genu corporis callosi and Columnae fornicis left in situ
For nomenclature see Fig. 172

FIG. 180

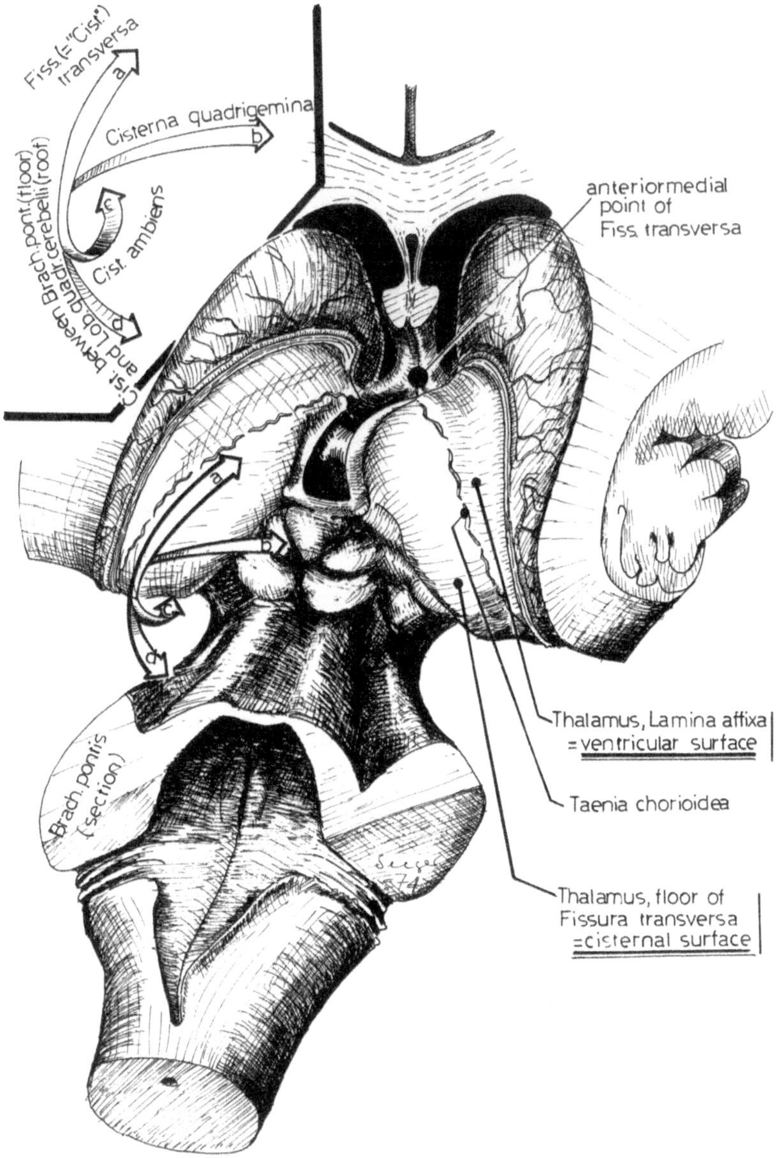
Fiss.(="Cist.") transversa
a
Cisterna quadrigemina
b
Cist. between Brach. pont. (floor) and Lob. quadr. cerebelli (root)
c
Cist. ambiens
d
anteriormedial point of Fiss. transversa
a
b
c
d
Brach. pontis (section)
Thalamus, Lamina affixa =ventricular surface
Taenia chorioidea
Thalamus, floor of Fissura transversa =cisternal surface

Fig. 181. View into the ventricular system from above. Plexus chorioideus removed. Medial ventricle wall under lateral retraction (arrows), causing Fissura chorioidea to gape wide open between Taenia fornicis and Taenia chorioidea. Arteries and veins of Fissura transversa become visible in Fissura chorioidea (branches of A. chorioidea post. and veins). The veins of the ventricle wall run subependymally, and the extraventricular veins run between arachnoidal trabeculae

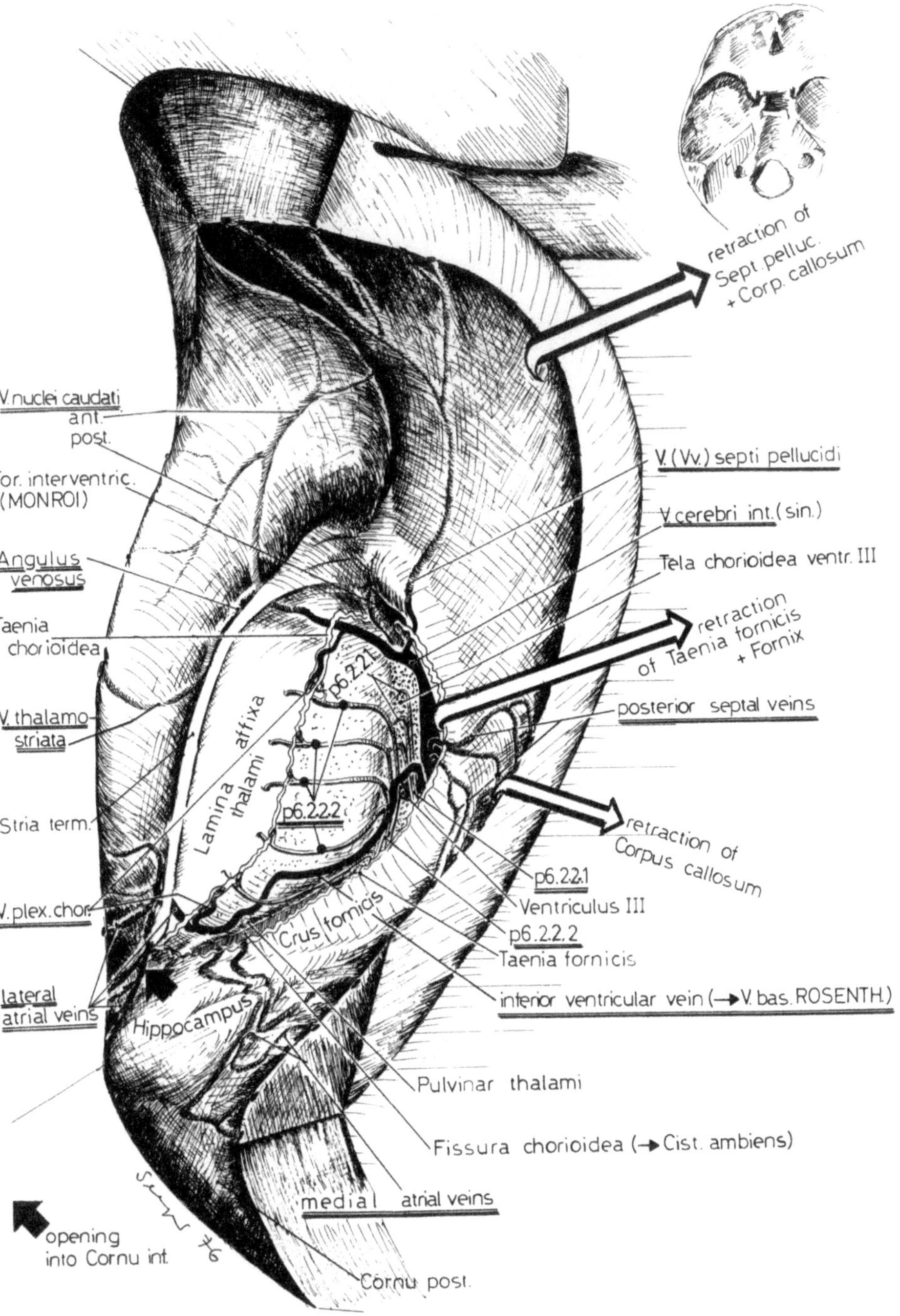
retraction of
Sept. pelluc.
+ Corp. callosum
V. nuclei caudati
ant.
post.
For. interventric.
(MONROI)
Angulus
venosus
Taenia
chorioidea
V. thalamo-
striata
Stria term.
V. plex. chor.
lateral
atrial veins
Hippocampus
Lamina affixa
thalami
p6.2.2.2
p6.2.2.2
Crus fornicis
V. (Vv.) septi pellucidi
V. cerebri int. (sin.)
Tela chorioidea ventr. III
retraction
of Taenia fornicis
+ Fornix
posterior septal veins
retraction of
Corpus callosum
p6.2.2.1
Ventriculus III
p6.2.2.2
Taenia fornicis
inferior ventricular vein (→ V. bas. ROSENTH.)
Pulvinar thalami
Fissura chorioidea (→ Cist. ambiens)
medial atrial veins
opening
into Cornu int.
Cornu post.

Fig. 182. Fissura transversa cerebri. View from above. Crura fornicis and Splenium corporis callosi have been cut through and pulled up in the rostral direction (arrow). The branches of A. chorioidea post. (*p6.2.2.2*) may run regularly and parallel (see right thalamus surface) or irregularly (see left thalamus surface). Irregular under- or overcrossing of large venous trunks by arteries in the region of the inner cerebral veins. Dorsal to the veins: A. corporis callosi (*p10*) (for arteries see also arterial catalogue, pages 3–4)

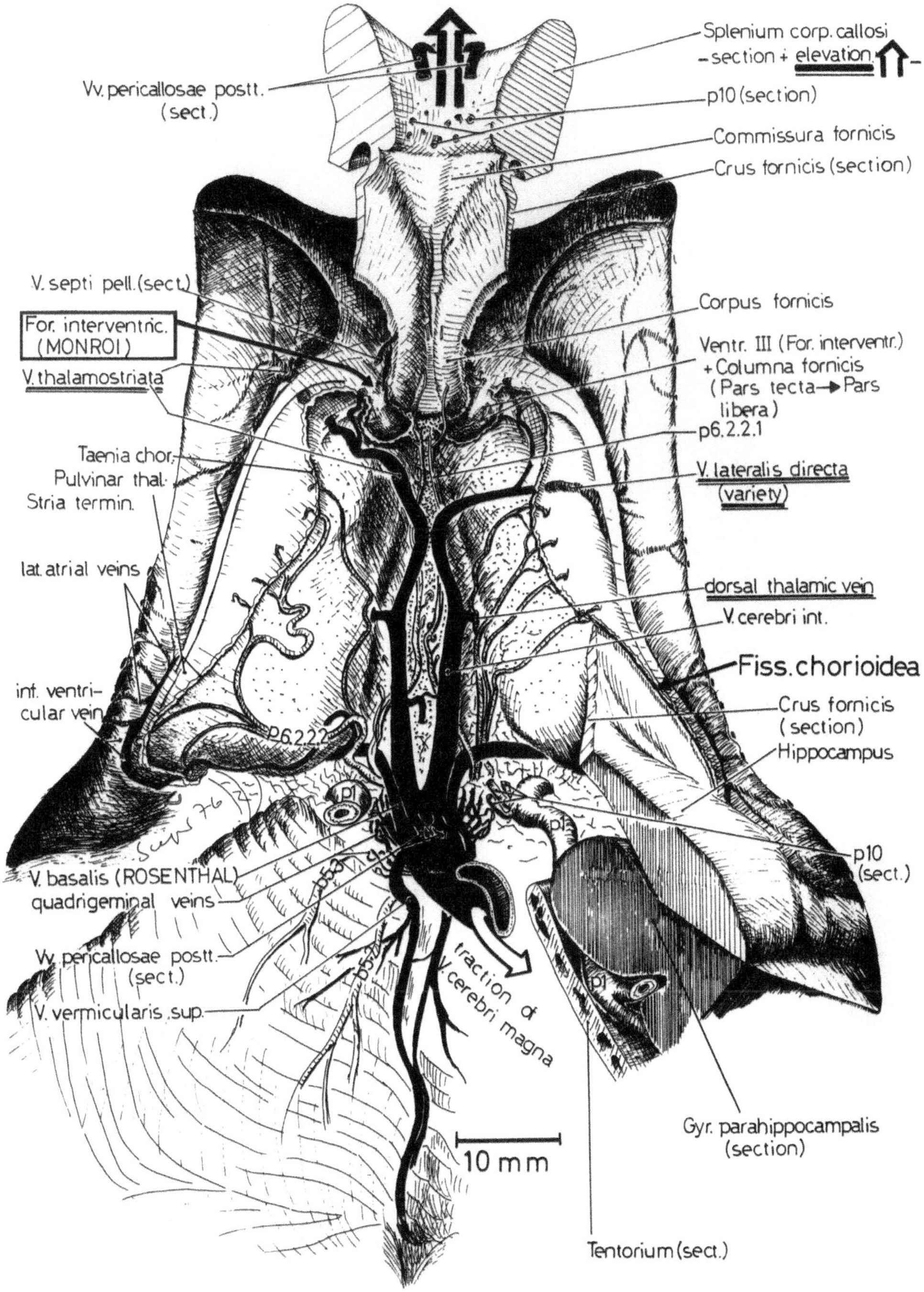
Splenium corp. callosi
- section + elevation
Vv. pericallosae postt. (sect.)
p10 (section)
Commissura fornicis
Crus fornicis (section)
V. septi pell. (sect.)
For. interventric. (MONROI)
V. thalamostriata
Corpus fornicis
Ventr. III (For. interventr.)
+ Columna fornicis
(Pars tecta → Pars libera)
p6.2.2.1
Taenia chor.
Pulvinar thal.
Stria termin.
V. lateralis directa (variety)
lat. atrial veins
dorsal thalamic vein
V. cerebri int.
Fiss. chorioidea
inf. ventri-cular vein
p6.2.2.2
Crus fornicis (section)
Hippocampus
p1
p10 (sect.)
V. basalis (ROSENTHAL)
quadrigeminal veins
Vv. pericallosae postt. (sect.)
V. vermicularis sup.
traction of V. cerebri magna
10 mm
Gyr. parahippocampalis (section)
Tentorium (sect.)

Fig. 183. Fissura transversa cerebri. View from above. Culmen and the divided large venous trunks retracted (arrows) in order to visualize Lamina quadrigemina.

A Floor area of Fissura transversa between the two Taeniae chorioideae after removal of Tela chorioidea ventriculi tertii, including whole Plexus chorioideus from lateral ventricle and 3rd ventricle. Quadrigeminal veins medially from different sources of cerebellar veins in front of Lobulus centralis cerebelli. Arteries of Lamina quadrigemina coming from lateral direction (*p4* A. quadrigemina, *p8* A. thalamo-geniculata, *p6* . . . branches of A. chorioidea post., *b5* A. cerebelli superior).

B Vessels of Tela chorioidea ventriculi tertii and adjacent vascular region at Culmen cerebelli

Arrow: V. cerebri magna (Galeni) retracted backwards

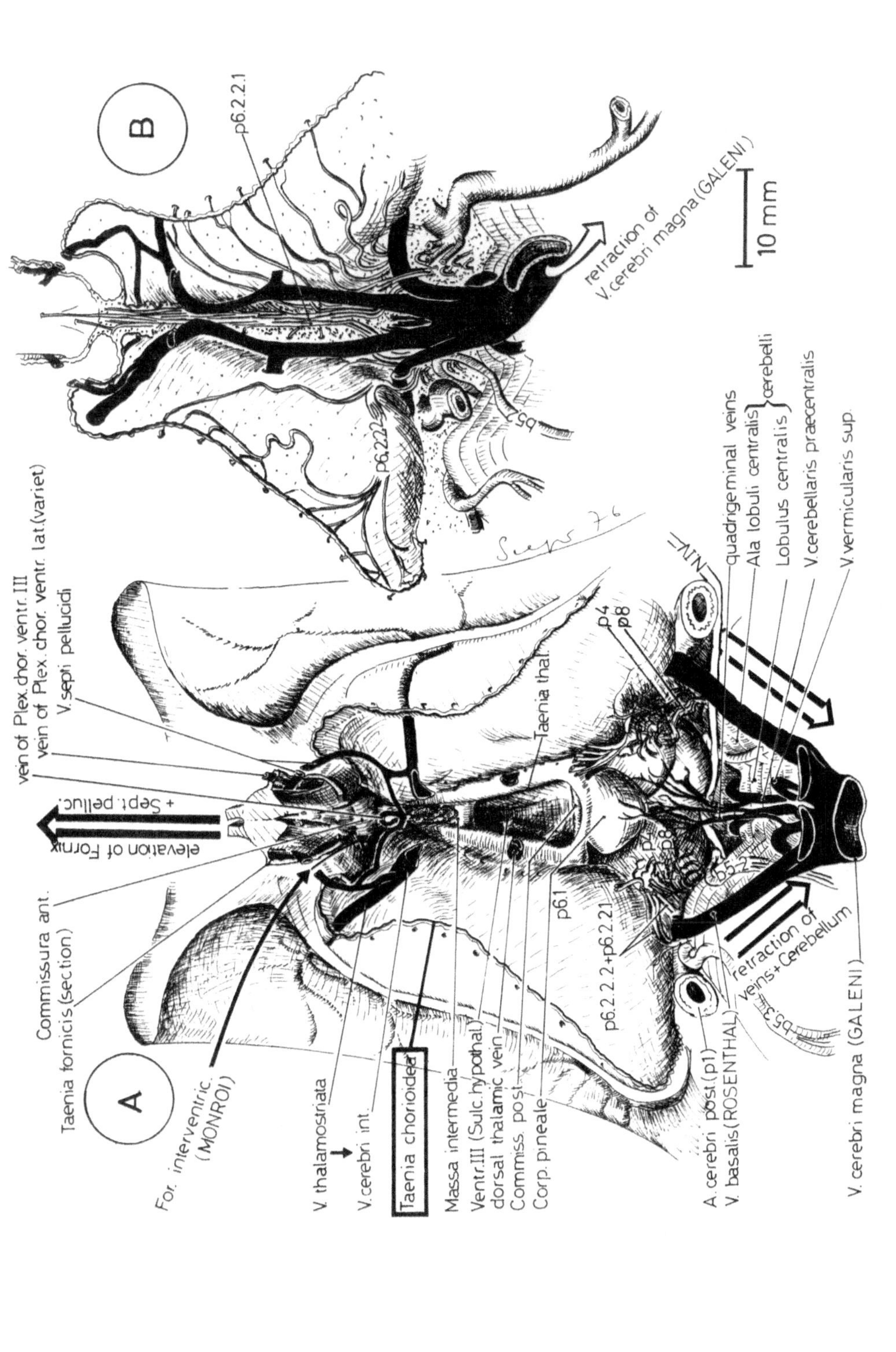
A
B
Taenia fornicis (section)
Commissura ant.
For. interventric. (MONROI)
V. thalamostriata
V. cerebri int.
Taenia chorioidea
Massa intermedia
Ventr.III (Sulc.hypothal.)
dorsal thalamic vein
Commiss. post.
Corp. pineale
A. cerebri post. (p1)
V. basalis (ROSENTHAL)
V. cerebri magna (GALENI)
vein of Plex. chor. ventr. III
vein of Plex. chor. ventr. lat. (variet)
V. septi pellucidi
elevation of Fornix + Sept. pelluc.
Taenia thal.
p6.1
p6.2.2.2+p6.2.2.1
p4
p8
b5.2
b5.3
N.IV
retraction of veins+Cerebellum
quadrigeminal veins
Ala lobuli centralis
Lobulus centralis
cerebelli
V. cerebellaris praecentralis
V. vermicularis sup.
p6.2.2.1
p6.2.2.2
b5
retraction of V. cerebri magna (GALENI)
10 mm

Fig. 184. Lobus temporalis with opening of Cornu inferius and Trigonum ventriculi lateralis. View of Cisterna ambiens through the gaping Fissura chorioidea

A General view

B Detail of preparation. The temporal lobe is dissected and unfolded (see both halves of Uncus). Plexus chorioideus removed. Between Taenia fornicis/Fimbria hippocampi and Taenia chorioidea the Cisterna ambiens with its vessels gapes wide open. V. basalis (Rosenthal) follows the surface of the brain more closely than the branches of A. chor. post. (*p6* ...), see also catalogue of arteries, pages 3–4. Vessels of Cornu inf. tip at Uncus: Arteries: A. chorioidea ant. (*c5*), also a sturdy terminal branch of A. chorioidea post. (*). Veins: lateral tip-vein, which may participate in drainage of roof of Cornu inf. and parts of Tractus opticus, Corpus geniculatum laterale, and of Crus cerebri at transition to internal capsule. It tears off easily at resection of Plexus chorioideus. The inferior ventricular vein may also run up to the tip of Cornu inferius

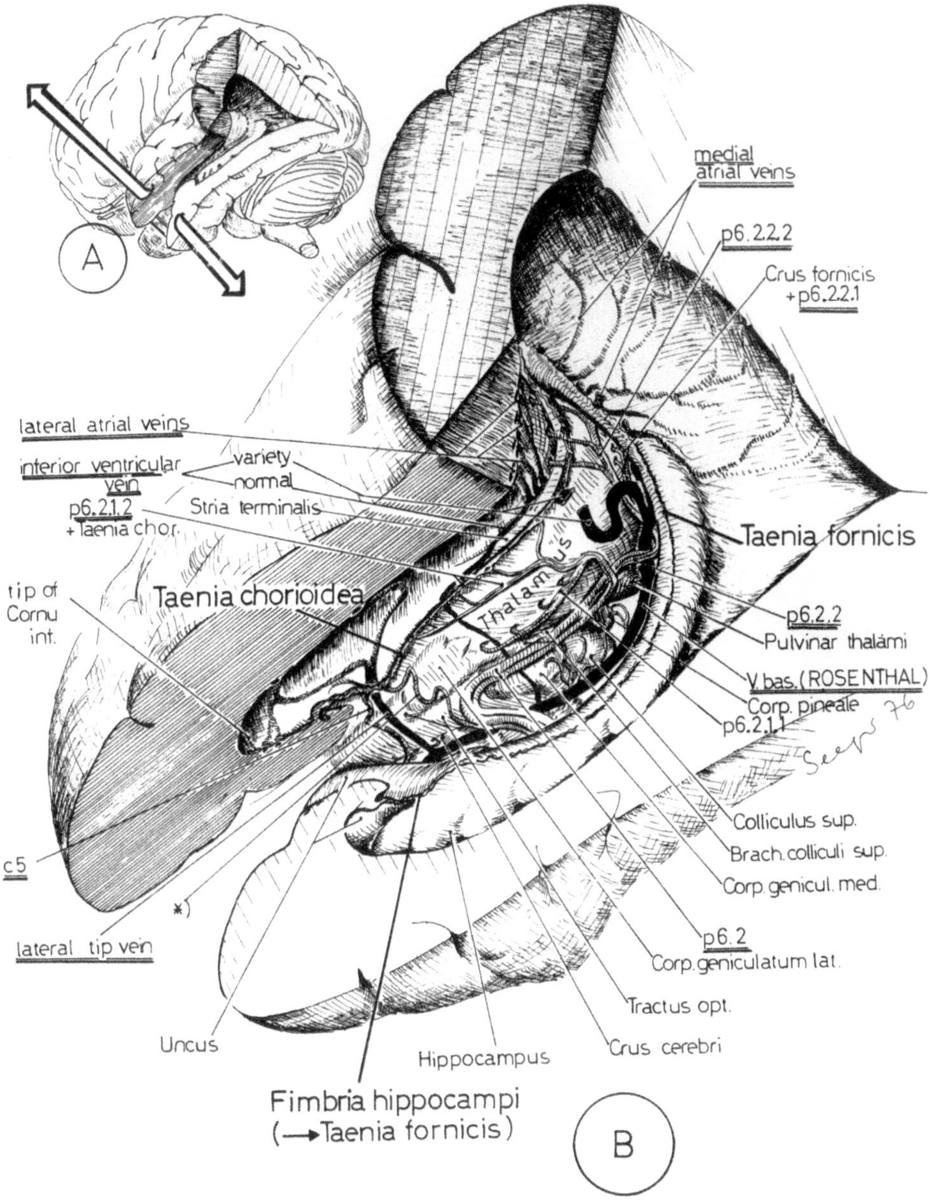
A
medial atrial veins
p6.2.2.2
Crus fornicis + p6.2.2.1
lateral atrial veins
interior ventricular vein
variety
normal
p6.2.1.2 + Taenia chor.
Stria terminalis
Taenia fornicis
tip of Cornu int.
Taenia chorioidea
Thalamus
p6.2.2
Pulvinar thalami
V. bas. (ROSENTHAL)
Corp. pineale
p6.2.1.1
Colliculus sup.
Brach. colliculi sup.
Corp. genicul. med.
c5
*)
lateral tip vein
p6.2
Corp. geniculatum lat.
Tractus opt.
Uncus
Hippocampus
Crus cerebri
Fimbria hippocampi (→Taenia fornicis)
B

Fig. 185. Vicinity of Foramen interventriculare (Monroi) seen from above and behind. Frontal section a few mm behind Foramen interventriculare (Monroi). Angulus venosus can posteriorly border Foramen interventriculare (Monroi). The positional relationship of V. thalamostriata with Angulus venosus to Stria medullaris is typical. Occasionally it lies superficially to Stria medullaris, but is more firmly connected to Thalamus than to Fornix. Plexus chorioideus is served by transversely entering arteries and by longitudinally running veins

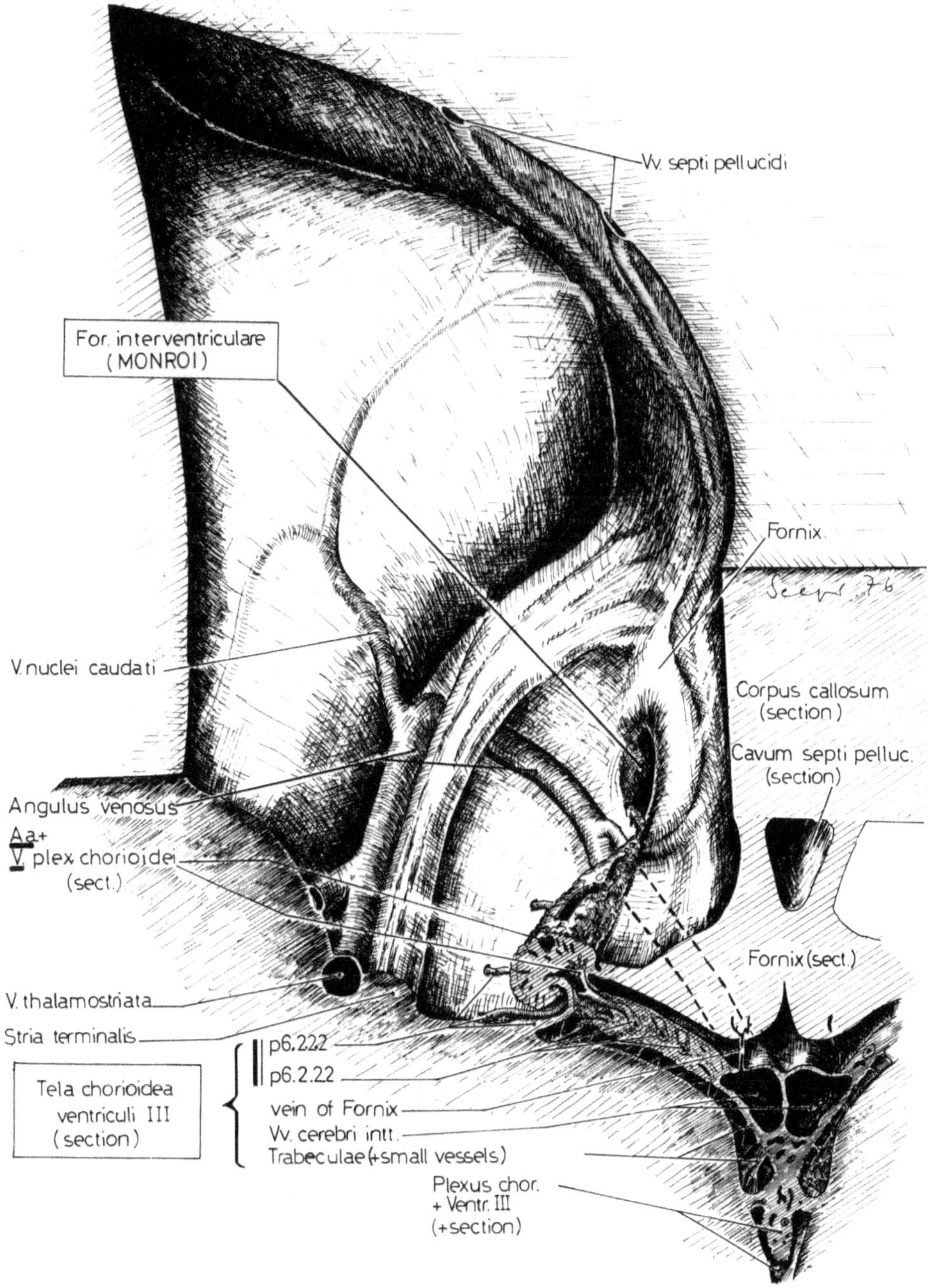

Vv. septi pellucidi
For. interventriculare (MONROI)
Fornix
V. nuclei caudati
Corpus callosum (section)
Cavum septi pelluc. (section)
Angulus venosus
Aa+ V. plex. chorioidei (sect.)
Fornix (sect.)
V. thalamostriata
Stria terminalis
p6.222
p6.2.22
Tela chorioidea ventriculi III (section)
vein of Fornix
Vv. cerebri intt.
Trabeculae (+small vessels)
Plexus chor. + Ventr. III (+section)

Fig. 186. Vicinity of Foramen interventriculare (Monroi), frontal sections

A Schematic drawing of transition from Plexus chorioideus of lateral ventricle into Plexus chorioideus of 3rd ventricle

B Enlarged detail from *A*. Foramen interventriculare (Monroi) bordered anteriorly by Columnae fornicis, posteriorly by transverse glial lamina strengthened with fibrous tissue (attachment point of Plexus chorioideus of lateral ventricle and 3rd ventricle). Arrow through Foramen interventriculare (Monroi) between Fornix and Plexus chorioideus to 3rd ventricle

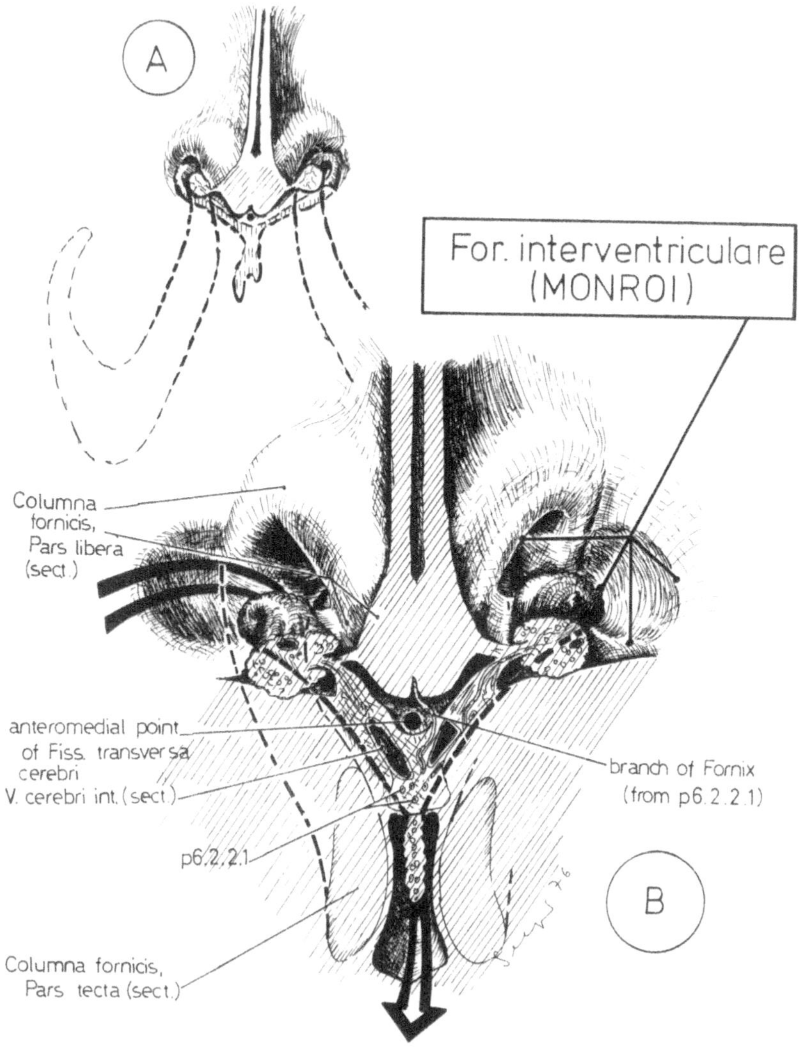
A
For. interventriculare (MONROI)
Columna fornicis, Pars libera (sect.)
anteromedial point of Fiss. transversa cerebri
V. cerebri int. (sect.)
p6.2.2.1
branch of Fornix (from p6.2.2.1)
B
Columna fornicis, Pars tecta (sect.)

Fig. 187. Relationships between Plexus chorioideus and Foramen interventriculare (Monroi) and to Fissura transversa cerebri, frontal section

A Plexus chorioideus of both lateral ventricles removed. Arrow in Foramen interventriculare (Monroi). Taenia fornicis terminates in fibrous-glial lamina (*a*), which borders both Foramina interventr. (Monroi) in posterior direction. Above this between the lamina (*a*) and Columnae fornicis is the rostrally narrowed Fissura transversa cerebri

B Exhibit *A* from oblique view

C Schematic oblique view of Plexus chorioideus of lateral ventricle and 3rd ventricle, with common point of attachment on posterior wall (*a*) of Foramina interventricularia (Monroi). Note the curving recess in Plexus chorioideus of the 3rd ventricle in the region of Massa intermedia. The longitudinal course of the veins of Plexus chorioideus with junction into V. basalis (Rosenthal) is typical. Larger venous connections in the region of Foramen interventriculare (Monroi) between Plexus chorioideus and V. thalamostriata are possible, also connections to the atrial veins, which tear easily at operative resection of Plexus chorioideus

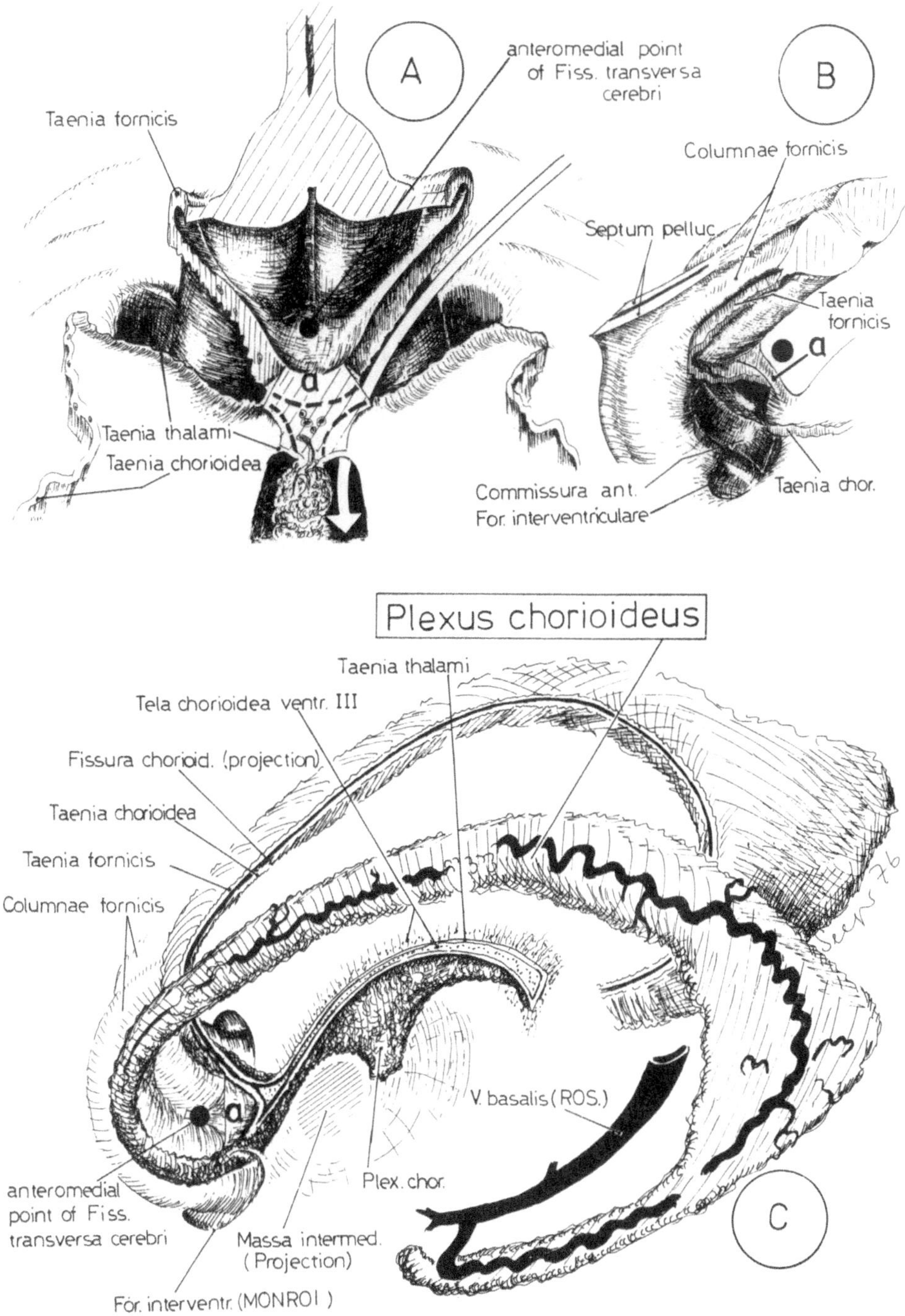
A
anteromedial point
of Fiss. transversa
cerebri
Taenia fornicis
a
Taenia thalami
Taenia chorioidea
B
Columnae fornicis
Septum pelluc.
Taenia
fornicis
a
Commissura ant.
For. interventriculare
Taenia chor.
Plexus chorioideus
Taenia thalami
Tela chorioidea ventr. III
Fissura chorioid. (projection)
Taenia chorioidea
Taenia fornicis
Columnae fornicis
a
V. basalis (ROS.)
anteromedial
point of Fiss.
transversa cerebri
Plex. chor.
Massa intermed.
(Projection)
För. interventr. (MONROI)
C

Fig. 188. Preparation with representation of 3rd ventricle, reproduced somewhat schematically and partly transparent (dorsal superior lateral view). Plexus chorioideus of Ventriculus lateralis and Ventriculus III removed. Tela chorioidea of 3rd ventricle with its fibrous-glial strengthening at posterior margin of Foramina interventricularia (Monroi) removed

Figs. 189 to 196. Same preparation with various views (oblique sections). Medial brain structures in vicinity of ventricular system. Particularly should be noted the relationships between Substantia perforata ant., Putamen, Radiatio rostri corporis callosi, Caput nuclei caudati, and Crus cerebri

Fig. 189

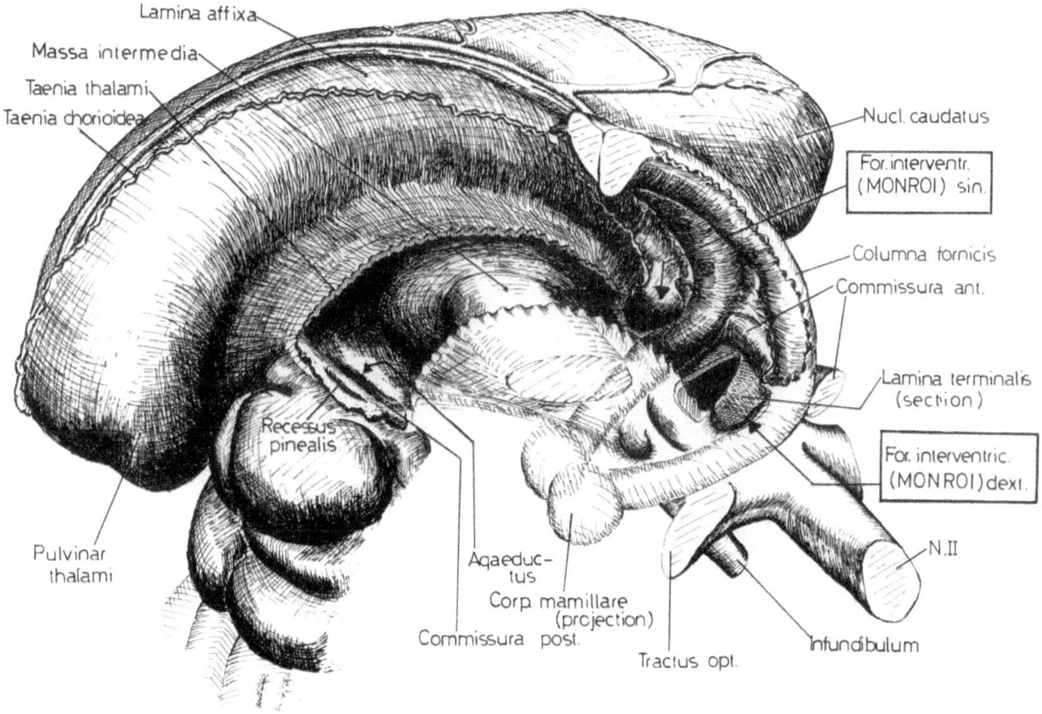
Lamina affixa
Massa intermedia
Taenia thalami
Taenia chorioidea
Nucl. caudatus
For. interventr. (MONROI) sin.
Columna fornicis
Commissura ant.
Lamina terminalis (section)
For. interventric. (MONROI) dext.
Recessus pinealis
Pulvinar thalami
Aqaeductus
Corp. mamillare (projection)
Commissura post.
Tractus opt.
Infundibulum
N. II

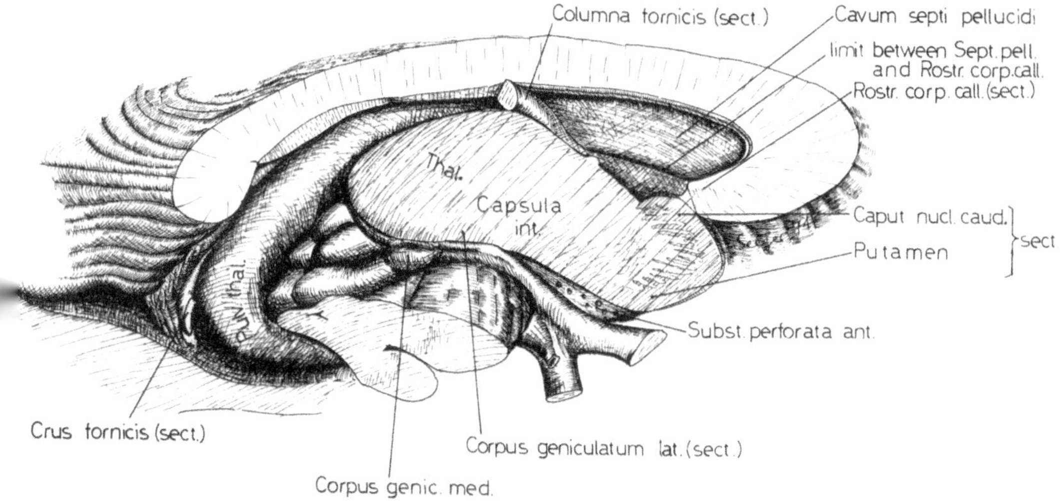
Columna fornicis (sect.)
Cavum septi pellucidi
limit between Sept. pell. and Rostr. corp. call.
Rostr. corp. call. (sect.)
Thal.
Capsula int.
Caput nucl. caud.
Putamen
sect
Pulv. thal.
Subst. perforata ant.
Crus fornicis (sect.)
Corpus geniculatum lat. (sect.)
Corpus genic. med.

Fig. 190

Fig. 191

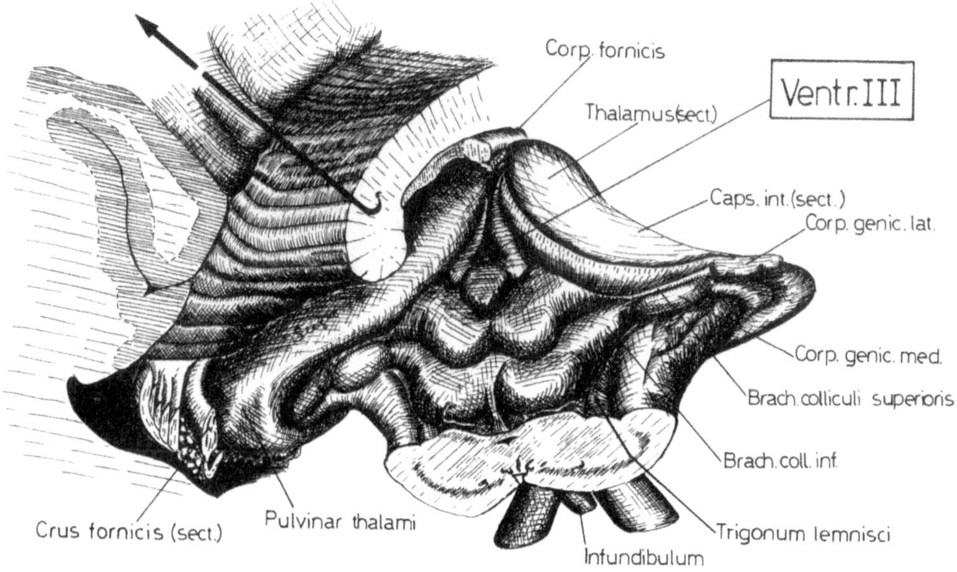
Corp. fornicis
Ventr. III
Thalamus(sect.)
Caps. int.(sect.)
Corp. genic. lat.
Corp. genic. med.
Brach. colliculi superioris
Brach. coll. inf.
Trigonum lemnisci
Infundibulum
Pulvinar thalami
Crus fornicis (sect.)

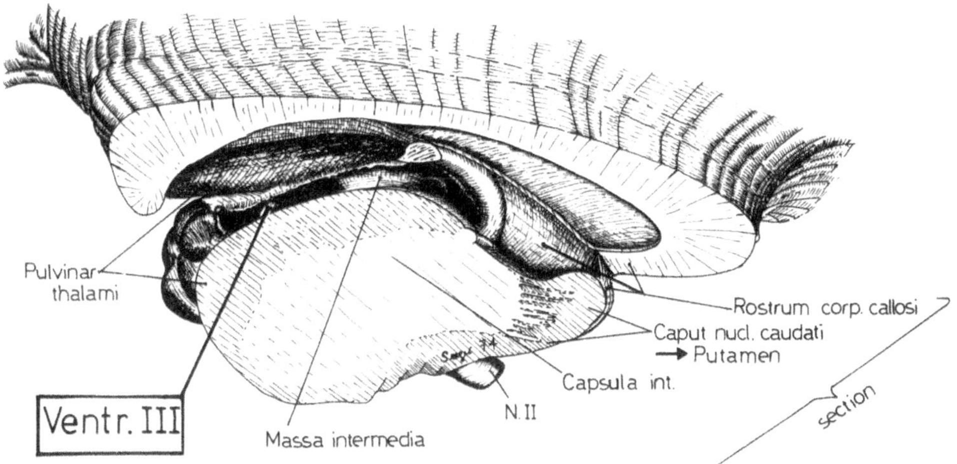
Pulvinar thalami
Rostrum corp. callosi
Caput nucl. caudati
→ Putamen
Capsula int.
N. II
section
Ventr. III
Massa intermedia

Fig. 192

Fig. 193

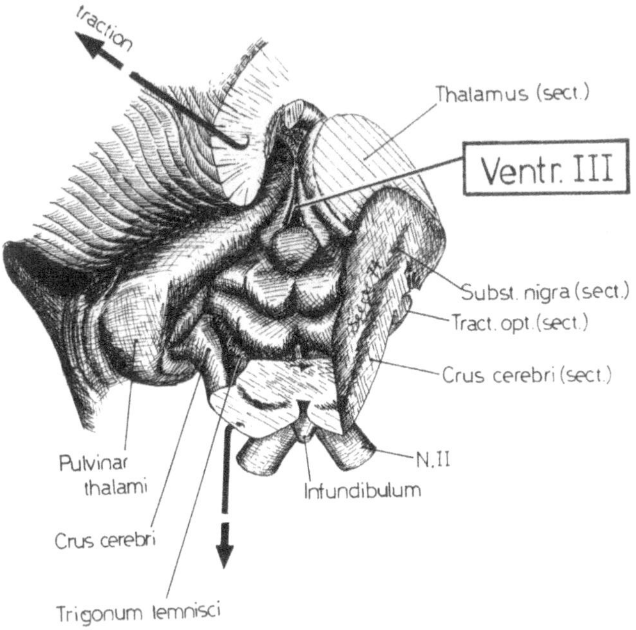
traction
Thalamus (sect.)
Ventr. III
Subst. nigra (sect.)
Tract. opt. (sect.)
Crus cerebri (sect.)
N. II
Infundibulum
Pulvinar thalami
Crus cerebri
Trigonum lemnisci

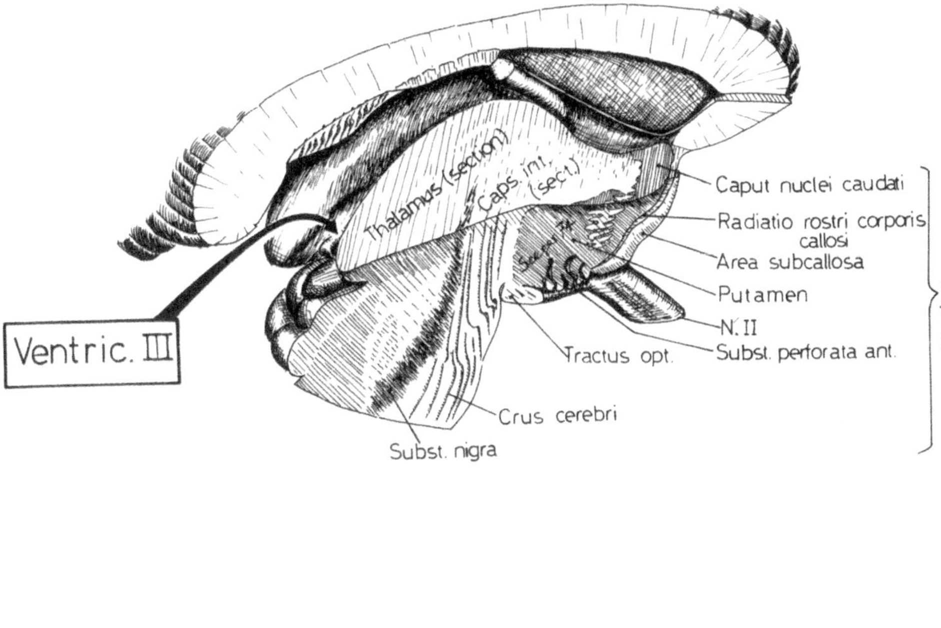
Thalamus (section)
Caps. int. (sect.)
Caput nuclei caudati
Radiatio rostri corporis callosi
Area subcallosa
Putamen
N. II
Subst. perforata ant.
section
Tractus opt.
Crus cerebri
Subst. nigra
Ventric. III

Fig. 194. The border between Septum pellucidum and the adjacent highest zone of Rostrum corporis callosi is hardly visible in the lumen of the ventricle. In the longitudinal fissure it lies in front of Commissura ant.

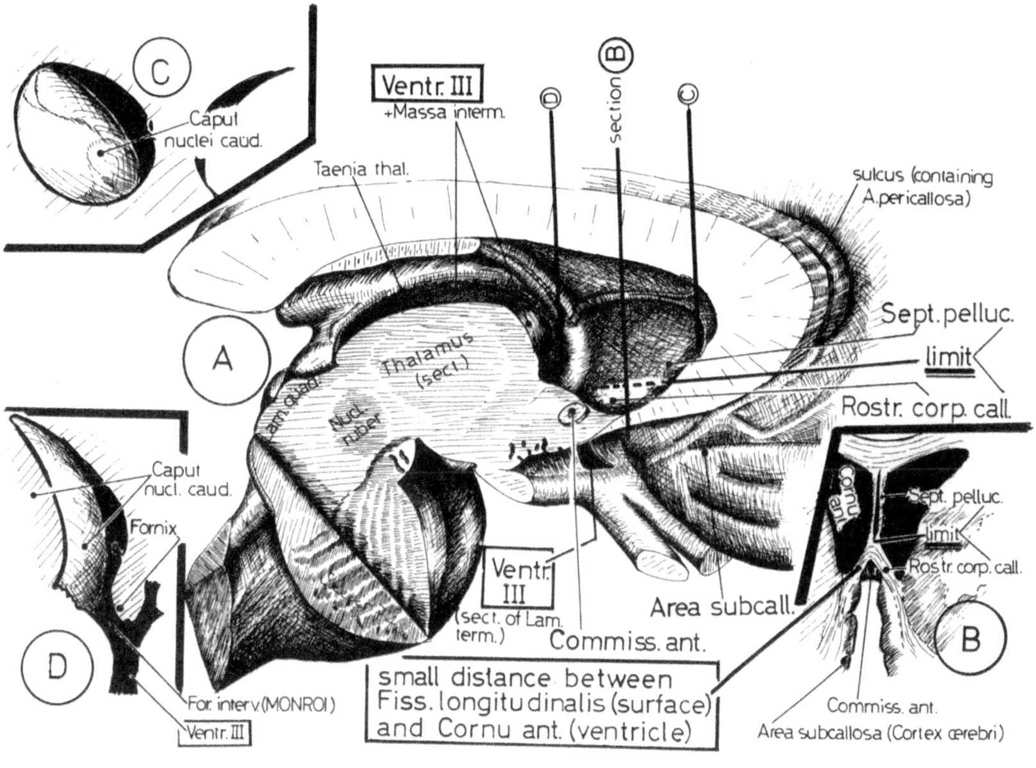
C
Caput
nuclei caud.
Ventr. III
+Massa interm.
D
section B
C
Taenia thal.
sulcus (containing
A.pericallosa)
Sept. pelluc.
limit
Rostr. corp. call.
A
Thalamus
(sect.)
Lam. quad.
Nucl.
ruber
Caput
nucl. caud.
Fornix
Ventr.
III
(sect. of Lam.
term.)
Commiss. ant.
Area subcall.
Cornu
ant.
Sept. pelluc.
limit
Rostr. corp. call.
B
D
For. interv.(MONROI)
Ventr. III
small distance between
Fiss. longitudinalis (surface)
and Cornu ant. (ventricle)
Commiss. ant.
Area subcallosa (Cortex cerebri)

Fig. 195

Fig. 196

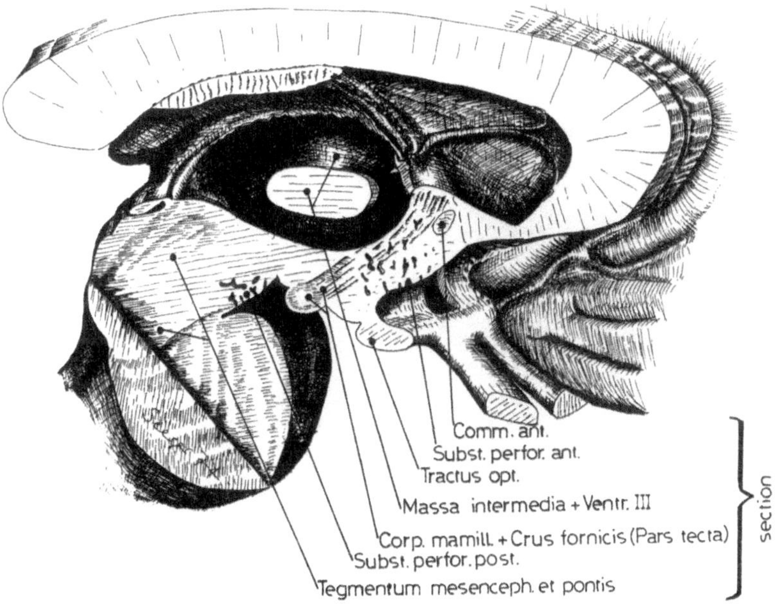

Comm. ant.
Subst. perfor. ant.
Tractus opt.
Massa intermedia + Ventr. III
Corp. mamill. + Crus fornicis (Pars tecta)
Subst. perfor. post.
Tegmentum mesenceph. et pontis
section

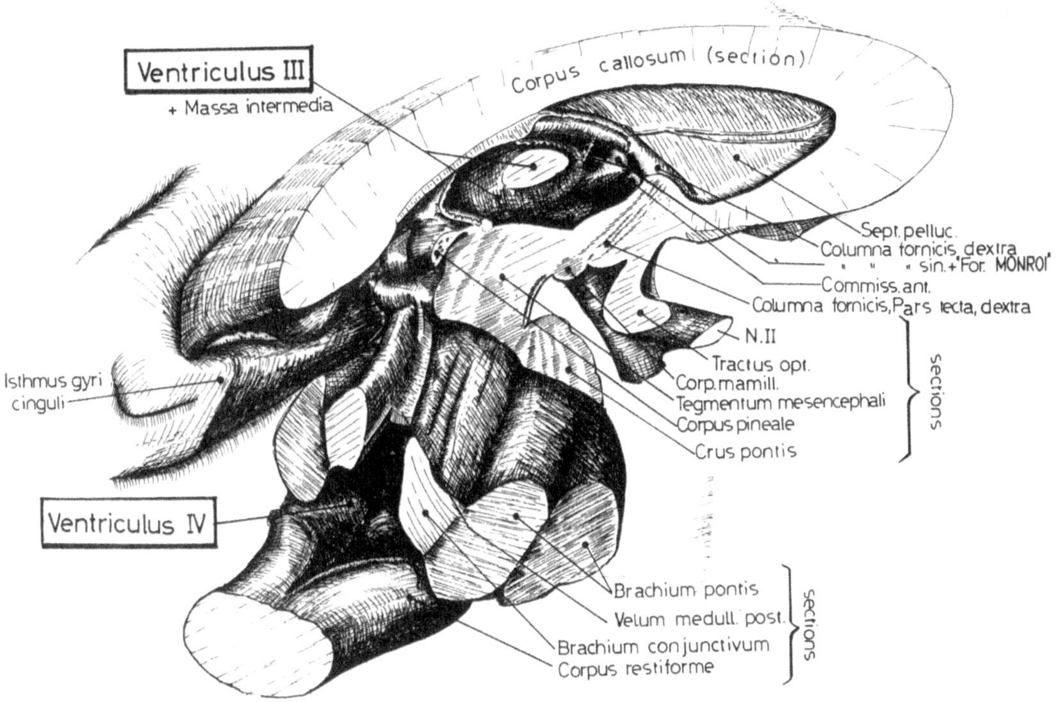

Ventriculus III
+ Massa intermedia
Corpus callosum (section)
Sept. pelluc.
Columna fornicis dextra
" " " sin. + 'For. MONROI'
Commiss. ant.
Columna fornicis, Pars tecta, dextra
N. II
Tractus opt.
Corp. mamill.
Tegmentum mesencephali
Corpus pineale
Crus pontis
sections
Isthmus gyri cinguli
Ventriculus IV
Brachium pontis
Velum medull. post.
Brachium conjunctivum
Corpus restiforme
sections

Figs. 197 and 198. Copy of model of ventricle (Retzius, 1900, quoted from Corrales and Torrealba, 1976). Nomenclature has been added, and rostral point of Fissura transversa cerebri shown in Fig. 198

Fig. 197

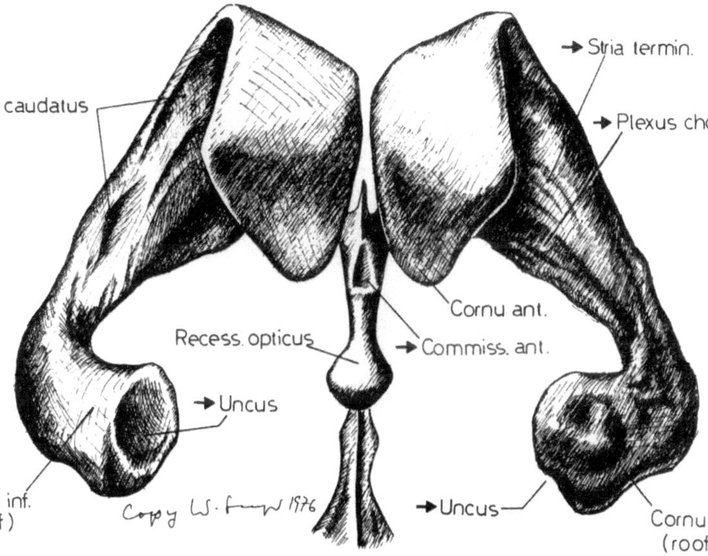
→ Nucl. caudatus
→ Stria termin.
→ Plexus chor.
Cornu ant.
Recess. opticus
→ Commiss. ant.
→ Uncus
Cornu inf.
(roof)
→ Uncus
Cornu inf.
(roof)

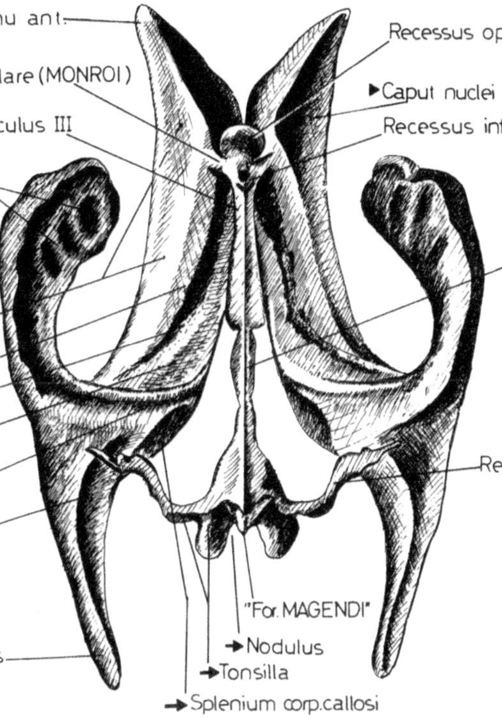
Cornu ant.
For. interventriculare (MONROI)
Ventriculus III
Recessus opt.
▸Caput nuclei caudati
Recessus infundibuli
→ Hippocampus
Aquaeductus cerebri
→ Nucl. caudatus
→ Lam. affixa thal.
→ Plexus chor.
→ Crus fornicis
→ Hippocampus
→ Calcar avis
Recessus lat. ventr. IV
"For. MAGENDI"
→ Nodulus
Cornu posterius
→ Tonsilla
→ Splenium corp. callosi

Fig. 198

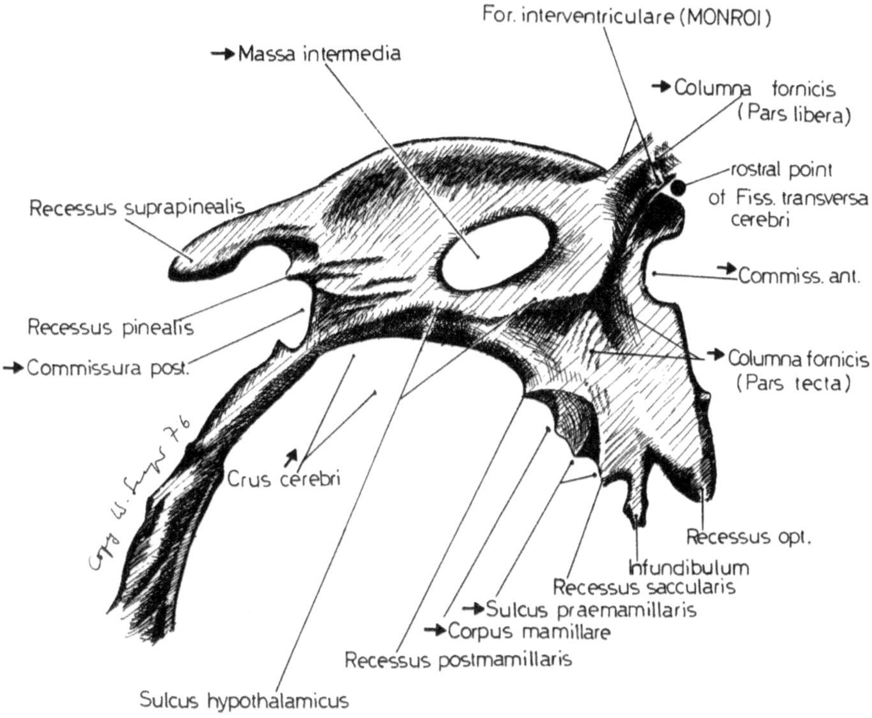
For. interventriculare (MONROI)
→Massa intermedia
→Columna fornicis (Pars libera)
rostral point of Fiss. transversa cerebri
Recessus suprapinealis
→Commiss. ant.
Recessus pinealis
→Commissura post.
→Columna fornicis (Pars tecta)
Crus cerebri
Recessus opt.
Infundibulum
Recessus saccularis
→Sulcus praemamillaris
→Corpus mamillare
Recessus postmamillaris
Sulcus hypothalamicus

Fig. 199. Distance measurements of structures of floor of lateral ventricle in millimetres (mm)

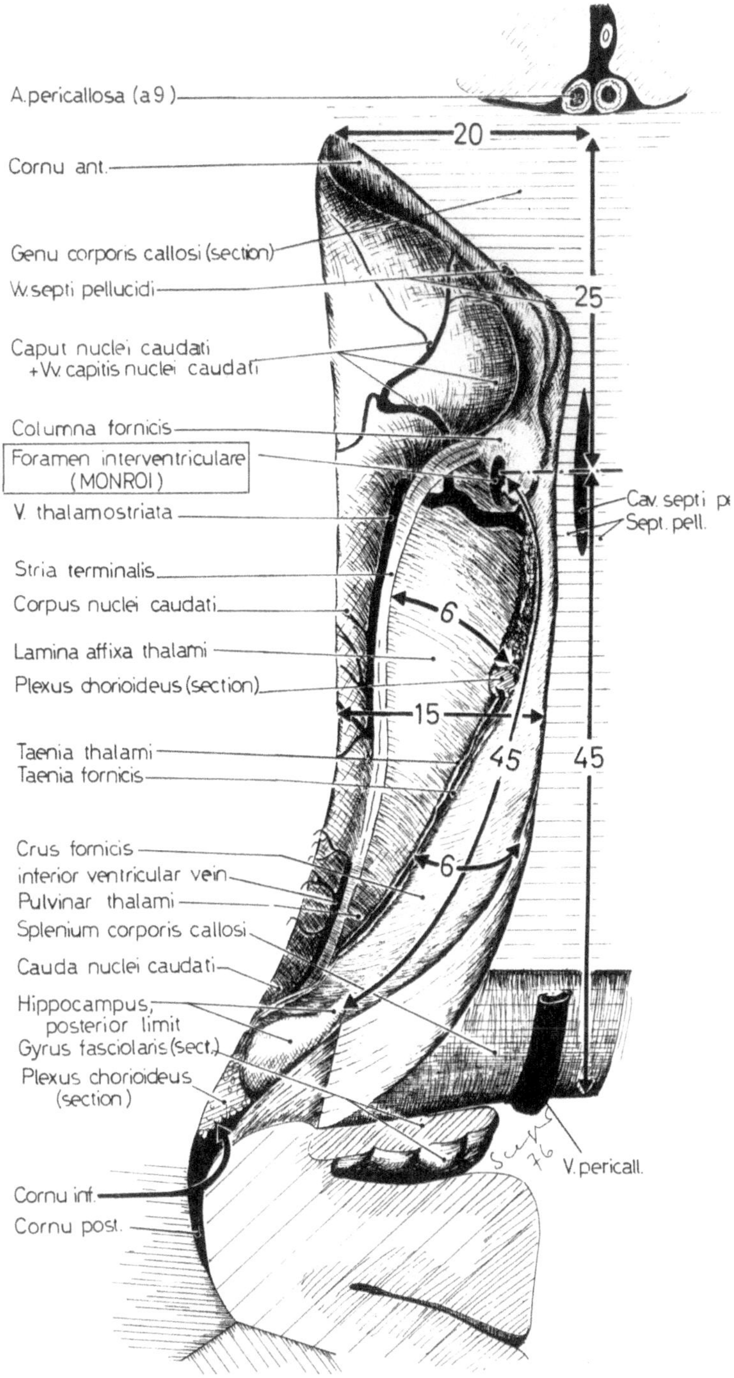
A.pericallosa (a9)
20
Cornu ant.
Genu corporis callosi (section)
Vv.septi pellucidi
25
Caput nuclei caudati
+Vv. capitis nuclei caudati
Columna fornicis
Foramen interventriculare
(MONROI)
V. thalamostriata
Cav. septi p
Sept. pell.
Stria terminalis
Corpus nuclei caudati
6
Lamina affixa thalami
Plexus chorioideus (section)
15
Taenia thalami
Taenia fornicis
45
45
Crus fornicis
interior ventricular vein
6
Pulvinar thalami
Splenium corporis callosi
Cauda nuclei caudati
Hippocampus,
posterior limit
Gyrus fasciolaris (sect.)
Plexus chorioideus
(section)
Cornu inf.
Cornu post.
V. pericall.

Fig. 200. Irregularities of structure of convexity of the skull, as seen on shaved head. Copy of historical exhibit of 1489 (Leonardo da Vinci). Inset quadrangles added (see Fig. 201)

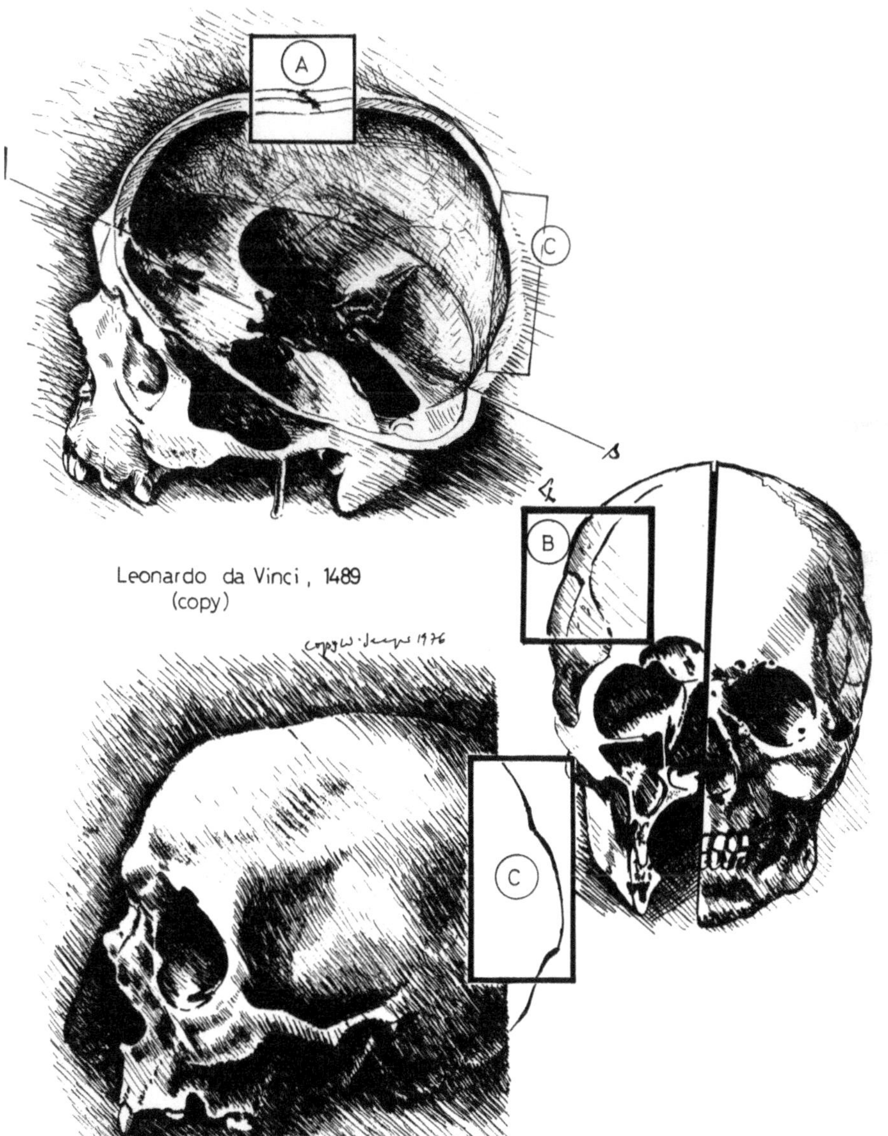

Leonardo da Vinci, 1489
(copy)

Fig. 201. *A B C* Structural peculiarities of convexity of the skull, according to historical examples (see Fig. 200)
D Projection of Sinus transversus and the often multiple Emissariae mastoideae on to the external surface of the skull.
E and *F* Variable vaulting of medial region of convexity, frontoparietally and parietooccipitally
to *B* Note the position of Pars orbitalis gyri frontalis III behind and below Linea temporalis superior

FIG. 201

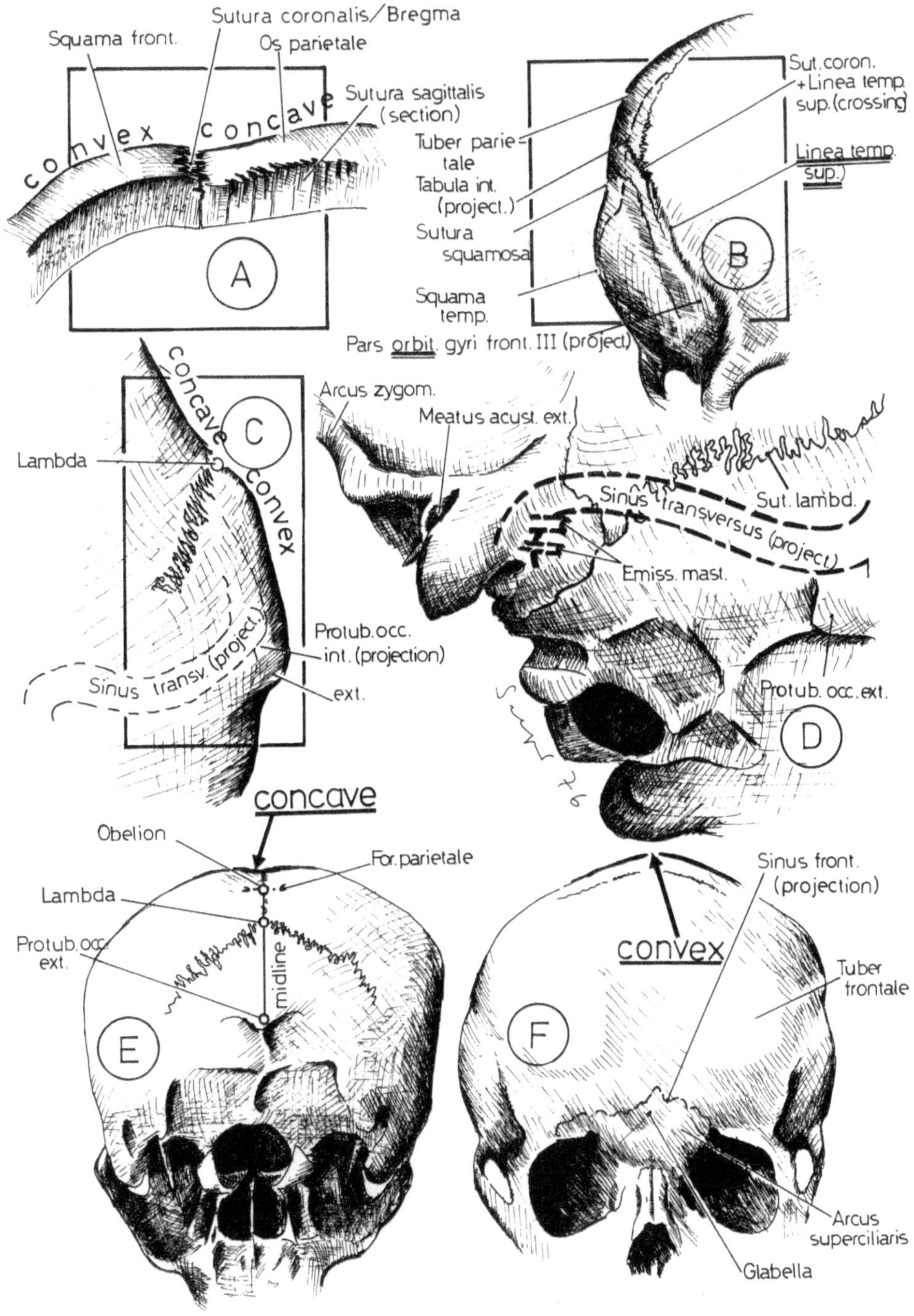
Sutura coronalis/Bregma
Squama front.
Os parietale
Sutura sagittalis (section)
convex
concave
A
Sut. coron. +Linea temp. sup. (crossing)
Tuber parietale
Tabula int. (project.)
Linea temp. sup.
Sutura squamosa
B
Squama temp.
Pars orbit. gyri front. III (project)
concave
C
Lambda
convex
Protub. occ. int. (projection)
ext.
Sinus transv. (project.)
Arcus zygom.
Meatus acust. ext.
Sinus transversus (project.)
Sut. lambd.
Emiss. mast.
Protub. occ. ext.
D
concave
Obelion
For. parietale
Lambda
Protub. occ. ext.
midline
E
convex
Sinus front. (projection)
Tuber frontale
F
Arcus superciliaris
Glabella

Fig. 202. Landmarks for ventricular puncture (prepared in collaboration with J. Gilsbach and H. Friedrich). Measurements in millimetres (mm)
Landmark *I:* to reach Cornu ant.
Landmark *II:* to reach Cornu post. and ventricular triangle.
Landmark *III:* to reach the ventricular triangle and Cornu inf. according to J. T. Robertson and I. C. Denton jr. Lambda is often inexactly localized due to irregularities of the sutures. It can be determined from the distance of Bregma from Inion (Protuberantia occipitalis externa) on external surface of head. If the skull surface is exposed, the connecting line between Foramina parietalia (Obelion) is an exact orientation point
A Puncture from lateral direction
B a-p direction of puncture. No puncture deeper than 60 mm! Puncture of Cornu post. not deeper than 25 mm (measured respectively from the surface of the dura)

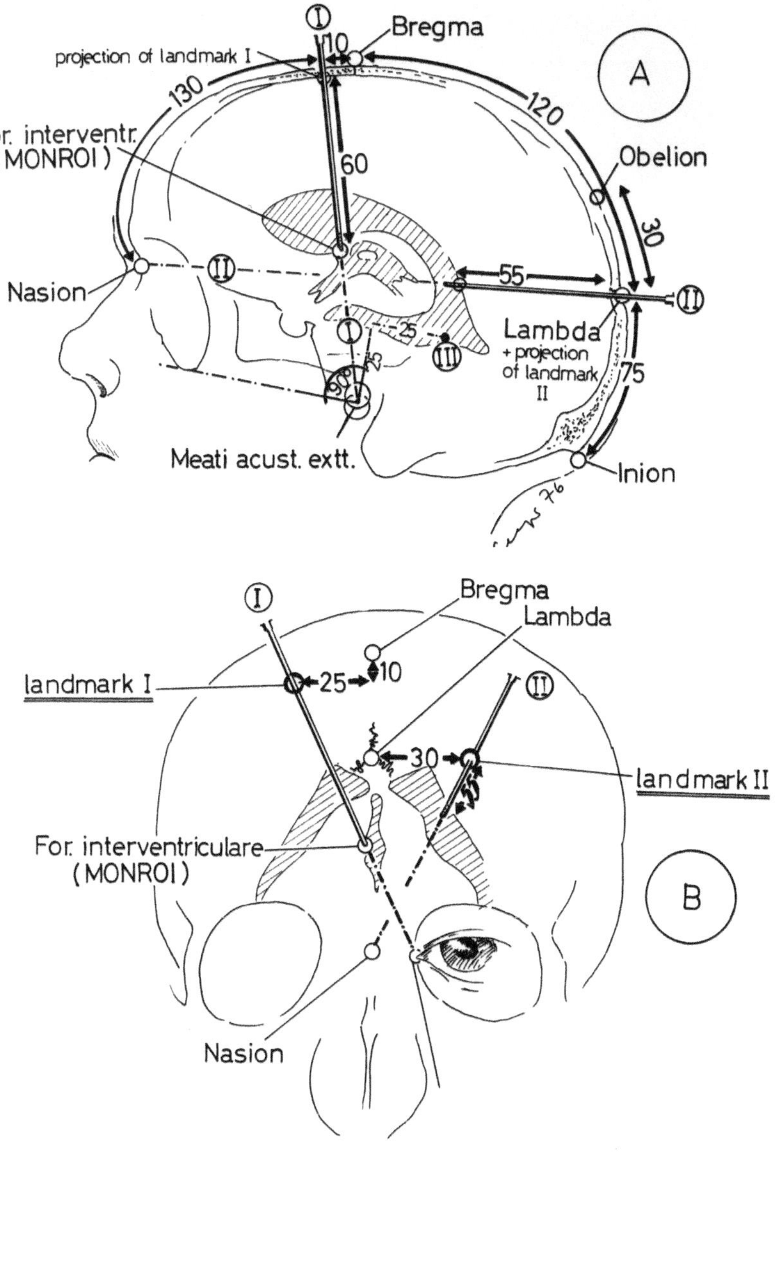

I
Bregma
10
projection of landmark I
A
130
120
For. interventr.
(MONROI)
60
Obelion
30
55
II
Nasion
Lambda
+ projection
of landmark
II
I
25
III
75
90°
Meati acust. extt.
Inion
I
Bregma
Lambda
landmark I
25
10
II
30
landmark II
For. interventriculare
(MONROI)
B
Nasion

Fig. 203. Possibilities of injury from faulty puncture of Cornu ant. Measurements in millimetres (mm)
A Medial view
B–D Oblique frontal section (see *A*)

Depth of puncture in mm	Structure reached
40	Corpus callosum, A. cerebri ant., Nucleus caudatus
50	Putamen, Capsula interna, Claustrum, Insula, Septum pellucidum
60	Foramen interventriculare (Monroi) (correct puncture), Columna fornicis, Rostrum corporis callosi, Thalamus, Globus pallidus, Genu corporis callosi
70	Area subcallosa with A. cerebri ant., Massa intermedia, Crus cerebri (upper portion), central region of Insula with main trunks of A. cerebri media
80	Chiasma and Tractus opticus, Cisterna optica, Cisterna interpeduncularis, Corpus mamillare, Crus cerebri, Tegmentum mesencephali, Cisterna quadrigemina, Pulvinar thalami, Uncus, tip of Cornu inferius

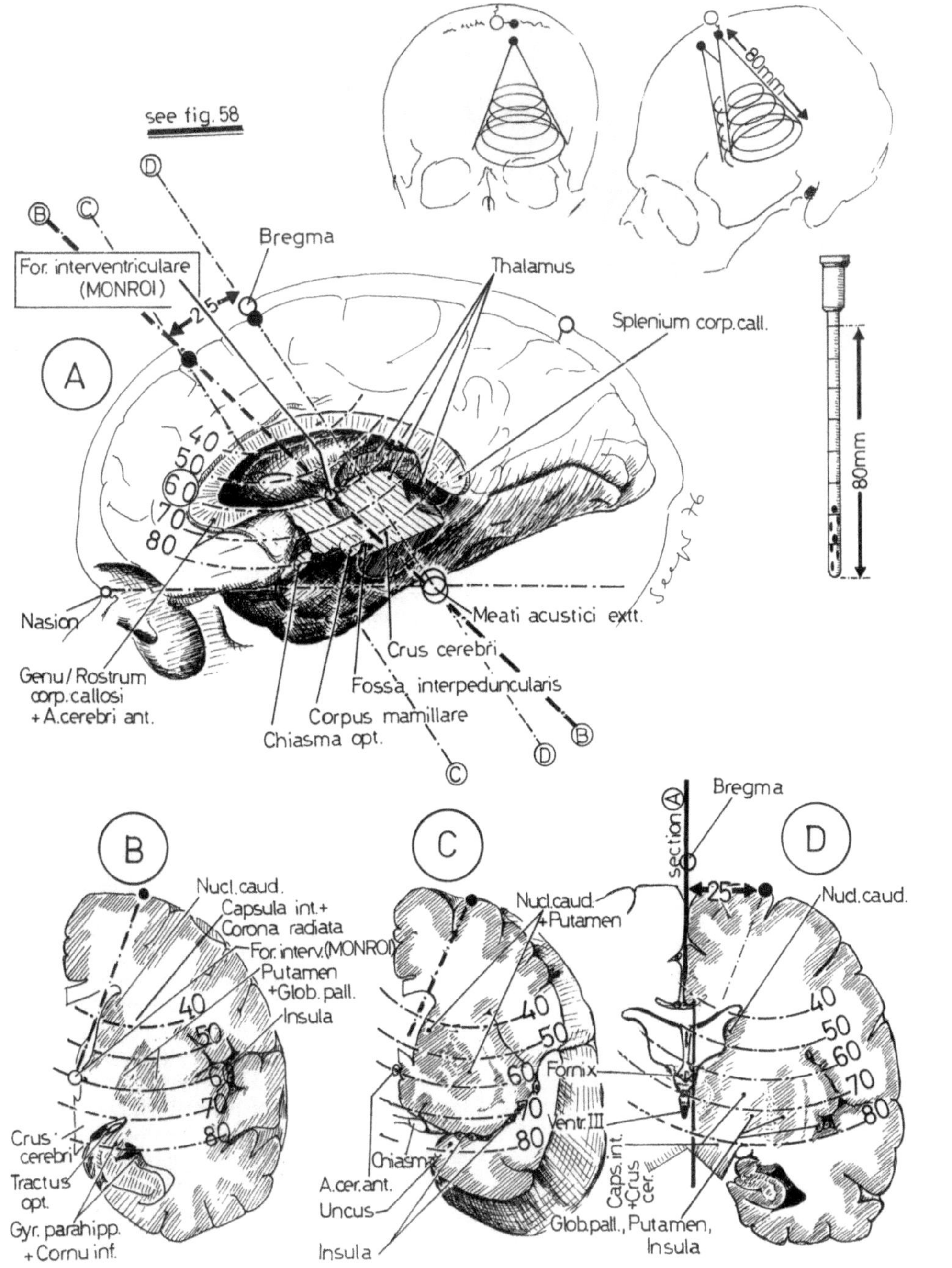

see fig. 58
80mm
Bregma
For. interventriculare (MONROI)
Thalamus
Splenium corp.call.
A
25
40
50
60
70
80
Nasion
Meati acustici extt.
Genu/Rostrum corp.callosi + A.cerebri ant.
Crus cerebri
Fossa interpeduncularis
Corpus mamillare
Chiasma opt.
B
C
D
Nucl.caud.
Capsula int.+ Corona radiata
For. interv.(MONROI)
Putamen +Glob. pall.
Insula
Crus cerebri
Tractus opt.
Gyr. parahipp. +Cornu inf.
Nucl.caud. +Putamen
A.cer.ant.
Chiasma
Uncus
Insula
section A
Nucl.caud.
Fornix
Ventr.III
Caps.int. +Crus cer.
Glob.pall., Putamen, Insula

Fig. 204. Possibilities of injury at occipital ventricular puncture. Puncture far outside the calcarina region (*a, b, c* in Fig. *A* to *C*). With correct puncture direction (*d-e*) important basal structures are reached earlier. Measurements in millimetres (mm)

A Puncture 1 cm laterally to the midline (see also Fig. *D*). Area striata endangered if puncture too steep

B Puncture 2 cm laterally to the midline. Ventricular system reached, Area striata endangered

C Puncture 3 cm laterally to the midline, correct puncture site.

Depth of puncture in mm	Structures reached (*A* to *C*)
40	Area striata, including Fissura calcarina (*1*)
50	Splenium corporis callosi (*2*), Cornu post. (*11*), Trigonum ventriculi lateralis
60	Commissura fornicis, Hippocampus, Splenium (*3*), Fascia dentata (*5*), Gyrus parahippocampalis (*4*), A. chor. post., anterior and posterior branches, Trigonum ventriculi lateralis, Fornix, posterior portions (*10*)
70	Pulvinar thalami (*6*)
80	Lamina quadrigemina (*7*), Aquaeductus (*8*), Corpus pineale (*9*), Fornix (anterior portion) (*10*)

FIG. 204

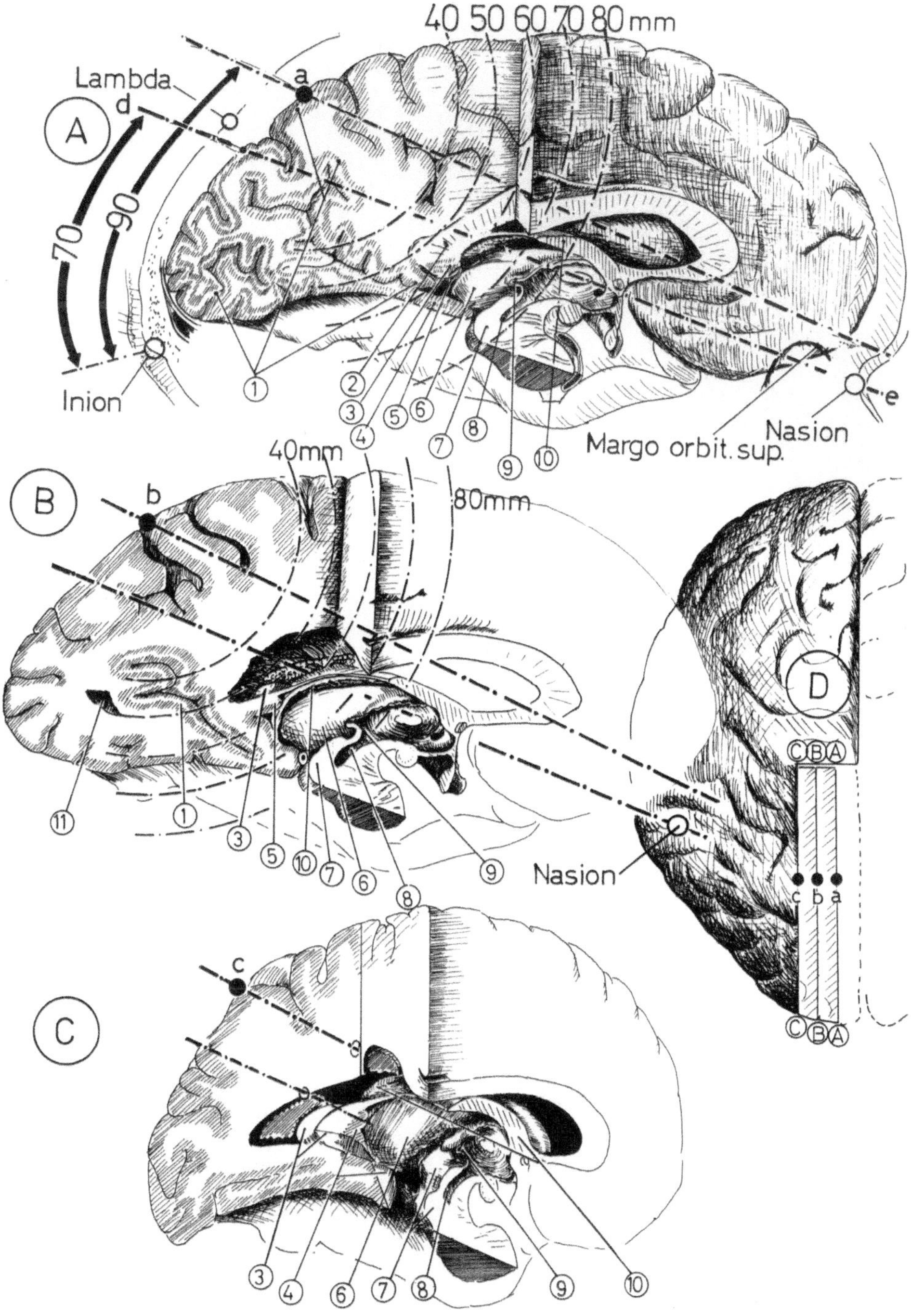

40 50 60 70 80 mm
Lambda
a
d
A
70
90
Inion
1
2
3
4
5
6
7
8
9
10
e
Nasion
Margo orbit. sup.
40mm
80mm
B
b
11
Nasion
D
C B A
c b a
C
c

Fig. 205. Close positional relationship between Foramina interventricularia (Monroi) (black arrows) and Genu capsulae internae (motor supply of contralateral upper extremity). Preparation with horizontal section at level of Massa intermedia right. Basal ganglion region preserved. 3rd ventricle pulled apart (white arrow)
Cave! Distortion effects at Genu capsulae internae in approach to the 3rd ventricle through Foramen interventriculare (Monroi)

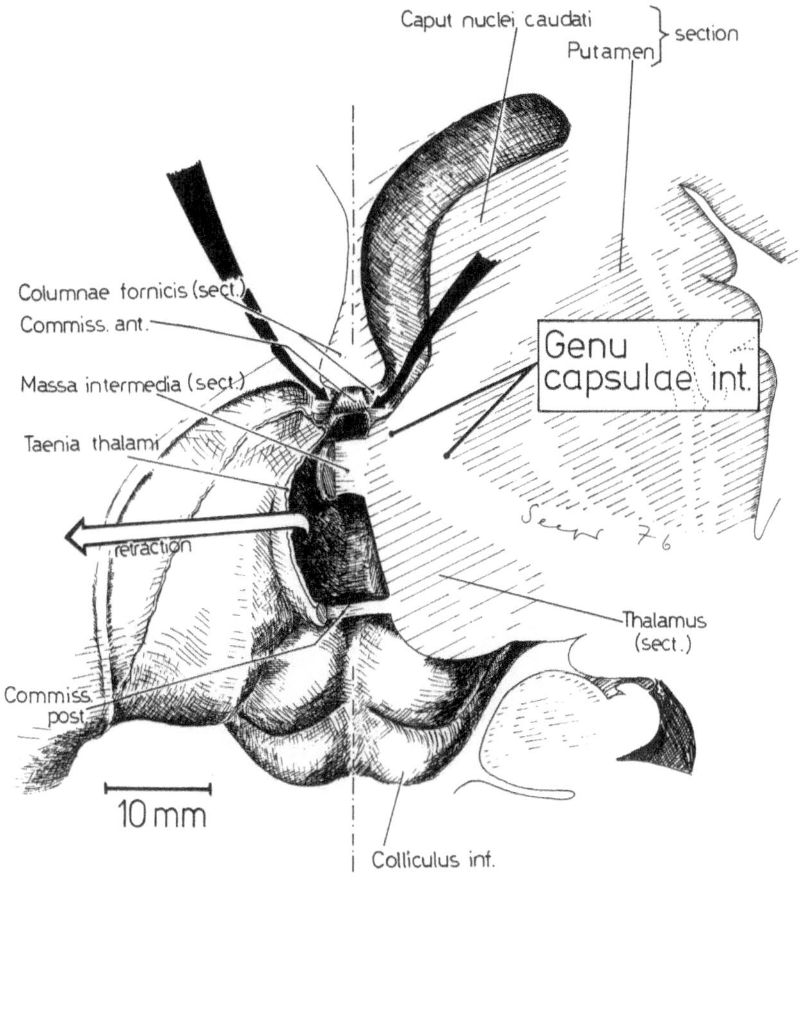
Caput nuclei caudati
Putamen
section
Columnae fornicis (sect.)
Commiss. ant.
Massa intermedia (sect.)
Taenia thalami
Genu capsulae int.
retraction
Thalamus (sect.)
Commiss. post.
10 mm
Colliculus inf.

Chapter 7
Cerebellum and Lower Brainstem

A. Outer and Inner Surface

All parts of Cerebellum are connected with the brainstem over the three cerebellar peduncles. All three form the white matter of Cerebellum, which is divided by the cerebellar Lobules into several segments. The preparations in Figs. 207 to 210, 213, and 215 are taken from successive resections of the cerebellar Lobules made from rostrally in the caudal direction. The preparation in Fig. 217 was used for the demonstration of vessels (Fig. 218). From the occipital viewpoint in Fig. 206 it can be seen that Lobulus semilunaris superior lies farther lateral and Lobulus semilunaris inferior farther medial (under Sinus transversus). The borders are difficult to recognize, also being hidden by the leptomeninges and vessels. Here, unlike at the basal surface, a dorsal demarcation of the tonsil from Lobulus biventer is easily possible. From Lobulus semilunaris superior the underlying white matter of Brachium pontis is soon reached. The white matter of Lobulus biventer is more voluminous. In Fig. 207 the relationships between Brachium pontis, Vermis cerebelli, and Lobulus semilunaris can be seen, after removal of Lobulus quadrangularis and Lobulus simplex. After Lobulus semilunaris superior and inferior have also been removed (Fig. 208), the deep fissure can be recognized that separates the lower vermis region (Uvula and Nodulus) from the upper.

Between Lingula cerebelli, Velum medullare ant., and Nodulus there remains only a narrow zone of white matter over Fastigium of the 4th ventricle. It becomes clear that the removed Lobulus quadrangularis had overlapped large parts of Brachium conjunctivum and Brachium pontis. This space is of practical importance: here the veins lie on Brachium pontis and Brachium conjunctivum (Fig. 218). If Brachium pontis is cut through when Lobulus biventer is removed, the stalk of the tonsil will be severed medially as well (Figs. 215 and 216). In the bed of Velum medullare post., into which the tonsil projects, Plexus chorioideus of the 4th ventricle still covered by thin Velum, can be recognized, and under it N. stato-acusticus attached to the brainstem. The narrow strip of white matter over which Nodulus is connected medially with the remaining region of Vermis (Figs. 209, 213, 214) also connects lateral cerebellar structures. In Fig. 210 only Flocculus is shown turned back. In an upward direction the zone of white matter merges into the tonsil. Velum medullare post. is fenestrated between its insertion at Nodulus and Plexus chorioideus of the 4th ventricle in Fig. 210. Here Plexus chorioideus is shown from the front, attached to Velum medullare post., whereas seen from behind (Fig. 209) it shimmers through the transparent Velum medullare post.

In Fig. 210 by removal of the tonsil and backward luxation of Flocculus the Recessus lateralis, which normally lies alongside Brachium pontis, has been opened wide. The author was not able to discover the so-called "Apertura lateralis" (Luschkae) although he examined 20 brains for this purpose.

The posterior surface of Fastigium is formed by the highest part of Velum medullare post., which projects from Uvula into the lumen of the 4th ventricle.

The section levels of the brainstem for the above preparation are shown in Figs. 211 and 212. Here it can also be seen that Nucleus dentatus (arrow) projects caudally beyond the level of the tonsil (*E* in Fig. 212), and that in a cranial direction (*D* in Fig. 212) it reaches Brachium conjunctivum. Its principal extension lies behind the level of Fastigium. After removal of the tonsil and Velum medullare posterius (Fig. 213) the positional relationships of the upper portions of Nucleus dentatus to Brachium conjunctivum and Brachium pontis can be recognized. Both are permeated by Nucleus dentatus. The fibres of Brachium conjunctivum push in between Nucleus dentatus and the dorsal wall of the 4th ventricle.

In the area of Pedunculus flocculi, the Brachium pontis, Pedunculus flocculi, and Pedunculus tonsillae are united. They form the roof of Recessus lateralis. N. stato-acusticus and the lateral portion of Velum medullare post. form its floor. Velum medullare post. closes off laterally Recessus lateralis of the 4th ventricle. In Fig. 214 the positional relationships between the 4th ventricle and its bordering structures are shown in a schematically simplified representation: the two tonsils and the Nodulus/Uvula-complex are connected transversely with one another by a zone of white matter, and laterally with Brachium pontis and is attached medially to the tonsil. The connection of the tonsil itself to Brachium pontis is situated farther dorsally. Velum medullare post. covers the tonsils and Nodulus anteriorly, and thus forms the lower half of the roof of the 4th ventricle. In the area of Fastigium the Velum medullare ant. and post. are still separated from each other by a narrow zone of white matter. At. operations on the 4th ventricle its Plexus chorioideus is often missed*. It is pushed away by the tonsil and Nodulus and is inserted into the rostral surface of Velum medullare post. On viewing from the usual, caudal, direction (Fig. 257) it becomes visible after removal of the tonsil, if Velum medullare post. is extremely thin or if a window is cut into it. The course of Plexus chor. is more clearly visible from an anterior direction (Fig. 210) if the cerebellar peduncles are dissected and Vermis severed medially. Recessus lateralis has been dissected below Pedunculus flocculi, and thus simulate a so-called Apertura lateralis ventriculi IV (Luschkae). Posterior medullary Velum and Plexus chor. form a unit which has been left in situ. Furthermore, from this direction the association between Pedunculus flocculi and Brachium pontis is clear.

B. Relations Between Cerebellum, Lower Brainstem, and Vessels

The structure of the vessels on the outer surface of Cerebellum (Culmen and declive of Vermis, Lobulus quadrangularis and Lobulus simplex) is the easiest to understand (Figs. 217 and 218). Anastomoses between A. cerebelli superior (R. lat.) and A. cerebelli inferior post. (Fig. 218 *A*, right) are rare in this form, but on injection preparations there are numerous connections with a diameter of less than 0.3 mm. In this regard the reader is referred to contributions by Newton and Mani, Margolis and Newton, Takahashi, Hoffmann, Margolis and Newton in Newton and Potts (1974). Scialfa et al. recently reported in detail that the peripheral ramifications of A. cerebelli inferior ant. and inferior post. may replace one another. If A. cerebelli inferior post. is hypoplastic, then A. cerebelli inferior ant. is dominant, and vice versa. The writer's own injection preparations confirm the variability of these vessels as described in the literature. The particularly frequent variant of A. cerebelli inferior ant. described by Naidich and Kricheff has been singled out in Fig. 220.

The courses of veins on the dorsal surface of Cerebellum often conform to the types described by Huang and Wolf, but of equal importance for the operator are the frequent irregular connections to the under-surface of Tentorium and thus to Lacunae of Sinus rectus and to the veins running at the edge of Lobulus semilunaris superior and passing directly to Sinus transversus. It can be established from injection preparations with such veins that occasionally only parts of the surface of Cerebellum show bigger veins. Adequate anastomoses with neighbouring regions are, therefore, uncertain and ligation of larger veins problematical. Together with Aa. vermiculares, solitary, double, or multiple Vv. vermiculares run near the midline, and in the upper region of Lobulus quadrangularis almost invariably take up contributory veins from the cerebellar hemispheres. V. vermicularis superior and supraculminalis are usually separate from V. cerebellaris praecentralis, which also runs near the midline, but deeper, and whose connection in a lateral direction to V. mesencephalica lateralis is overlapped by Lobulus quadrangularis. Brachium pontis overlapped by Lobulus quadrangularis and Brachium conjunctivum may be covered by large veins. The main drainage routes – medially to V. cerebri magna (Galeni), and laterally to V. basalis (Rosenthal) – are extremely variable. In the writer's specimens these drainage routes are partly missing. In one operative case V. mesencephalica lateralis was dominant and had no connection to V. basalis (Rosenthal).

Fig. 220 *B* demonstrates the venous supply of Cerebellum and lower brainstem. An example has been selected in which the right cerebellar hemisphere

* Or pushed in a posterior direction by tumours – e.g. overlying tumours of Nodulus vermis visible near the surface of Uvula and Pyramis vermis.

has mainly direct drainage over Sinus transversus, and the left hemisphere, together with the brainstem, is drained over V. petrosa superior to Sinus petrosus superior. The inconstant veins from the region of the pons are of practical importance. They may penetrate the dura directly over Clivus, and then enter the extradurally situated Plexus basilaris; rostrally the originate from the anterior median pontine vein and caudally they run more laterally to V. petrosa inferior. The latter may reach Sinus petrosus inferior (Fig. 220 *B*, after Duvernoy). These venous connections could not be demonstrated in our own injection preparations by filling through V. petrosa superior. Remarkably often the ventral veins of the pons were only filled on one side in the correct injection preparation. This, too, indicates an inadequate collateral circulation with corresponding risks associated with the elimination of larger veins.

C. Preoperative Radiology – Some Aspects

The variability of the basilar arterial system has attracted increased attention in recent years. The most important data given in the literature are evaluated in Figs. 221 to 232. The illustrations of the authors named in the legends have been considerably modified. In particular, it follows from the variability of A. cerebelli inferior ant. that in future before operations in the region of the base of the brain and the posterior cranial fossa angiography with a basal projection will be indispensable, since only by this means can an analysis of the course of A. cerebelli inf. ant. be made. This is particularly important for processes in the cerebellopontine angle.

D. Operative Techniques – Some Aspects

Apart from the traditional suboccipital, osteoclastic exposure from a gridiron incision with and without resection of the atlas arch (Fig. 233 *A*), Yaşargil uses the modified osteoplastic* method of Fedor Krause, with trepanation to beyond the level of Sinus transversus and Confluens sinuum (Fig. 233 *B*) in order to expose Lobulus quadrangularis up to Lamina quadrigemina. Laterally situated processes, for example in the cerebellopontine angle, can be approached along the furrow between the under-surface of Tentorium and the posterior surface of the petrous bone. For this purpose exposure up to the knee of the sinus is necessary. In order to avoid haemorrhages one must be familiar with the direction of the course of the emissaries through the bone in the vicinity, and bear in mind that Emissarium mastoideum may be split up into several emissaries.

A second lateral approach from the basal direction with resection up to Condylus occipitalis and Fossa condylaris (Drake, Yaşargil) is adequate for deep-seated cerebellar processes. Processes at the basal surface of Medulla oblongata – e.g., aneurysms – cannot always be reached. From preparation of a fresh cadaver, using a midbrain section and leaving the lower brainstem and Cerebellum untouched, it can easily be recognized that the reclination of the temporal lobe must be considerable, and that an approach from the suboccipital direction is also associated with a dangerous reclination of the lower brainstem.

For this reason a new method with resection of Tuberculum jugulare, shown in Figs. 234 and 235, was developed in collaboration with Gilsbach*, in order to reach in the straight sagittal direction from behind to the basal surface of Medulla oblongata and Pons (a method which has since been successfully tried out on a medially situated A. vertebralis aneurysm between the two Nn. abducentes). The principle is that A. vertebralis is freed from Sulcus arteriae vertebralis of the atlas and Arcus atlantis post. is resected up to Condylus atlantis superior. After preparation of A. vertebralis, an narrow medial zone of Condylus occipitalis is drilled out as far as Canalis hypoglossi. After visualization of the dural sheath of N. hypoglossus the Tuberculum jugulare in the roof of Canalis hypoglossi is also drilled out extradurally. Stretching of the dura should be avoided because Nn. IX to XI are stretched over it intradurally. The dura now sinks down between Meatus acusticus internus and Canalis hypoglossi, as can be seen when the dura is subsequently opened. The deep clivus groove is now shallow in the lateral direction, and a direct approach into the premedullary cisterns is possible without reclination of Medulla oblongata. Only Lobulus biventer and the cerebellar tonsil must be raised.

Since the introduction of computer tomography the approach shown at *A* in Fig. 233 has become rarer.

* Personal operative demonstration and Yaşargil, G. (1976).

* Neurosurgical Clinic of the University Freiburg i. Br., Federal Republic of Germany.

since processes of the cerebellar hemispheres can be approached directly from a paramedian incision. But because large parts of both cerebellar hemispheres are no longer exposed as in the past, intracerebellar orientation has become more difficult.

The positional relationships between the 4th ventricle, the cerebellar peduncle, and Nucleus dentatus (Fig. 236) are of particular importance. Here it is clear that Nucleus dentatus is at risk in resections in the area of the lateral roof of the 4th ventricle (arrow in Fig. 236).

Figs. 238 to 241 show the relationships between the pons and clivus groove. The clivus groove is filled laterally by the vault of the pons. Brachium pontis hugs the anterior half of the posterior surface of the petrous bone and thus projects over Tuberculum jugulare.

In opening the dura the possibility of the sinus variants must be considered (Fig. 237). An atypical Sinus occipitalis usually possesses extended accompanying Lacunae, which can easily be under control if bone is immediately resected to ensure better access. The traditional approach routes make such anomalies dangerous. In operations for intracerebellar processes atypical veins in the vicinity of Lobuli semilunares can easily be bypassed. When more extensive cerebellar resection is necessary, Brachium pontis, Brachium conjunctivum, Nucleus dentatus, and Flocculus must be conserved as far as possible, insofar as they have not already been destroyed by the disease process. *B* in Fig. 237 shows such a situation as it might occur, for example, at resection of an angioma in a cerebellar hemisphere. Knowledge of the positional relationships and distances (Fig. 239) facilitates the careful dissection. It is important to know that larger resections of Lobulus biventer are possible without approaching the pons. In Lobuli semilunares the farther medial or in a parasagittal direction the resection is positioned, the sooner will Brachium pontis and Pons be reached (*A* in Fig. 238).

Difficulties of orientation are to be expected mediobasally in the extracerebral space since Pons and Medulla oblongata lie deeply in the groove of Clivus and can only be slightly raised at operation. The approach to the ventral side of Medulla oblongata is facilitated by the described resection in the region of Foramen jugulare (Fig. 234). The medial pons region projects farther into the clivus groove. The border of Pons with Medulla oblongata, the junction of Aa. vertebrales with A. basilaris (variants see Fig. 221), and the posterior border of Porus acusticus internus lie almost in one plane perpendicular to the longitudinal axis of Clivus. A deviation of only 40° in a medial direction from the approach direction (Sinus knee - Dorsum sellae) would lead to Foramen occipitale magnum instead of reaching Dorsum sellae (*B* in Fig. 239). Orientation can be difficult with the patient in an oblique sitting position. A big extension is not unusual for tumours in the cerebellopontine angle and in front of the pons (Friedrich and Seeger, 1976).

The course of N. trigeminus is important for an evaluation of the pons and Brachium pontis (Figs. 238 and 239). Medial to its exit lies the pons, and lateral to it, partly covered by Lobulus quadrangularis, Brachium pontis. The projection onto the bony base (*B* in Fig. 239) shows that the pons projects laterally far beyond the clivus groove, and covers medial parts of Pars petrosa. The depth of the clivus groove increases caudally, due to the increasing bilateral projection of Tuberculum jugulare. The anterior part of Foramen occipitale is narrowed by Condyli occipitales. Condylus occipitalis and Tuberculum jugulare form a strong bony block, which in its medial surface has a recess in a lateral direction to Canalis hypoglossi. Consequently the distance between Canales hypoglossi is larger than the distance of the anterior edges of Foramen occipitale. It is equal to the maximal transverse diameter of Foramen occipitale approximately 5 mm behind Canalis hypoglossi (*B* in Fig. 239 and *A* in Fig. 241).

Flocculus deserves special attention for two reasons: first, its loss means irreversible impairment of optokinetic nystagmus; secondly, a knowledge of its topographical relations to Brachium pontis, N. stato-acusticus and N. facialis, and Lobulus simplex is important for operations at the cerebellopontine angle. Porus acusticus internus borders immediately on the lateral edge of Flocculus. At operations in the area of the cerebellopontine angle the spatula touches Lobulus quadrangularis if placed dorsally to Porus acusticus internus.

Under normal conditions Flocculus is also reached by the spatula. In the presence of neurinomas of N. acusticus the Flocculus is pressed below Lobulus quadrangularis into Brachium pontis and together with it is rolled out widely. Identification of these structures is no longer possible if Arachnoidea is cloudy. Orientation should, therefore, be taken from Plexus chorioideus, which can easily be seen.

The situation illustrated in Fig. 241 (*C* is seen, for example, after removal of epidermoid tumours in the presence of a falling back Cerebellum with stretching of the cranial nerves V and VII to XII. The cranial nerves VII to XI cover Tuberculum jugulare. The connection between Canalis hypoglossi and Porus acusticus internus (posterior wall), and the connection between Porus acusticus internus and the lateral border of Dorsum sellae almost form a right angle (*A* in Fig. 241). Of the numerous measurements in Fig. 241, the distance between Porus acusticus internus and the dural penetration of the cranial nerves IX to XII is of great practical significance (less than 10 mm). The typical enlargement of Porus acusticus internus by neurinomas may reduce this distance to zero. The bone may also shrink as far as Sinus petrosus superior (neurinomal invasions of Sinus petrosus superior and adhesions of the capsule at Tentorium are not uncommon). In drilling open the internal auditory meatus, therefore, only the zone between the posterior border of Porus acusticus internus and the anterior border of Sinus sigmoideus is without risk, apart from that of opening pneumatic spaces (Yaşargil), which must be accordingly closed.
V. petrosa superior passes between N. trigeminus and N. facialis to Sinus petrosus superior. As it is usually of small calibre it can be coagulated without risk in the presence of tumours. If it is of large calibre, the fact that it drains both V. mesencephalica lateralis and V. cerebellaris ant. must be taken into consideration. In one operative case of the author the coagulation and clipping of an unusually large V. petrosa superior led to a fatal malacia of the neighbouring pontine area.
In Fig. 242 (modified after Rhoton) the relationships between the 7th and 8th cranial nerves and A. cerebelli inferior ant. are illustrated. In opening the porus, particular attention should be paid to A. petrosa in the roof of the porus. It can be coagulated. The proximal segment of A. cerebelli inf. ant. itself must, however, be preserved. Aa. labyrinthi can often not be preserved. In operations for neurinomas of N. acusticus attempts have recently been made to conserve N. cochleae. Fisch* points out, however, that if only minimal residual hearing will be left, the preservation of the nerve is not justified (if the nerve on the opposite side is healthy), since there is a risk that abnormal ear noises will develop. A further source of bleeding in opening Porus acusticus internus is Sinus petrosus superior (particularly the variant *D* in Fig. 243), as described by Rhoton. In widening Meatus acusticus, Yaşargil recently recommended drilling off large parts of the posterior surface of Pars petrosa which often protrude into the interior of the skull. Since Sinus sigmoideus is difficult to recognize through the tough dura, the distances to the knee of the sinus must be known (Fig. 244 *B*). The posterior wall of Porus acusticus is 35 mm distant from the sinus knee. Sinus sigmoideus is maximally 15 mm wide. Thus there remains a zone of maximally 20 mm which can be drilled out in a posterior direction; however it should not usually exceed 10 mm.
More important than to preserve N. facialis – a procedure that recently has been so widely propagated – is to conserve the vitally important cranial nerves IX and X. If Porus and Meatus acusticus int. are enlarged, the positional relationships of the cranial nerves VII to XI will be altered (Fig. 246): Porus acusticus int. and canals of cranial nerves IX to XI at the exit touch each other directly. They are therefore at risk during operative opening of Meatus acusticus int. The distance between the widened Meatus acusticus and Sinus petrosus sup. and/or Tentorium is also shortened (Fig. 246).
If the posterior cranial fossa is entered laterally and basally from the sinus knee, Flocculus is already reached 20 to 25 mm from the posterior limit of Sinus sigmoideus. The posterior edge of Flocculus borders on the anterior edge of Lobulus biventer. In this furrow there are terminal branches of A. cerebelli inferior ant. (Fig. 244 *A*). The two main branches of A. cerebelli inferior ant. may form a circle of arteries around Flocculus, in which case the rostrolateral branch is the more frequent one and larger (b 4.1). This area is shown in Fig. 245: in half of the cases the meatal loop lies in the immediate vicinity of the porus, in 31% it plunges deeply into the porus (normal meatal length 8 mm). The positional relationships and distances are summarized with several important variants in Figs. 247 to 251. The distance of the sinus knee from N. trigeminus anteriorly is approximately equal to that in a basal direction under Lobulus biventer to Recessus lateralis (marked by Plexus chorioideus). The direct distance of N. trigeminus from Recessus lateralis is less than half of this (Fig. 247 *A*). The close relationships of Brachium pontis to Flocculus, Lobulus quadrangularis, Lobulus semilunaris

* Personal communication.

superior, and Lobulus biventer are portrayed in Fig. 247 *B*; they make it understandable why deficits in Brachium pontis are also to be expected if distal parts of A. cerebelli inferior ant. are ligated (Fig. 247 *C*). The pulling apart of Flocculus, Lobulus biventer, Lobulus quadrangularis/simplex, and Lobulus semilunaris superior at this point should only be carried out under microsurgical conditions with big magnification. The arteries of this region pass partly under the arachnoidal layer of the above-named cerebellar structures, and partly freely through the cisternal space in the vicinity of the VII/VIII and IX/XII cranial nerves.

Injection preparations may demonstrate variants as shown in Figs. 248 and 249, in which an inner and an outer circle of arteries surrounds the flocculus. The outer circle consists of the rostrolateral branch of A. cerebelli inferior ant., which is recognizable at the lower border of Lobulus quadrangularis during exposure of cerebellopontine arteries, covered by Arachnoidea, or free in the cisterna in the vicinity of cranial nerves VII and VIII. The rostrolateral branch may make connection between Flocculus and Lobulus biventer with the caudomedial branch of A. cerebelli inferior ant. or with arteries of Plexus chorioideus, which is surrounded by an inner circle of arteries (Fig. 249). Thus, with careful conservation of Plexus chorioideus there is a possibility here of sufficient collateral vascularization, but this is inconstant.

Flocculus and Plexus chorioideus normally cover the proximal portion of cranial nerves VII to XI. If they are raised (Figs. 248 and 249), it is possible to recognize only the exit of N. facialis from the pontomedullary border and the immediately adjacent exit of cranial nerves IX to XI from Medulla oblongata behind the olive, but not the course of N. stato-acusticus. Fig. 248 *B* gives a schematic representation of the dorsolateral region of Medulla oblongata to Recessus lateralis and Plexus chorioideus, and to Pedunculus flocculi; it crosses below Plexus chor. and Pedunculus flocc. and appears again in front of Flocculus. In other cases it covers the rostral flocculus region from the lateral direction. Janetta in 1977 quoted the variants of the three cerebellar arteries as possible causes of trigeminal neuralgia (Figs. 221 to 232). The variants observed by Janetta at operation have been redrawn in Figs. 250 and 251, since the original illustrations do not exhibit the exact positional relationships to the surface of the brain. A knowledge of such variants is important when an approach to the ventral surface of Medulla oblongata is carried out (Fig. 252). The approach from the lateral direction (Fig. 252) shows the exit area of cranial nerves IX to XI from the brainstem and the dural penetration sites in front of Bulbus venae jugularis superior. Rhoton showed that only N. IX penetrated the anterior niche of Foramen jugulare (Figs. 241 *C*, 243, 245 *B* and 252). It is separated by a bridge of the dura from N. X in Foramen jugulare. N. X and XI pass through the anterior inferior part of Pars venosa of Foramen jugulare (Fig. 252 *A* and *B*). After drilling off Tuberculum jugulare above N. XII the clivus groove is shallower and an approach size of approximately 1 cm² to the pons (exit of Nn. VI) is possible.

This approach may in some circumstances be hampered by variants of A. vertebralis. If the approach is free, Cisterna is penetrated by a curtain of numerous perforating arteries from A. vertebralis or A. cerebelli inferior post. The exposure of the exit and proximal course of N. facialis and N. statoacusticus are possible from the basal direction. The temporary facialis paresis described by Drake is no doubt also possible here.

Our only operative case (aneurysm at the junction of Aa. vertebrales in the midline) also presented a temporary incomplete paresis of N. facialis. The approach above N. statoacusticus and facialis to the ventral pons under the flocculus is easier. A. cerebelli inferior ant. is visible from both approaches. In the basal approach it lies in front of the pons and crosses under or over N. abducens before passing from above to run alongside N. facialis. In the laterobasal approach it appears above the meatal loop. The trigeminal loop is usually less clearly visible in the region of Brachium pontis than in Fig. 252 *B*. Distally from the trigeminal loop the sturdy trunk is almost always recognizable under the arachnoid membrane in its course between Flocculus and Lobulus quadrangularis and farther back between Lobulus biventer and Lobulus semilunaris superior. It has already been specified that even beyond this stretch branches may go off to Brachium pontis, deeply between Flocculus and Tonsilla.

The well-known dangers of resection of the tonsil (e.g., in Arnold-Chiari syndrome) make it necessary to provide a special demonstration of the structure and connections of the cerebellar tonsil (Figs. 253 to 258). The relationships to the lower vermis region medially and to the flocculus as well as to the 4th ventricle were schematically illustrated in Fig. 214. They can also be seen in Figs. 209 and 210 and on the section drawings in Figs. 211 and 212. In Fig. 243 the relationship to the posterior medullary velum and to its encircling vessel trunks is illustrated as it would be seen at operation (there with conservation of the arteries). It can easily be recognized that conservation of the arteries is only possible if the tonsil is not luxated in toto, but resected subpially. The tonsil has contact surfaces with Velum medullare post., Uvula, and Nodulus, as well as with Medulla oblongata and Flocculus.

The white matter of the tonsil is firmly joined to Brachium pontis and to Pedunculus flocculi. In Figs. 254 to 258 an attempt has been made to demonstrate these relationships from above, below, medially, and laterally. At extirpation of the tonsil it is particularly important to preserve Pedunculus flocculi. Its elimination results in the abolishment of optokinetic nystagmus to the opposite side. This damage can be avoided if at reduction of the tonsil its area of attachment (5 in Figs. 254 and 255) is not approached too closely. If all the cerebellar peduncles are sectioned (Fig. 257), the relationships between the anterior and posterior medullary velum, the 4th ventricle, and the cerebellar peduncles can be seen. From the dorsal direction one may expect to find caudally the large arterial trunks in the region of Medulla oblongata, and the large venous connections in the rostral part near the brainstem (Fig. 258). Here regions are reached which only rarely are the subject of neurosurgical intervention.

E. References

Caille, J. M., Piton, J., Boussens, J.: In: Advances in Cerebral Angiography, edited by Salamon, G. Part I, Anatomy: Anatomic-Radiologic Study of the Cerebello-Labyrinthi Arterial System. Normal Aspect. Connections with Internal Auditory Canal, p. 62. Berlin–Heidelberg–New York: Springer. 1975.

Drake, C. G.: Surgical treatment of ruptured aneurysms of the basilar artery. Experience with 14 cases. J. Neurosurg. **23,** 457–473 (1965).

Drake, C. G.: The surgical treatment of vertebral-basilar aneurysms. Clin. Neurosurg. **16,** 114–169 (1969).

Duvernoy, H. M.: The Superficial Veins of the Human Brain. Veins of the Brain Stem and of the Base of the Brain. Berlin–Heidelberg–New York: Springer. 1975.

Huang, Y. P., Wolf, B. S.: In: Advances in Cerebral Angiography, edited by Salamon, G., Part I, Anatomy: Variations of Basal Cerebral Veins: Embryologic Considerations, p. 82. Berlin–Heidelberg–New York: Springer. 1975.

Jannetta, J. P.: Observations on the etiology of trigeminal neuralgia, hemifacial spasm. acoustic nerve dysfunction and glossopharyngeal neuralgia. Neurochirurgia **20,** 145–154 (1977).

Krause, F., Schum, H.: Die spezielle Chirurgie der Gehirnkrankheiten. Stuttgart: F. Enke. 1932.

Naidich, T. P., Kricheff, I. I.: In: Advances in Cerebral Angiography, edited by Salamon, G., Part I, Anatomy: The Anterior Inferior Cerebellar Artery in Profile Anatomic-Radiographic Correlation in the Lateral Projection, p. 74. Berlin–Heidelberg–New York: Springer. 1975.

Newton, Th., Potts, D. G.: Radiology of the Skull and Brain Angiography. St. Louis: The C. V. Mosby Company. 1974.

Rhoton, A. L., Jr.: Microsurgical removal of acoustic neuromas. Surg. Neurol. **6,** 211–219 (1976).

Rhoton, A. L., Jr., Buza, R.: The microsurgical anatomy of the jugular foramen. J. Neurosurg. **42,** 541–550 (1975).

Rhoton, A. L., Jr.: Microsurgery of the internal acoustic meatus Surg. Neurol. **2,** 311–318 (1974).

Scialfa, G., Michotey, P., Bank, W., Salamon, G.: Anatomic Variations of the Vertebrobasilar System. In: Salamon, G., Huang, Y. P., Radiological Anatomy of the Human Brain. Berlin–Heidelberg–New York: Springer. 1976.

Scialfa, G., Bank, W., Megret, M., Corbaz, J. M.: In: Advances in Cerebral Angiography, edited by Salamon, G. Part I, Anatomy: The Posterior Fossa Arteries: 1. The Morphology and Variations of the Anterior Inferior Cerebellar Artery. 2. The Arteriographic Localization of the Fourth Ventricle, p. 55. Berlin–Heidelberg–New York: Springer. 1975.

Takahashi, M., Okudera, T., Fukui, H., Kitamura, K.: Choroidal and nodular branches of the posterior inferior cerebellar artery: Their value in diagnosis of medulloblastomas. Radiology **103,** 347 (1972).

Wende, S., Nakayama, N.: In: Advances in Cerebral Angiography, edited by Salamon, G., Part. I, Anatomy: Anatomical Variations of the Internal Auditory Artery, p. 69. Berlin–Heidelberg–New York: Springer. 1975.

Yaşargil, G. M., Fox, J. L.: The microsurgical approach to acoustic neurinomas. Surg. Neurol. **2,** 393–398 (1974).

Yaşargil, M. G., So, S. C.: Cerebellopontine angle meningioma presenting as subarachnoid haemorrhage. Surg. Neurol. **6,** 3–6 (1976).

Yaşargil, M. G.: Intracranial microsurgery. Clin. Neurosurg. **17,** 250–255 (1970).

Yaşargil, M. G., Smith, R. D.: Association of middle cerebral artery anomalies with saccular aneurysms and moyamoya disease. Surg. Neurol. **6,** 39–43 (1976).

Yaşargil, M. G., et al.: Arteriovenous Malformations of the Splenium of the Corpus Callosum: Microsurgical Treatment. Surg. Neurol. **5,** 5–13 (1976).

Yaşargil, M. G., De Preux, J.: Expériences microchirurgicales dans 21 cas d'hémangioblastomes intramédullaires. Neuro-Chirurgie **21,** N° 6, 425–434 (1975).

Yaşargil, M. G., et al.: Arteriovenous Malformations of Vein of Galen: Microsurgical Treatment. Surg. Neurol. **6,** 195–200 (1976).

Yaşargil, M. G., Antic, M. D. J., Laciga, R., Jain, K. K., Hodosh, R. M., Smith, R. D.: Microsurgical Pterional Approach to Aneurysms of the Basilar Bifurcation. Surg. Neurol. **6,** 83–91 (1976).

Literature for Further Reading

Drake, C. G.: The surgical treatment of vertebral-basilar aneurysm. Clin. Neurosurg. **16,** 114–169 (1969).

Drake, C. G.: Surgical treatment of ruptured aneurysms of the basilar artery. Experience with 14 cases. J. Neurosurg. **23,** 457–473 (1965).

Drake, C. G.: The surgical treatment of aneurysms of the basilar artery. J. Neurosurg. **29,** 436–446 (1968).

Drake, C. G.: Further experience with surgical treatment of aneurysms and their surgical treatment. J. Neurosurg. **29,** 372–392 (1968).

Huang, Y. P., Wolf, B. S., Antin, S. P., Okudera, T., Kim, I. H.: Angiographic features of aqueductal stenosis. Amer. J. Roentgenol. **104,** 90–108 (1968).

Huang, Y. P., Wolf, B. S.: The vein of the lateral recess of the fourth ventricle and its tributaries. Amer. J. Roentgenol. **101,** 1–21 (1967).

Jamieson, K. G.: Aneurysms of the vertebrobasilar system. Further experience with nine cases. J. Neurosurg. **28,** 544–555 (1967).

Lazorthes, G., Poulhes, J., Espagno, J.: Les artères du cervelet. Comp. Ren. Ass. Anat. **62,** 275–287 (1951).

Lazorthes, G., Gouaze, A., Salamon, G.: Vascularisation et circulation cérébrales. In press. Paris: Masson et Cie.

Salamon, G., Huang, Y. P.: Radiological Anatomy of the Human Brain. Berlin–Heidelberg–New York: Springer. 1976.

Stopford, J. B. S.: The arteries of the pons and medulla oblongate. J. Anat. and Physiol. **50,** 130–164 (1916).

Takahaski, M.: The Anterior Inferior Cerebellar Artery. In: Radiology of the Skull and Brain – Angiography, vol. 2, pp. 1796–1807, edited by Newton, Th., Potts, D. G. St. Louis: The C. V. Mosby Company. 1974.

F. Illustrations
(Figs. 206 to 258)

Fig. 206. Dorsal view of Cerebellum

Fig. 207. Upper and middle vermis region split sagittally, with removal of Lobulus quadrangularis and simplex. Cut surface of Brachium pontis at transition to Medulla of Cerebellum

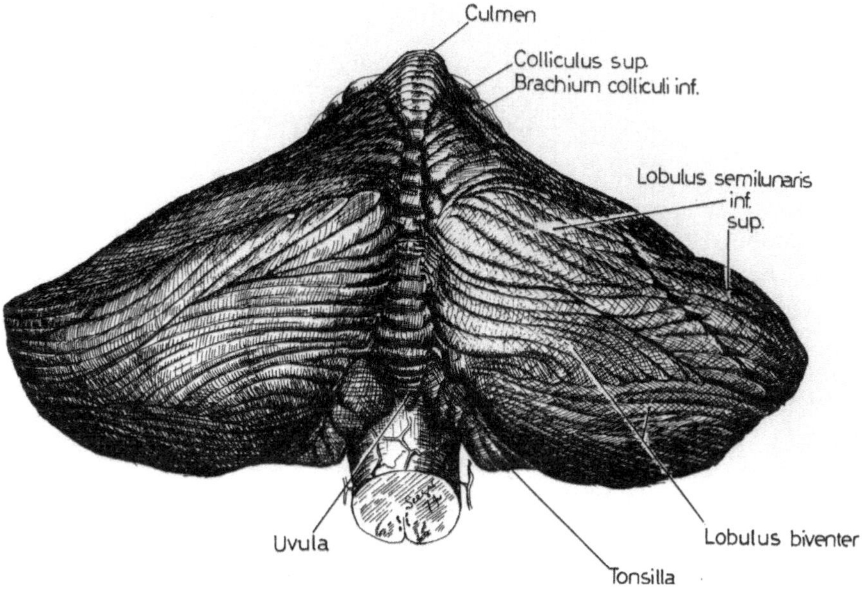
Culmen
Colliculus sup.
Brachium colliculi inf.
Lobulus semilunaris
inf.
sup.
Uvula
Lobulus biventer
Tonsilla

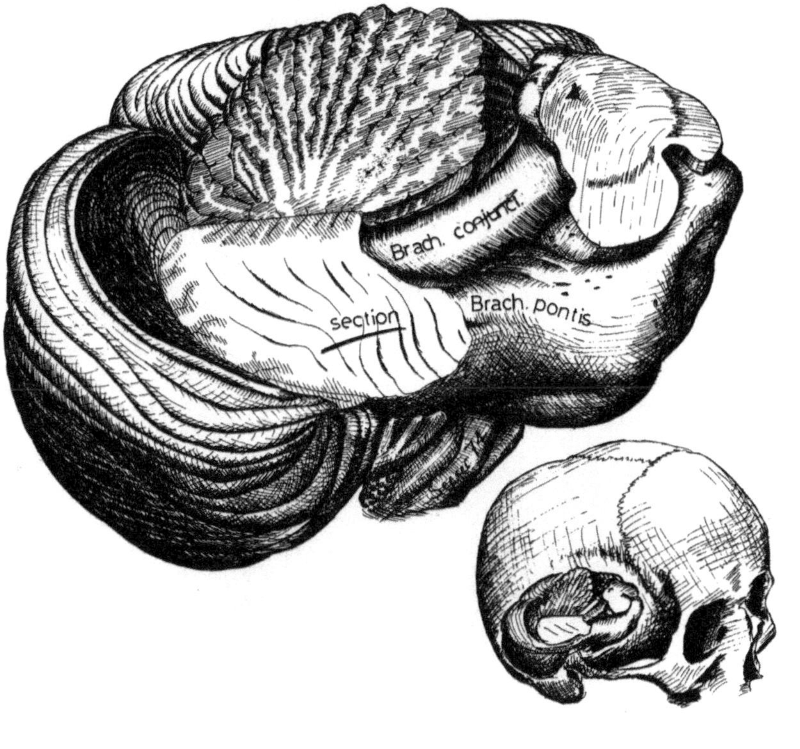
Brach. conjunct.
Brach. pontis
section

Fig. 208. Preparation of Fig. 207 with additional removal of Lobulus semilunaris superior and inferior, oblique view: connection between Nodulus/Uvula complex, Tonsilla, Lobulus centralis, Lingula cerebelli, and Velum medullare ant. = Fastigium point of 4th ventricle (*)

Fig. 209. Median section of upper and middle vermis region, division of Uvula/Nodulus-complex right parasagittally at the tonsil insertion. Complete section at right of Brachium pontis with removal of Lobulus biventer and tonsil. Velum medullare post. freed at tonsil insertion. Recessus lateralis and exit of N. stato-acusticus covered by Velum medullare post. Transition of Velum medullare post. into the paper-thin layer

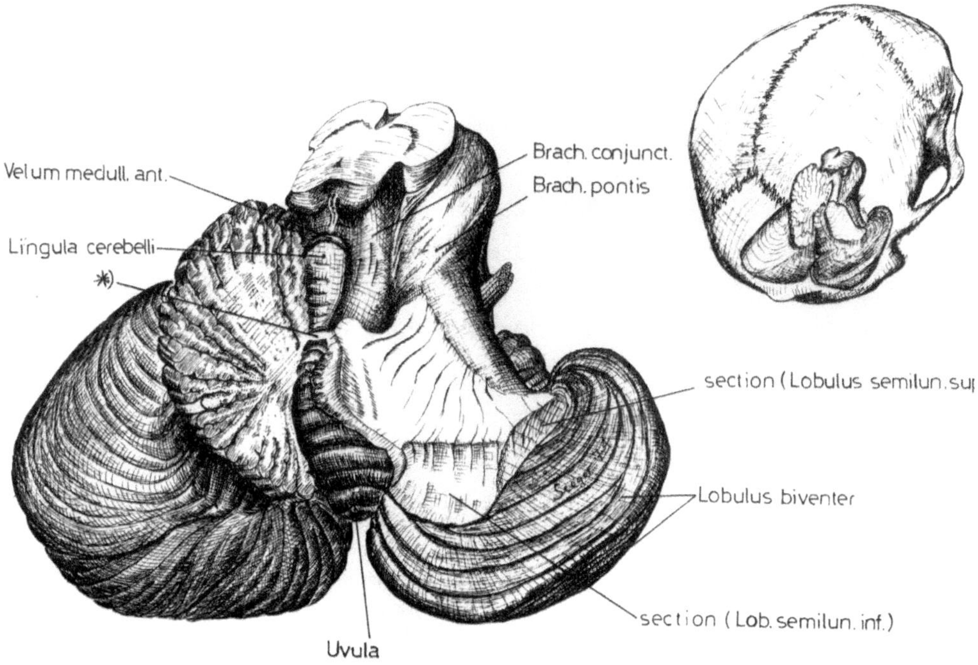
Velum medull. ant.
Lingula cerebelli
*)
Brach. conjunct.
Brach. pontis
section (Lobulus semilun. sup
Lobulus biventer
section (Lob. semilun. inf.)
Uvula

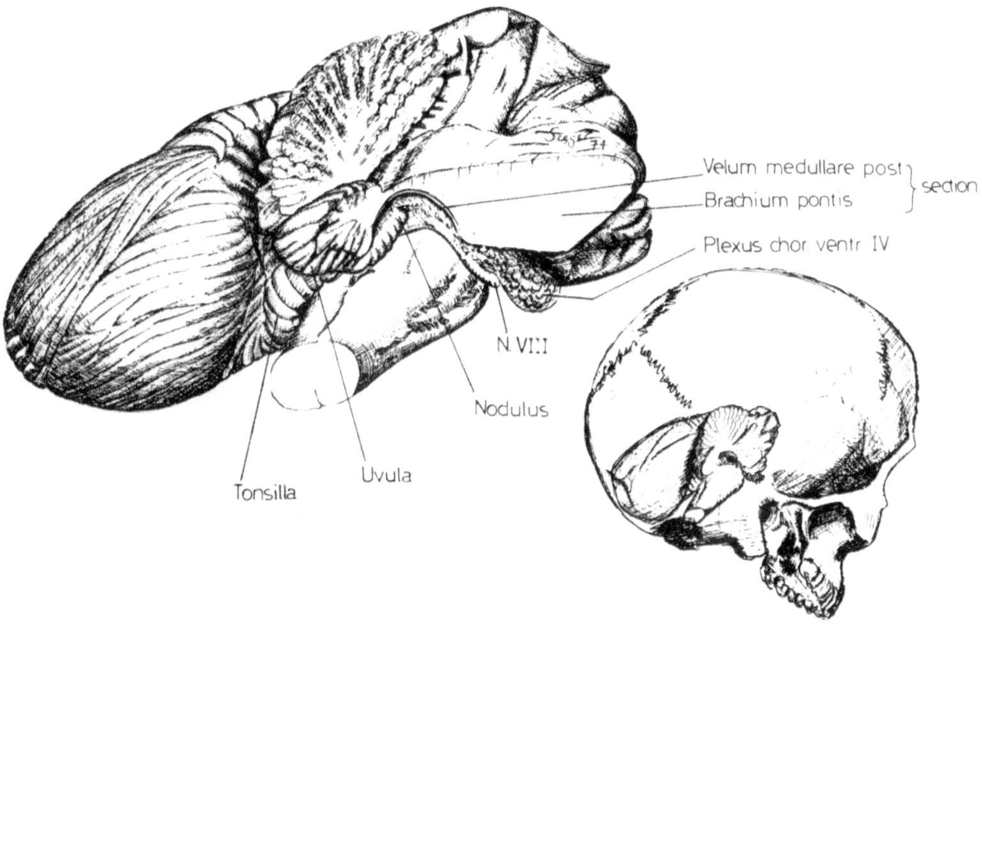
Velum medullare post
Brachium pontis
section
Plexus chor. ventr. IV
N. VIII
Nodulus
Tonsilla
Uvula

Fig. 210. Rostral view after section of left Brachium pontis, removal of left cerebellar hemisphere and of left half of Velum medullare ant. Flocculus with tonsil pushed towards caudal direction and freed from Brachium pontis. View into left half of 4th ventricle from rostral direction. Velum medullare post. fenestrated over rostral surface of tonsil
* Cut surface of tonsil insertion at Brachium pontis

Fig. 211. Preparation of Fig. 210 with section lines of Fig. 212

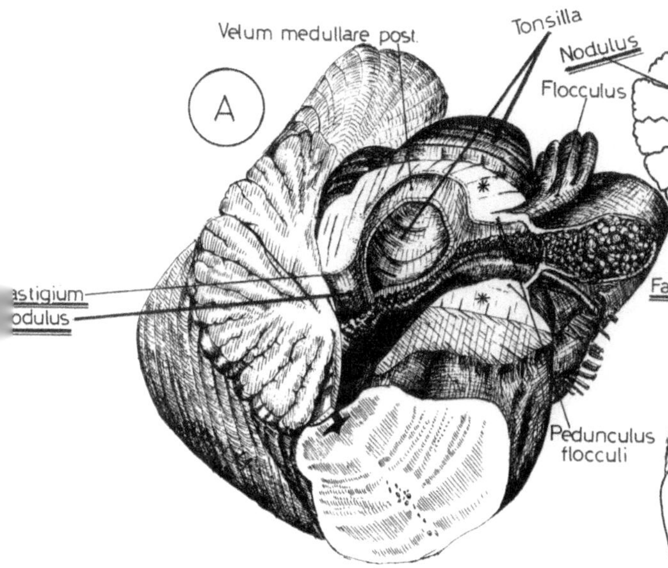
A
Velum medullare post.
Tonsilla
Flocculus
astigium
odulus
Pedunculus
flocculi

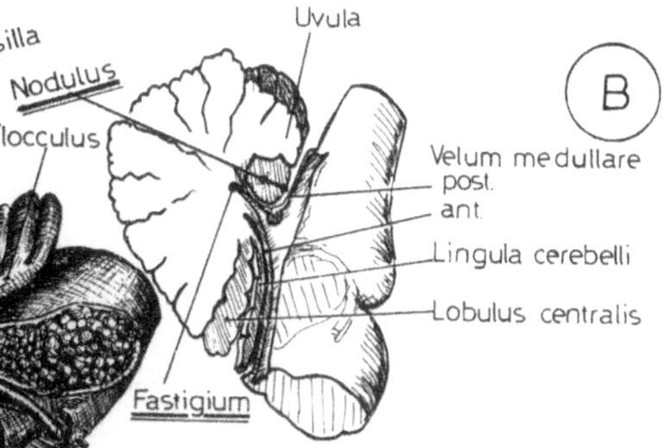
B
Uvula
Nodulus
Velum medullare
post.
ant.
Lingula cerebelli
Lobulus centralis
Fastigium

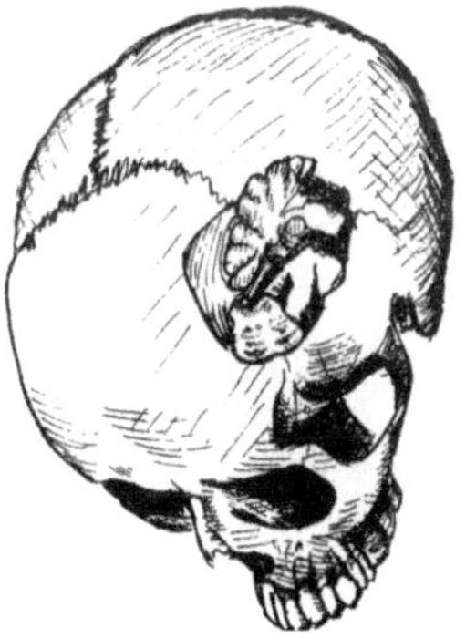

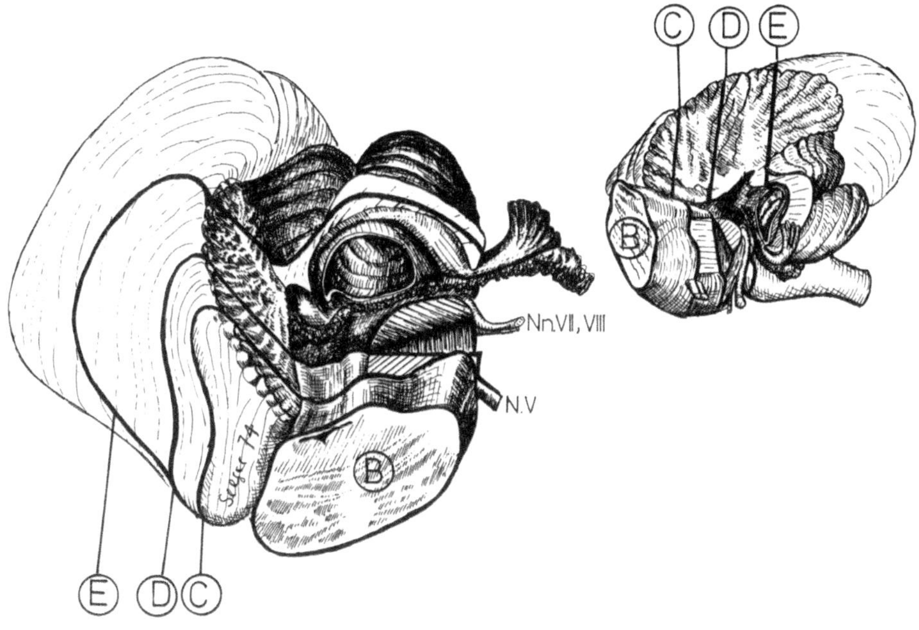
C
D
E
B
Nn.VII, VIII
N.V
E
D
C

Fig. 212. Section planes of preparation of Fig. 210
For position of section planes see Fig. 211
Arrow: Nucleus dentatus

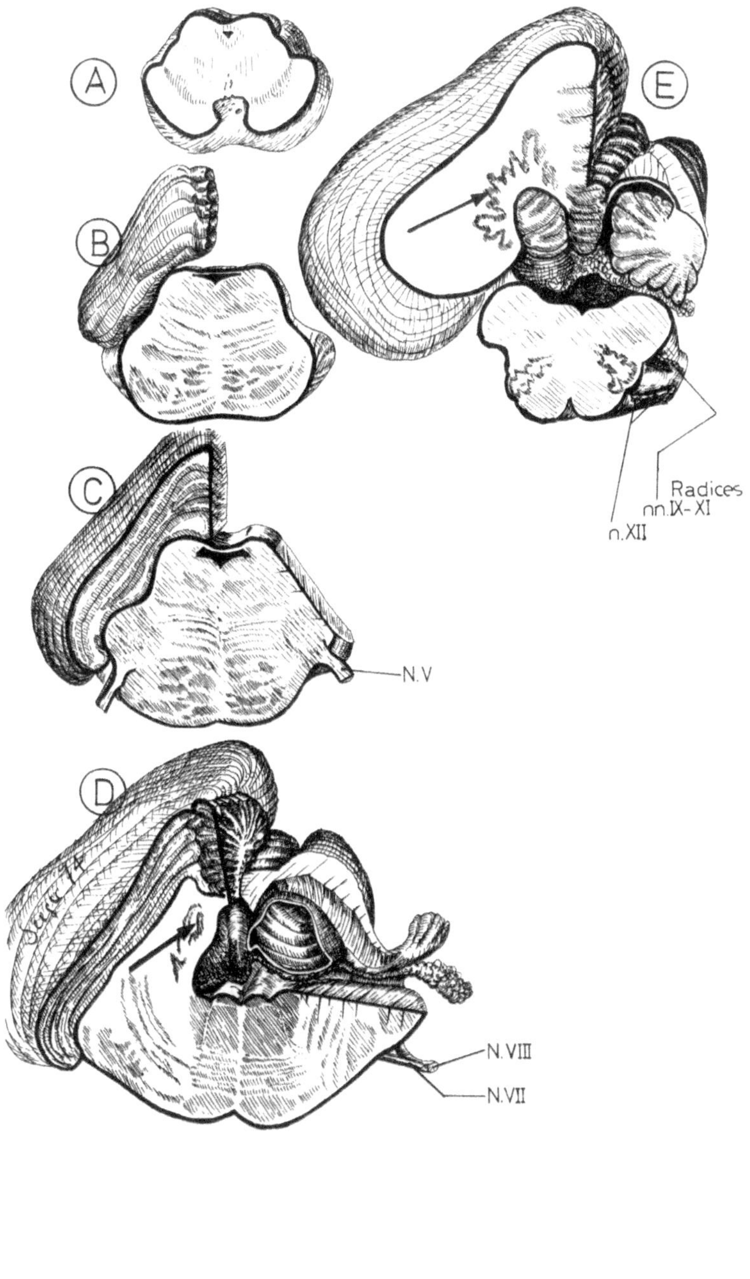
A
B
C
D
E
N.V
N.VIII
N.VII
Radices
nn.IX- XI
n.XII

Fig. 213. Caudal view into 4th ventricle after removal of right cerebellar hemisphere and sagittal section of Vermis. Contralateral cerebellar tonsil also removed
Arrow: Recessus lateralis of 4th ventricle, Lobulus centralis, Lingula cerebelli (and underlying Velum medullare ant.) merge in front of Fastigium to form homogeneous zone of white matter

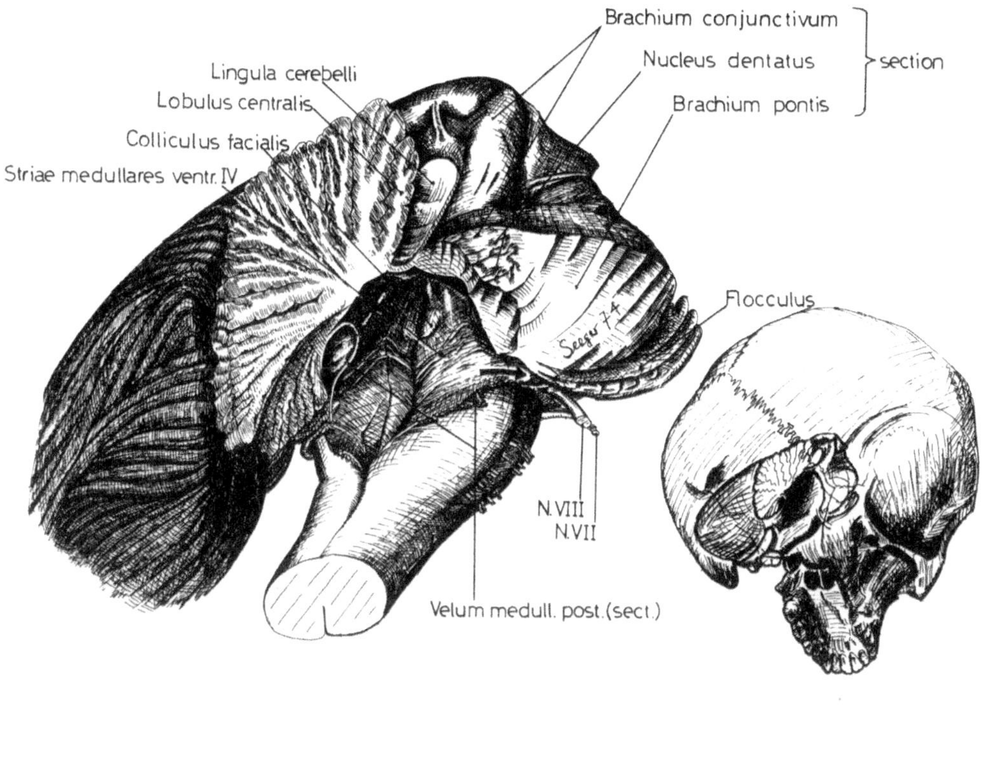
Brachium conjunctivum
Nucleus dentatus
Brachium pontis
section
Lingula cerebelli
Lobulus centralis
Colliculus facialis
Striae medullares ventr. IV
Flocculus
N. VIII
N. VII
Velum medull. post. (sect.)

Fig. 214 a. Schematic representation of connection between Brachium pontis, Flocculus, Tonsilla, and Uvula/Nodulus complex. Velum medullare ant. and post. are at the highest point of the 4th ventricle – Fastigium – still separated by a narrow zone of white matter (*)

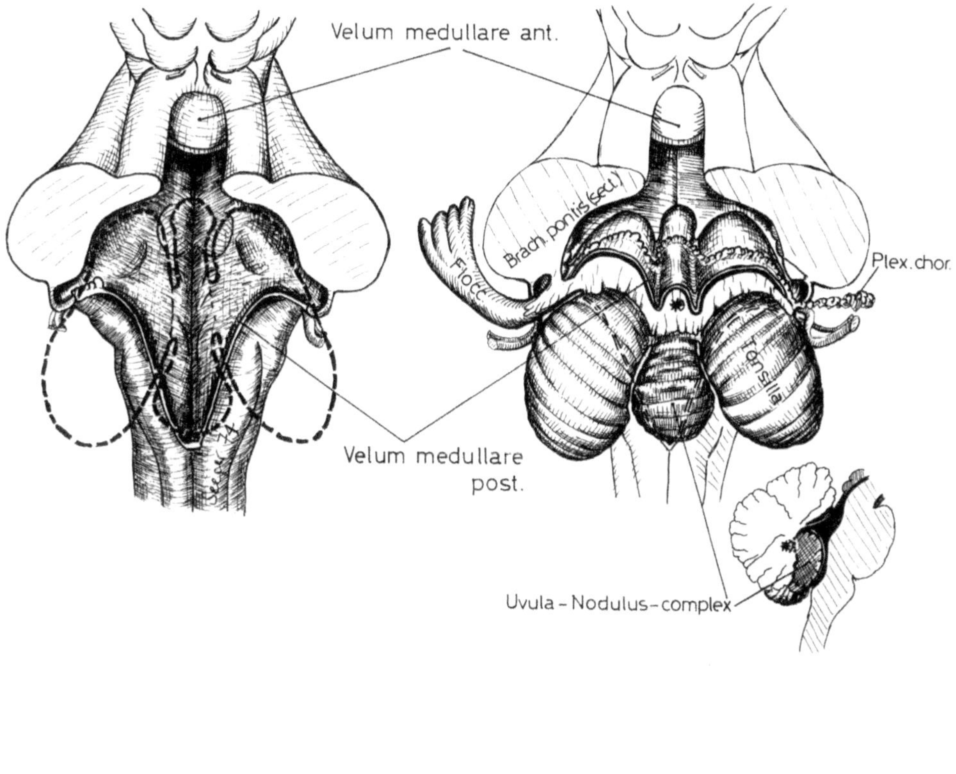
Velum medullare ant.
Brach. pontis (sect.)
Flocc.
Plex. chor.
Tonsilla
Velum medullare post.
Uvula - Nodulus - complex

Fig. 214 b. Relationships between Velum medullare posterius and Ventriculus IV
A, B, C Brain structures
D Cast of Ventriculus IV (schematically drawn)

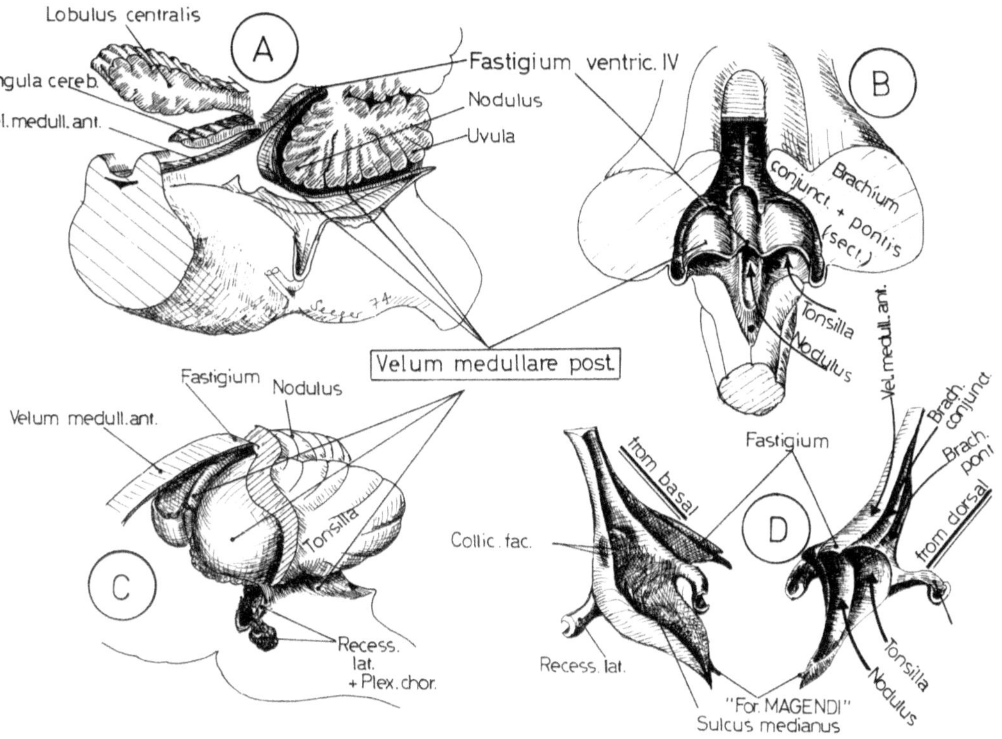
Lobulus centralis
A
Lingula cereb.
Vel. medull. ant.
Fastigium ventric. IV
Nodulus
Uvula
B
Brachium conjunct. + pontis (sect.)
Tonsilla
Nodulus
Velum medullare post.
Fastigium
Nodulus
Velum medull. ant.
Tonsilla
C
Recess. lat. + Plex. chor.
Vel. medull. ant.
Brach. conjunct.
Brach. pont.
Fastigium
from basal
from dorsal
D
Collic. fac.
Recess. lat.
"For. MAGENDI"
Sulcus medianus
Tonsilla
Nodulus

Fig. 215. Contents of posterior cranial fossa without vessels. After section of Brachium pontis and removal of both tonsils, median section of Culmen and longitudinal section of Uvula/Noduluscomplex lateral to the midline. Velum medullare post. is fenestrated behind Plexus chorioideus in order to show Plexus chorioideus

Fig. 216. Isolated left cerebellar hemisphere

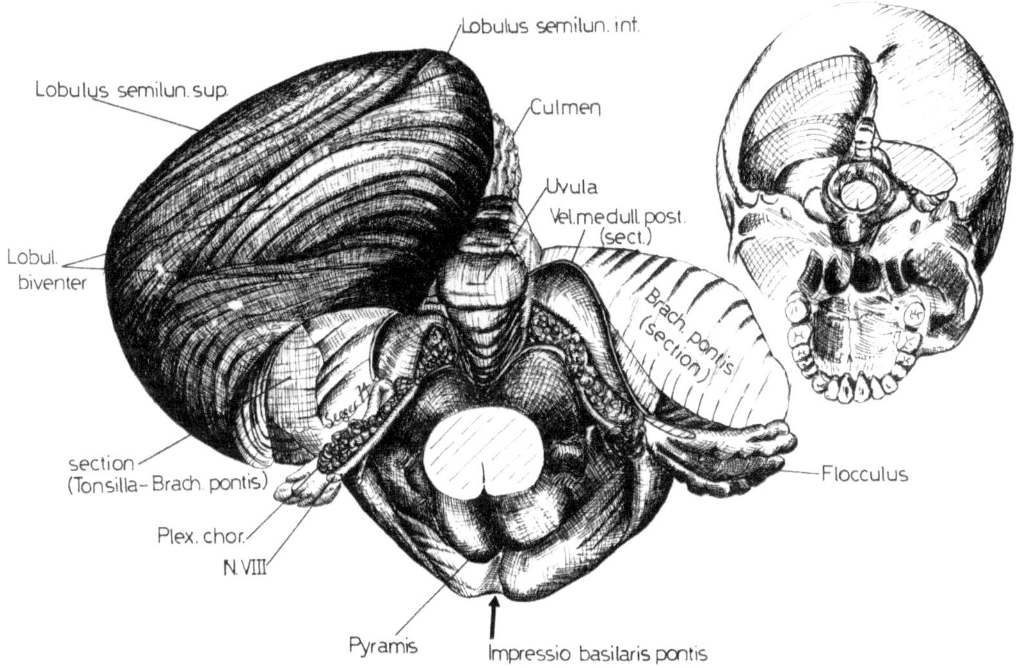
Lobulus semilun. inf.
Lobulus semilun. sup.
Culmen
Uvula
Vel. medull. post. (sect.)
Lobul. biventer
Brach. pontis (section)
section (Tonsilla-Brach. pontis)
Flocculus
Plex. chor.
N. VIII
Pyramis
Impressio basilaris pontis

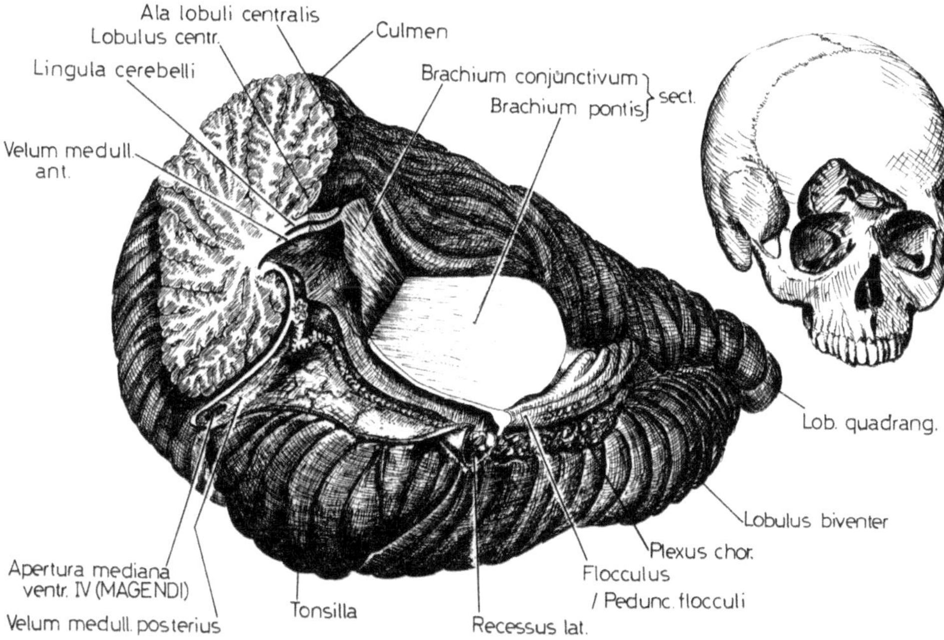
Ala lobuli centralis
Lobulus centr.
Culmen
Lingula cerebelli
Brachium conjunctivum
Brachium pontis
sect.
Velum medull. ant.
Lob. quadrang.
Lobulus biventer
Plexus chor.
Apertura mediana ventr. IV (MAGENDI)
Flocculus
/ Pedunc. flocculi
Tonsilla
Velum medull. posterius
Recessus lat.

Fig. 217.
A Brainstem section and Cerebellum from above (for vessels see *A* in Fig. 218)
B The same preparation as *A* after removal of Lobulus quadrangularis with Lobulus simplex in situ (for vessels see *B* in Fig. 218)

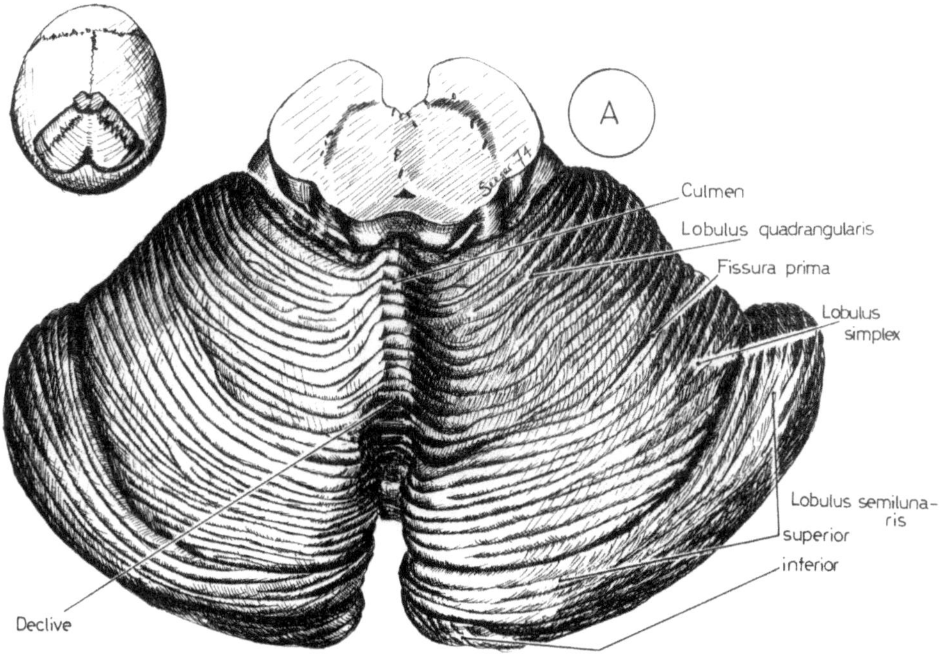
A
Culmen
Lobulus quadrangularis
Fissura prima
Lobulus simplex
Lobulus semiluna-ris
superior
interior
Declive

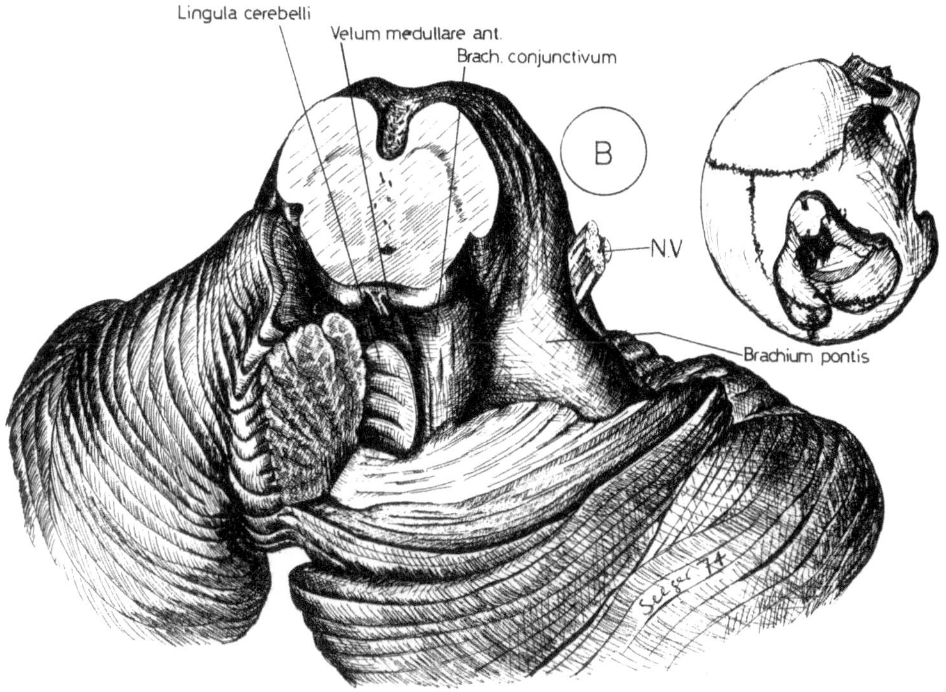
Lingula cerebelli
Velum medullare ant.
Brach. conjunctivum
B
N.V
Brachium pontis

Fig. 218.
A Preparation of Fig. 217 *A* with vessels
B Preparation of Fig. 217 *B* with vessels
The arteries cross over the veins (see A. cerebelli sup.)

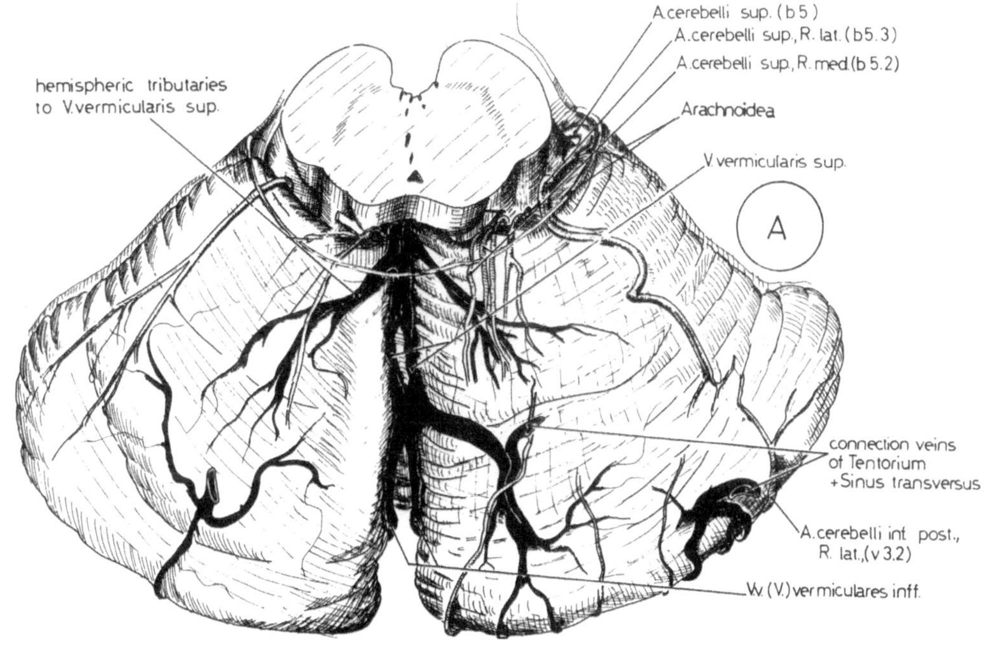
A.cerebelli sup. (b5)
A.cerebelli sup., R. lat. (b5.3)
A.cerebelli sup., R. med.(b 5.2)
hemispheric tributaries to V.vermicularis sup.
Arachnoidea
V.vermicularis sup.
A
connection veins of Tentorium +Sinus transversus
A.cerebelli int. post., R. lat.,(v 3.2)
Vv. (V.) vermiculares inff.

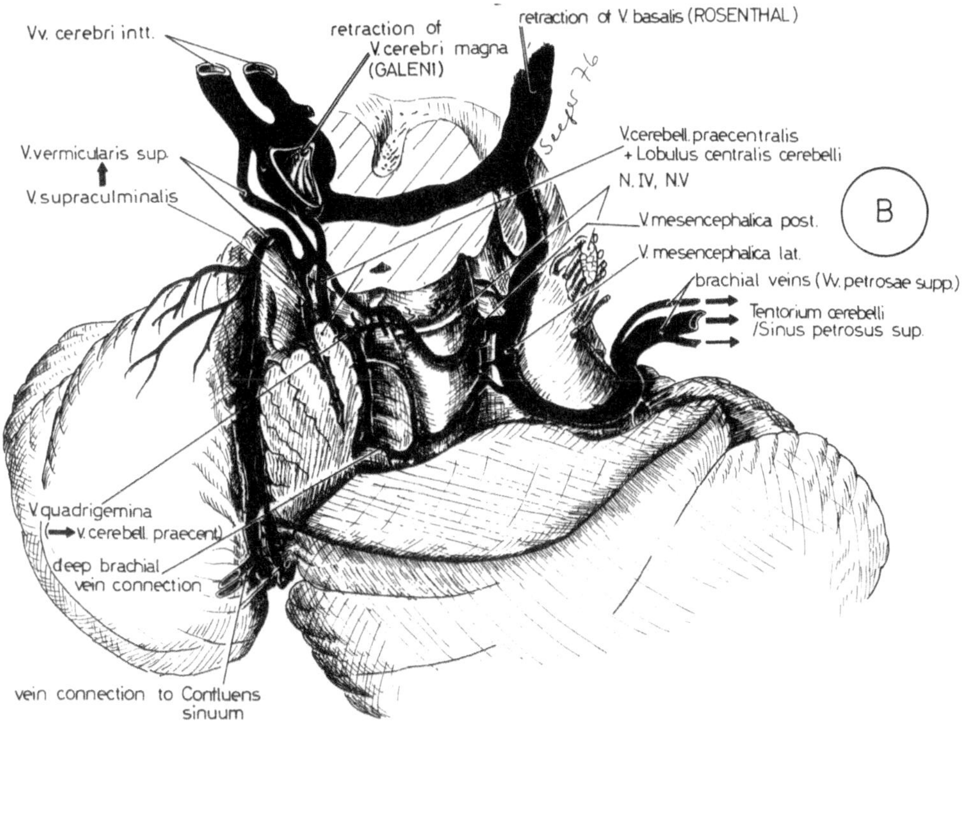
Vv. cerebri intt.
retraction of V.cerebri magna (GALENI)
retraction of V. basalis (ROSENTHAL)
V.vermicularis sup.
V.supraculminalis
V.cerebell. praecentralis + Lobulus centralis cerebelli
N. IV, N.V
V.mesencephalica post.
B
V. mesencephalica lat.
brachial veins (Vv. petrosae supp.)
Tentorium cerebelli /Sinus petrosus sup.
V.quadrigemina (→ v. cerebell. praecent.)
deep brachial vein connection
vein connection to Confluens sinuum

Fig. 219. Brainstem and Cerebellum from basal view
With vessels drawn in, see Fig. 220 *A* and *B*

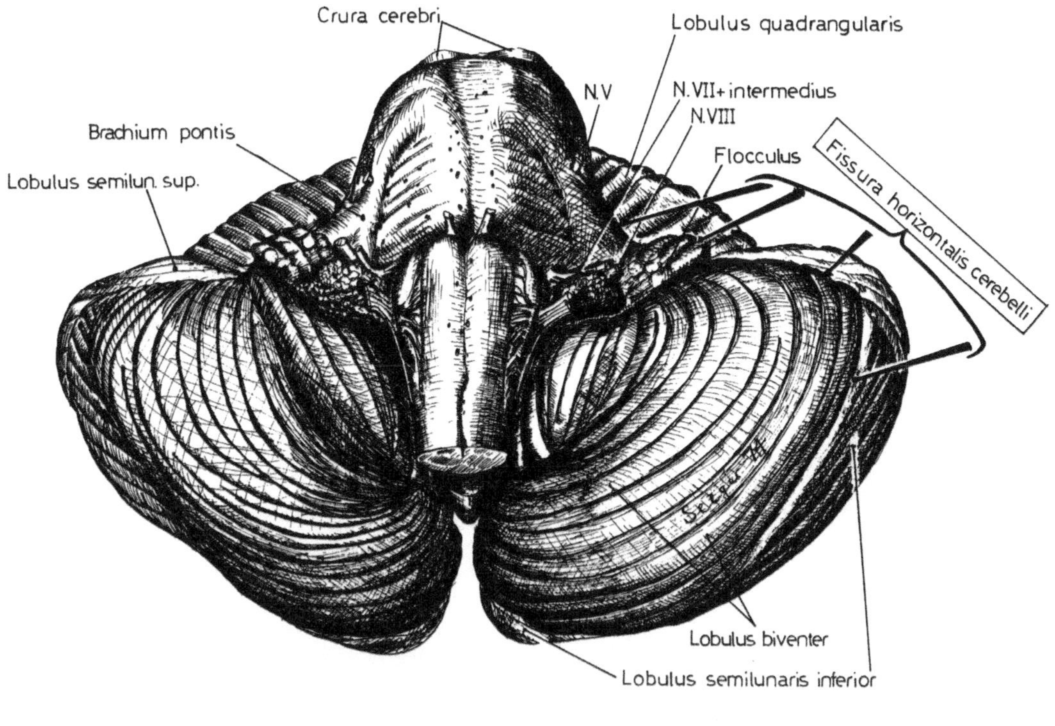
Crura cerebri
Lobulus quadrangularis
N.V
N.VII+ intermedius
N.VIII
Brachium pontis
Flocculus
Lobulus semilun. sup.
Fissura horizontalis cerebelli
Lobulus biventer
Lobulus semilunaris inferior

Fig. 220. See Fig. 219
A * Rami perforantes between Flocculus and Lobulus biventer, to Brachium pontis
B Veins lie close to the surface of the brain and are crossed over by arteries
For arterial nomenclature see catalogue of arteries, pages 3–4

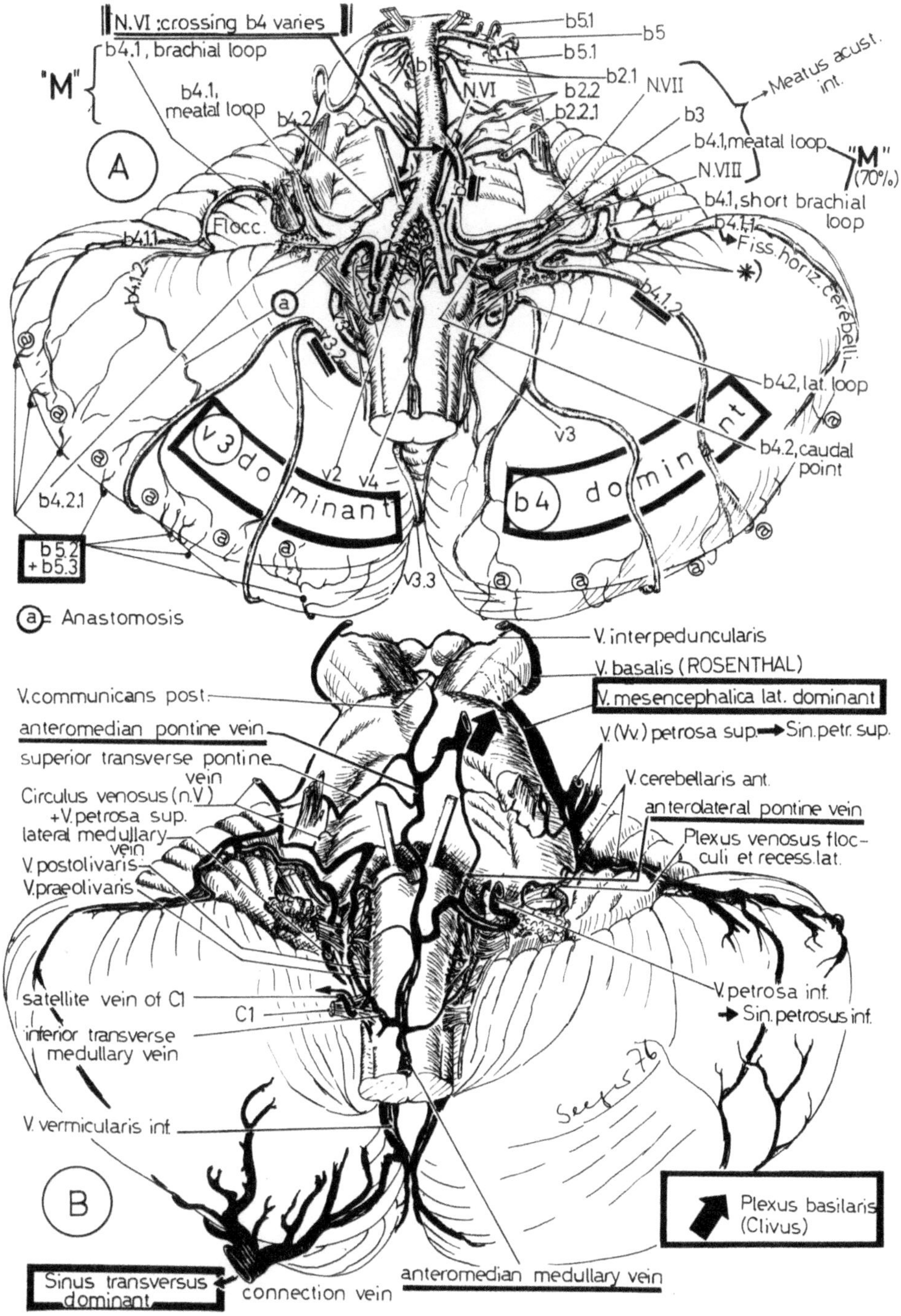
N.VI :crossing b4 varies
"M"
b4.1, brachial loop
b4.1, meatal loop
b4.2
A
Flocc.
b4.1.1
b4.1.2
b5.1
b5
b5.1
b1
N.VI
b2.1
b2.2
b2.2.1
N.VII
Meatus acust. int.
b3
b4.1, meatal loop
"M" (70%)
N.VIII
b4.1, short brachial loop
b4.1.1
Fiss. horiz. cerebelli
*)
b4.1.2
b4.2, lat. loop
b4.2, caudal point
v3
v3.2
v3 dominant
v2
v4
b4.2.1
b4 dominant
b5.2 + b5.3
v3.3
a = Anastomosis
V. interpeduncularis
V. basalis (ROSENTHAL)
V. communicans post.
V. mesencephalica lat. dominant
anteromedian pontine vein
V. (Vv.) petrosa sup. → Sin. petr. sup.
superior transverse pontine vein
V. cerebellaris ant.
Circulus venosus (n.V) + V. petrosa sup.
anterolateral pontine vein
lateral medullary vein
Plexus venosus flocculi et recess. lat.
V. postolivaris
V. praeolivaris
V. petrosa inf. → Sin. petrosus inf.
satellite vein of C1
C1
inferior transverse medullary vein
V. vermicularis inf.
B
Plexus basilaris (Clivus)
Sinus transversus dominant
connection vein
anteromedian medullary vein

Fig. 221. Variants of A. vertebralis (according to Scialfa et al., 1976)
A Variants of course
B Variants of calibre
C Varying localization of junction with A. basilaris

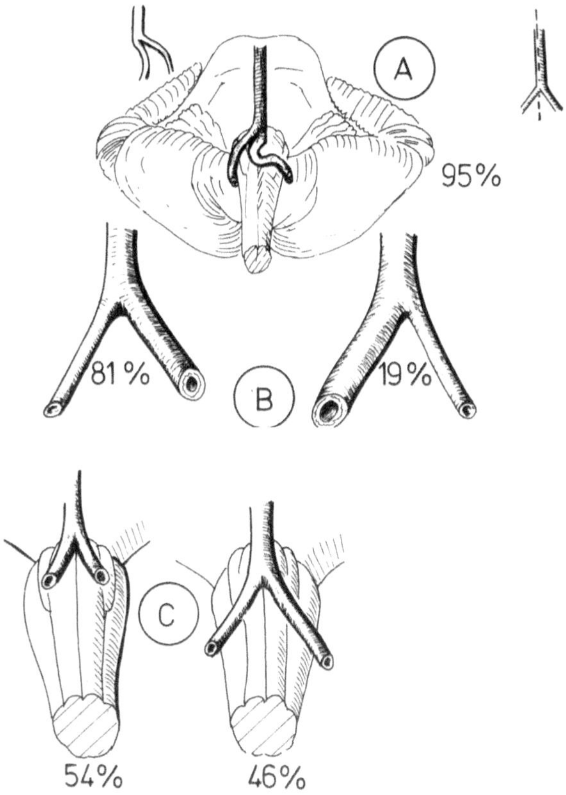
A
95%
81%
B
19%
C
54%
46%

Fig. 222. Variants of A. basilaris (according to Scialfa et al., 1976)
D Deviations of trunk from midline
E Deviations of bifurcation point from midline
F Duplication

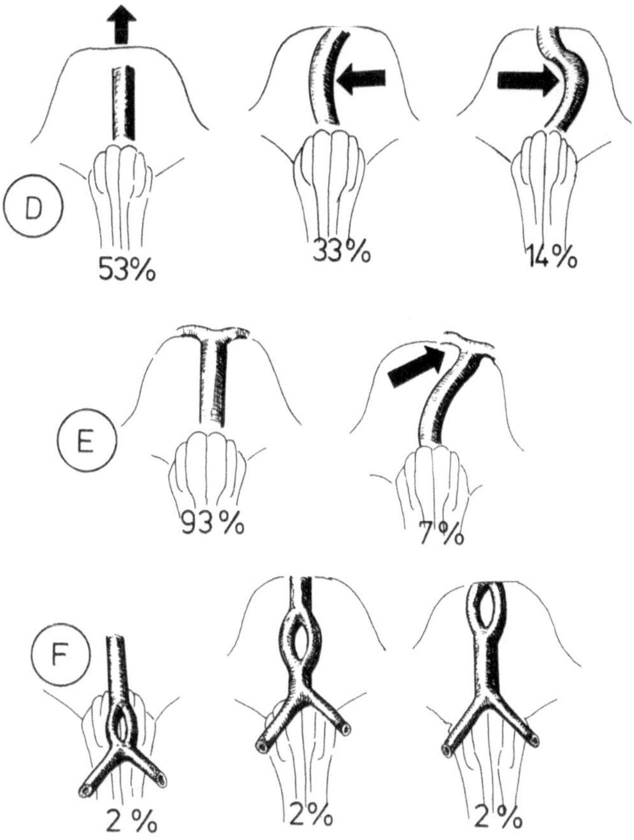
D
53%
33%
14%
E
93%
7%
F
2 %
2%
2 %

Fig. 223. Variants in number of A. cerebelli inferior ant. (according to Scialfa et al., 1976)

 FIG. 223

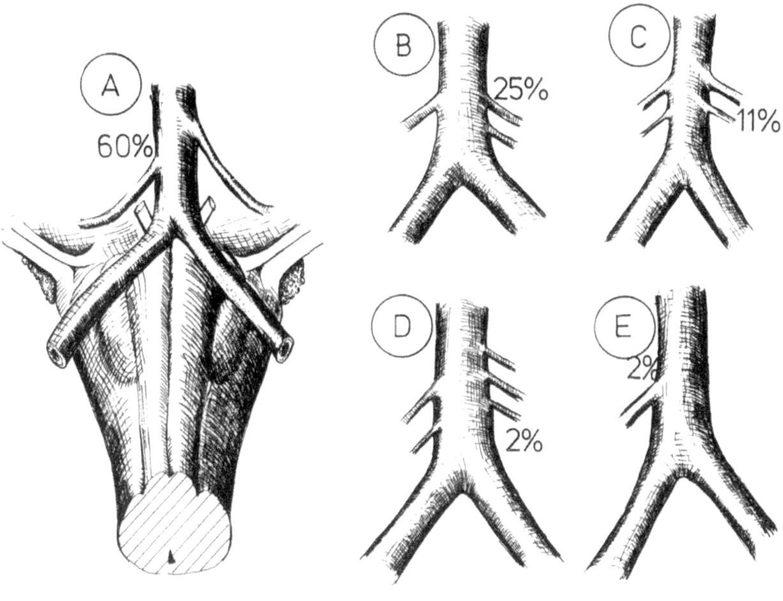

Fig. 224. Level of origin of A. cerebelli inferior ant ("Aica") from A. basilaris (according to Scialfa et al., 1976): caudal *F*, cranial *G*, middle region *H, I* from A. vertebralis (designated A. cerebelli inferior ant. by Naidich and Kricheff)

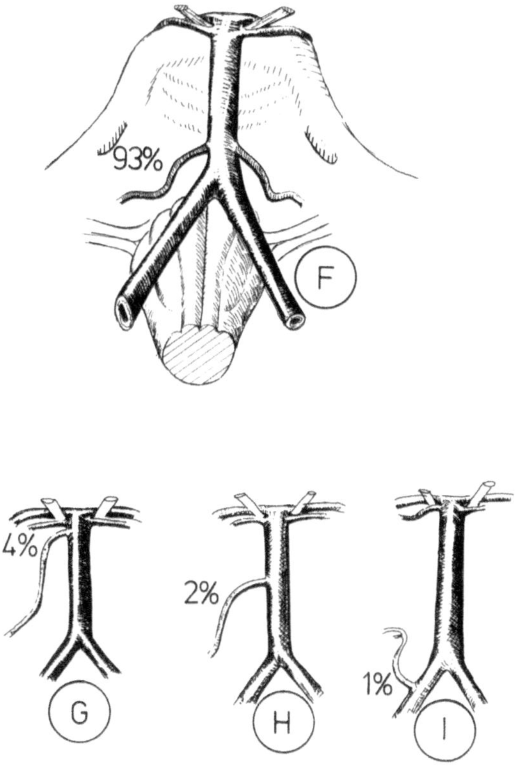
93%
F
4%
G
2%
H
1%
I

Fig. 225. Variants of A. cerebelli inferior ant. and A. auditiva interna:
I-III Origin of A. auditiva interna, according to Wende et al. (1975)
IV Origin of A. cerebelli inferior ant., according to Caillé et al. (1975)
V-VI Types of A. cerebelli inferior ant., according to Scialfa et al. (1975)

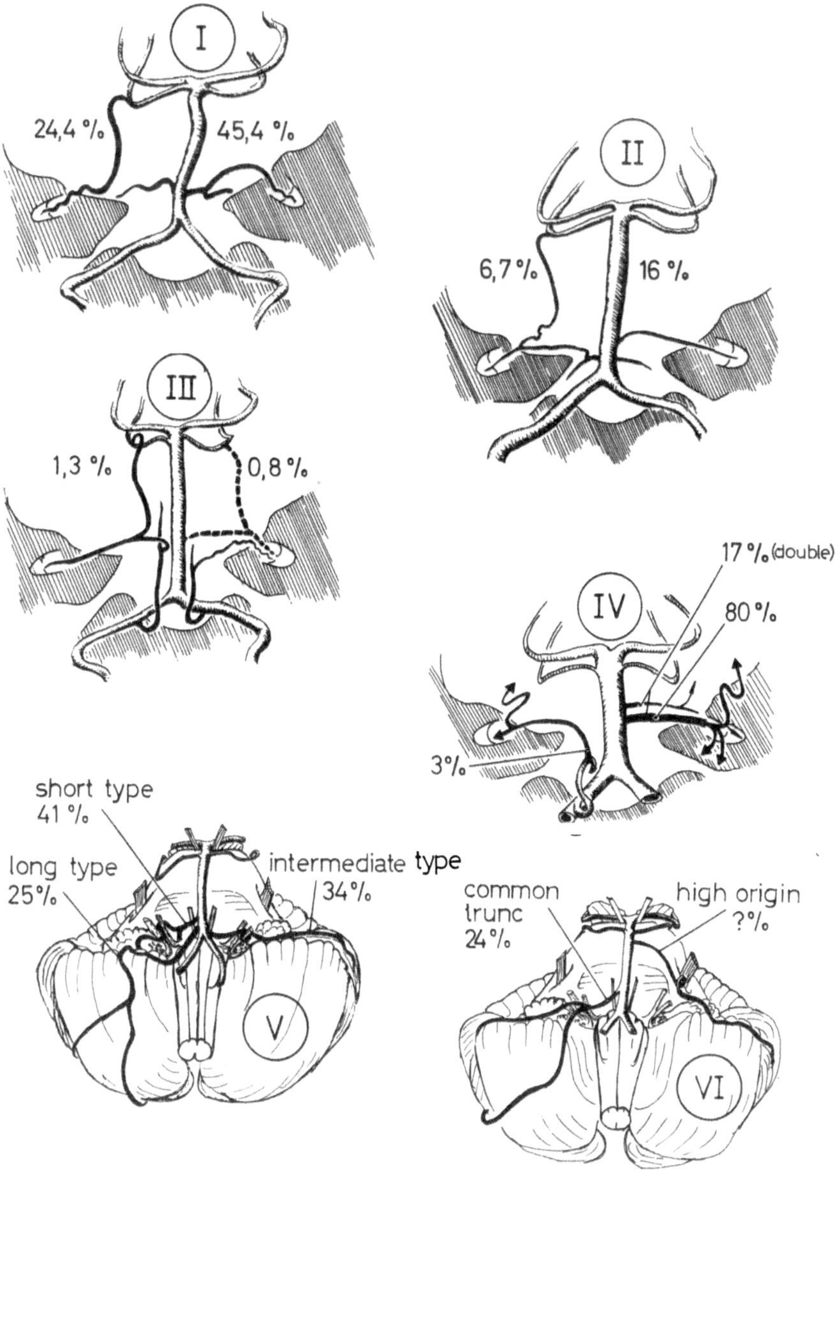
I
24,4 %
45,4 %
II
6,7 %
16 %
III
1,3 %
0,8 %
17 %(double)
IV
80 %
3%
short type
41 %
long type
25%
intermediate type
34%
V
common
trunc
24%
high origin
?%
VI

Fig. 226. Types of A. cerebelli inferior ant. (according to Scialfa et al., 1976)

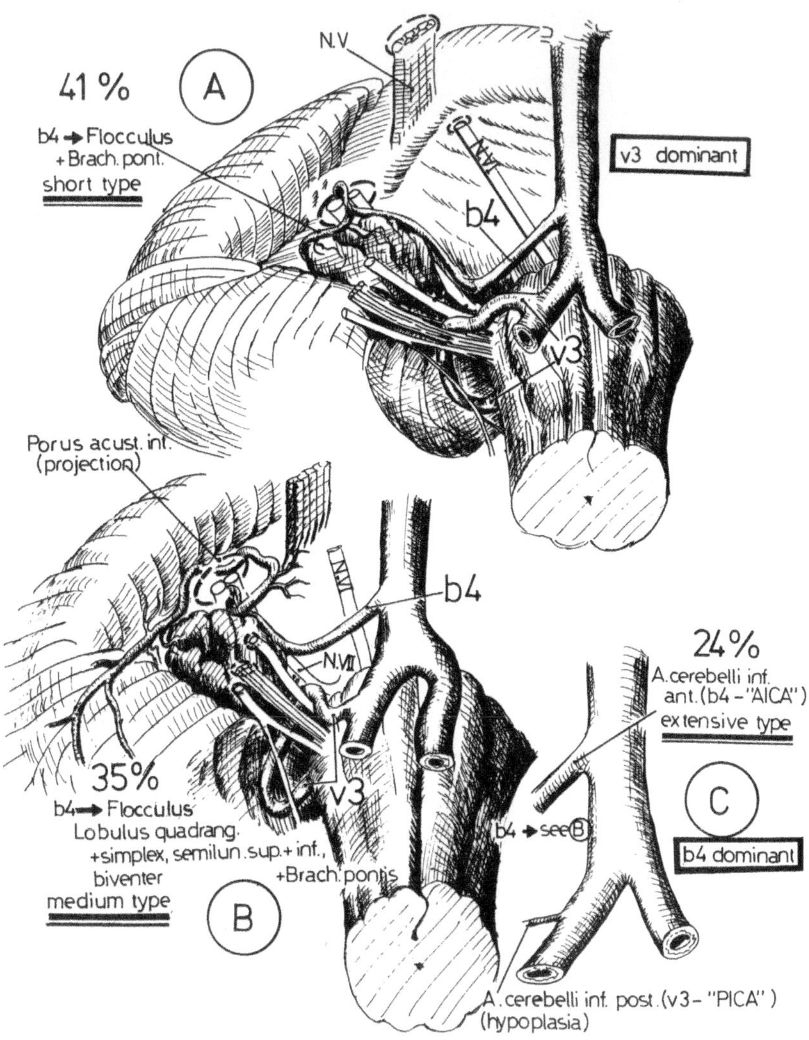

N.V
41 %
A
b4 → Flocculus
+ Brach. pont.
short type
v3 dominant
b4
v3
Porus acust. inf.
(projection)
b4
N.VII
24%
A. cerebelli inf.
ant. (b4 - "AICA")
extensive type
35%
v3
b4 → Flocculus
Lobulus quadrang.
+simplex, semilun. sup. + inf.,
biventer
medium type
+Brach. pontis
b4 → see B
C
b4 dominant
B
A. cerebelli inf. post. (v3 - "PICA")
(hypoplasia)

Fig. 227. Variants of A. cerebelli superior (according to Scialfa et al., 1976)
A Number of trunks
B and *C* Variants of bifurcation

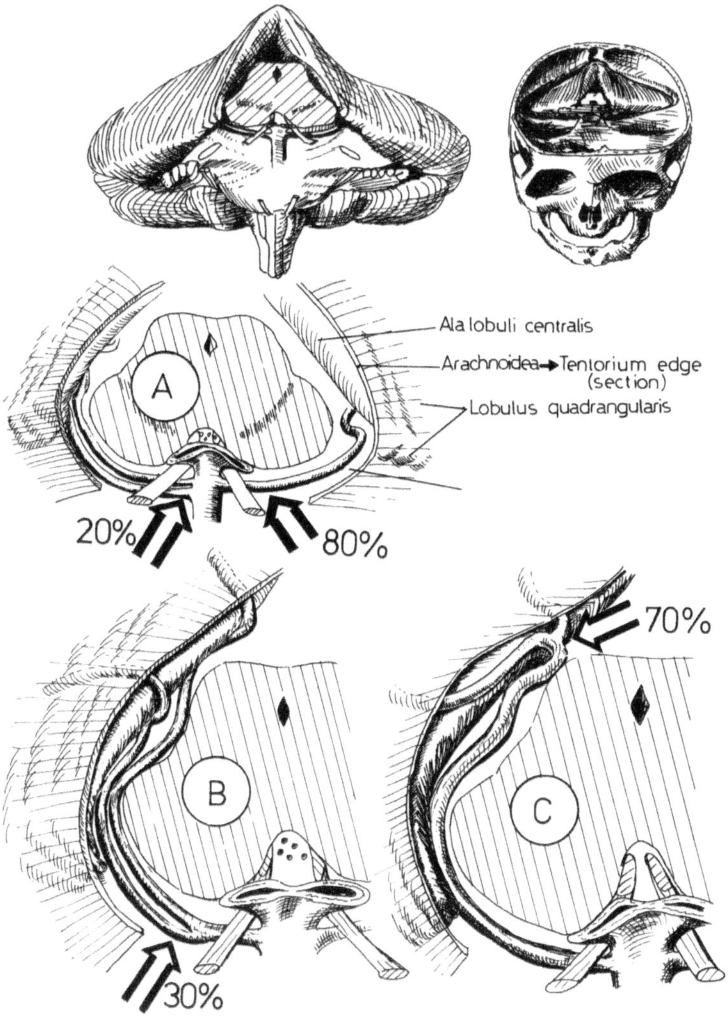
Ala lobuli centralis
Arachnoidea → Tentorium edge (section)
Lobulus quadrangularis
A
20%
80%
B
30%
C
70%

Fig. 228. Variants of A. cerebelli superior (according to Scialfa et al., 1976)
D Variants of course
E Exit point from A. basilaris or A. cerebri post.

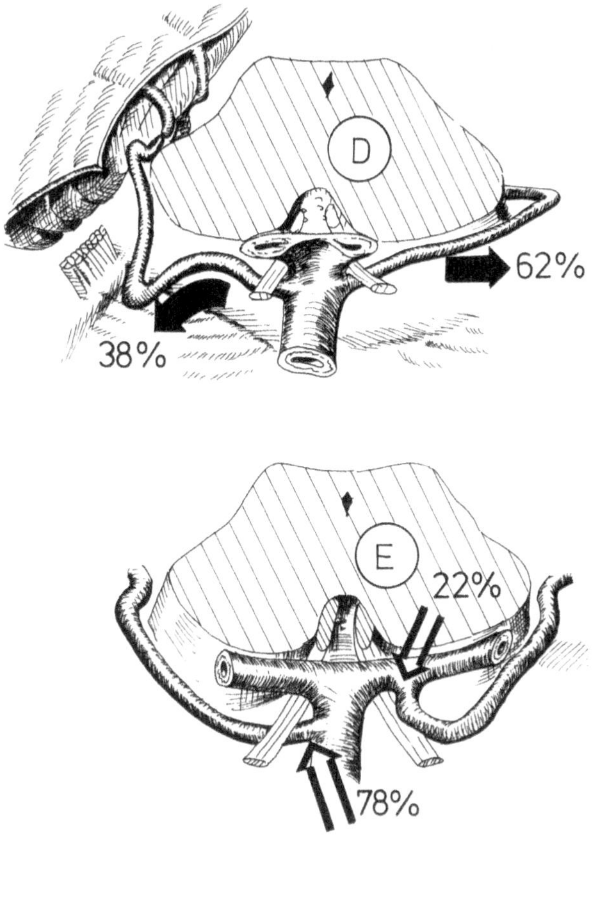
D
62%
38%
E
22%
78%

Fig. 229. Variants of A. cerebelli superior (according to Scialfa et al., 1976)
F Distribution of lateral branch groups
G Arborization types of medial terminal branches

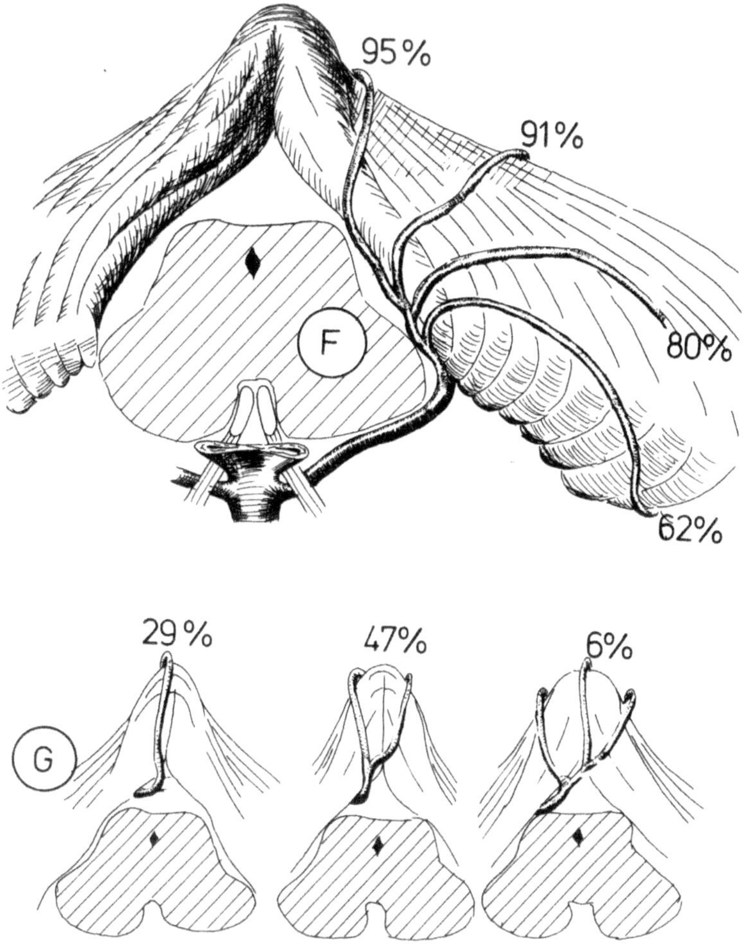
95%
91%
80%
62%
F
29%
47%
6%
G

Fig. 230. A. cerebelli inferior post. (according to Scialfa et al., 1976)
A to *C* Variants of origin
D to *F* Atresia or congenital anomaly of A. cerebelli inferior post.

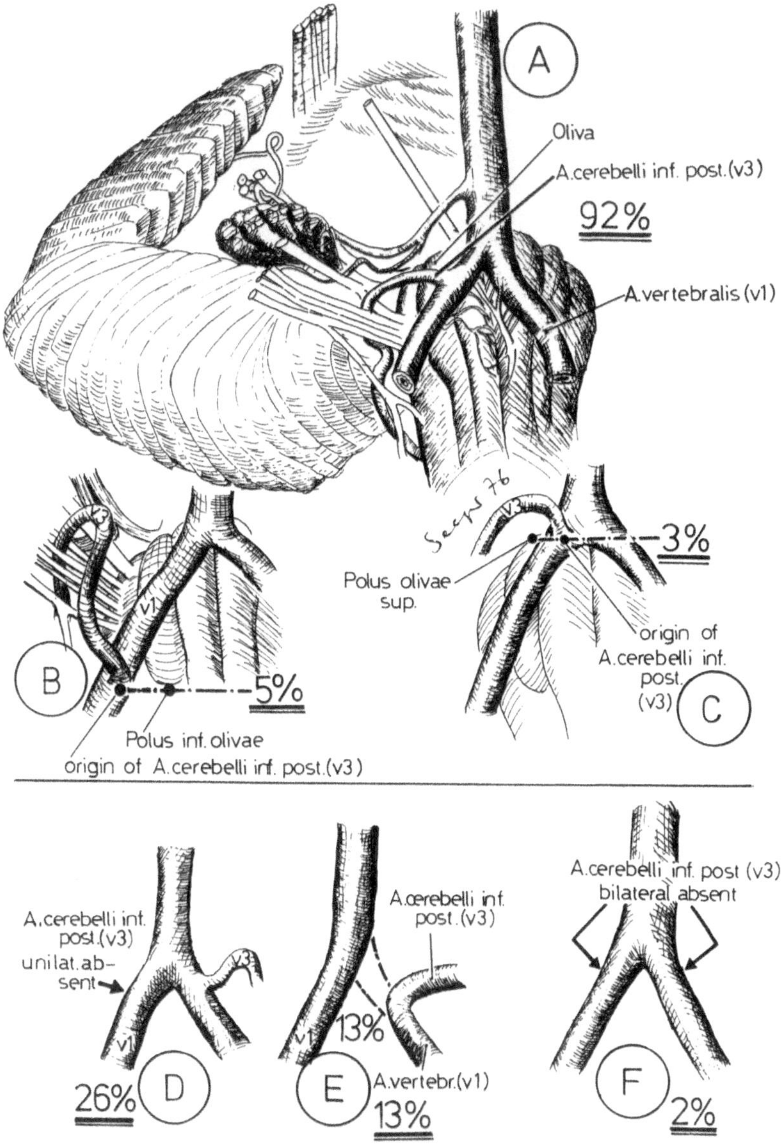
A
Oliva
A.cerebelli inf. post.(v3)
92%
A.vertebralis (v1)
B
v3
v1
5%
Polus inf. olivae
origin of A.cerebelli inf. post.(v3)
v3
3%
Polus olivae sup.
origin of A.cerebelli inf. post. (v3)
C
A.cerebelli inf. post.(v3) unilat. ab-sent
v3
v1
26%
D
A.cerebelli inf. post.(v3)
v1
13%
E
A.vertebr.(v1)
13%
A.cerebelli inf. post (v3) bilateral absent
F
2%

Fig. 231. Main arterial supply of convexity of Cerebellum. Course of lateral terminal branches of A. cerebelli inferior post. (according to Scialfa et al., 1976):
Various combinations of medial and lateral branches are possible. Variable overlapping with A cerebelli sup. and A. cerebelli inf. ant.

FIG. 231

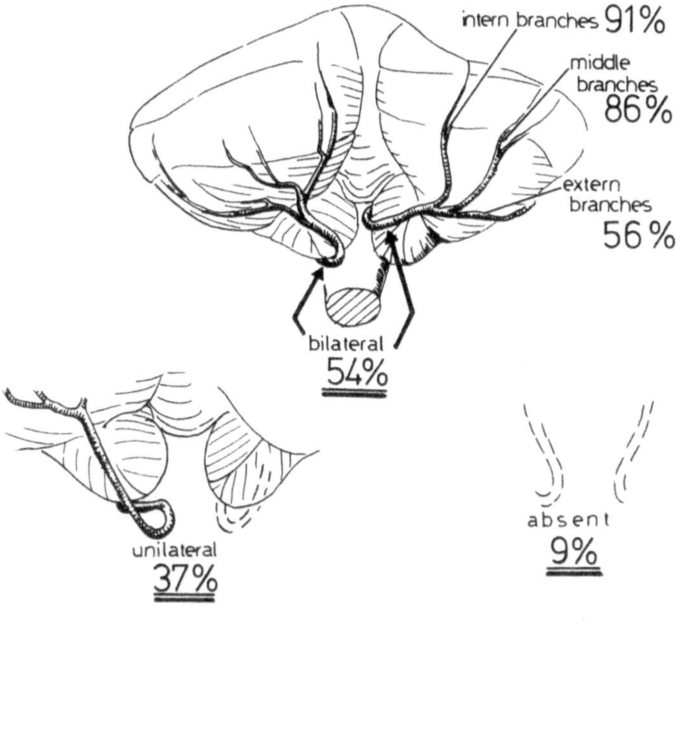
intern branches 91%
middle branches 86%
extern branches 56%
bilateral 54%
unilateral 37%
absent 9%

Fig. 232. Various types of medial terminal branches (A. vermicularis) of A. cerebelli inferior ant. (according to Scialfa et al., 1976)

FIG. 232

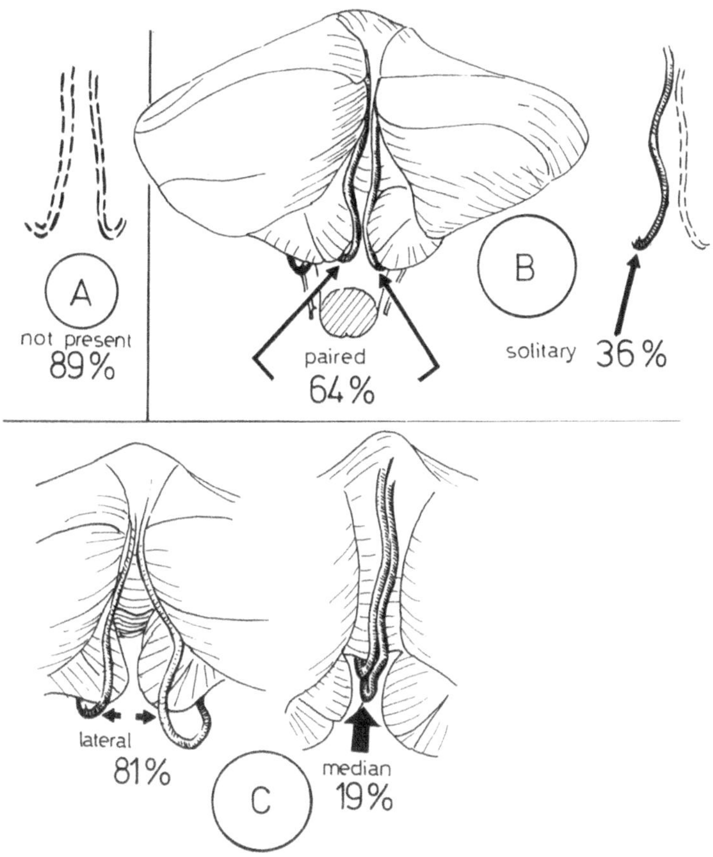
A
not present
89%
paired
64%
B
solitary
36%
lateral
81%
C
median
19%

Fig. 233. Suboccipital exposure
A With and without resection of atlas
B Yaşargil's method, also used unilaterally
C Cave air embolism in the region of the thin-walled Sinus sigmoideus!
D Position of emissaries to Sinus sigmoideus

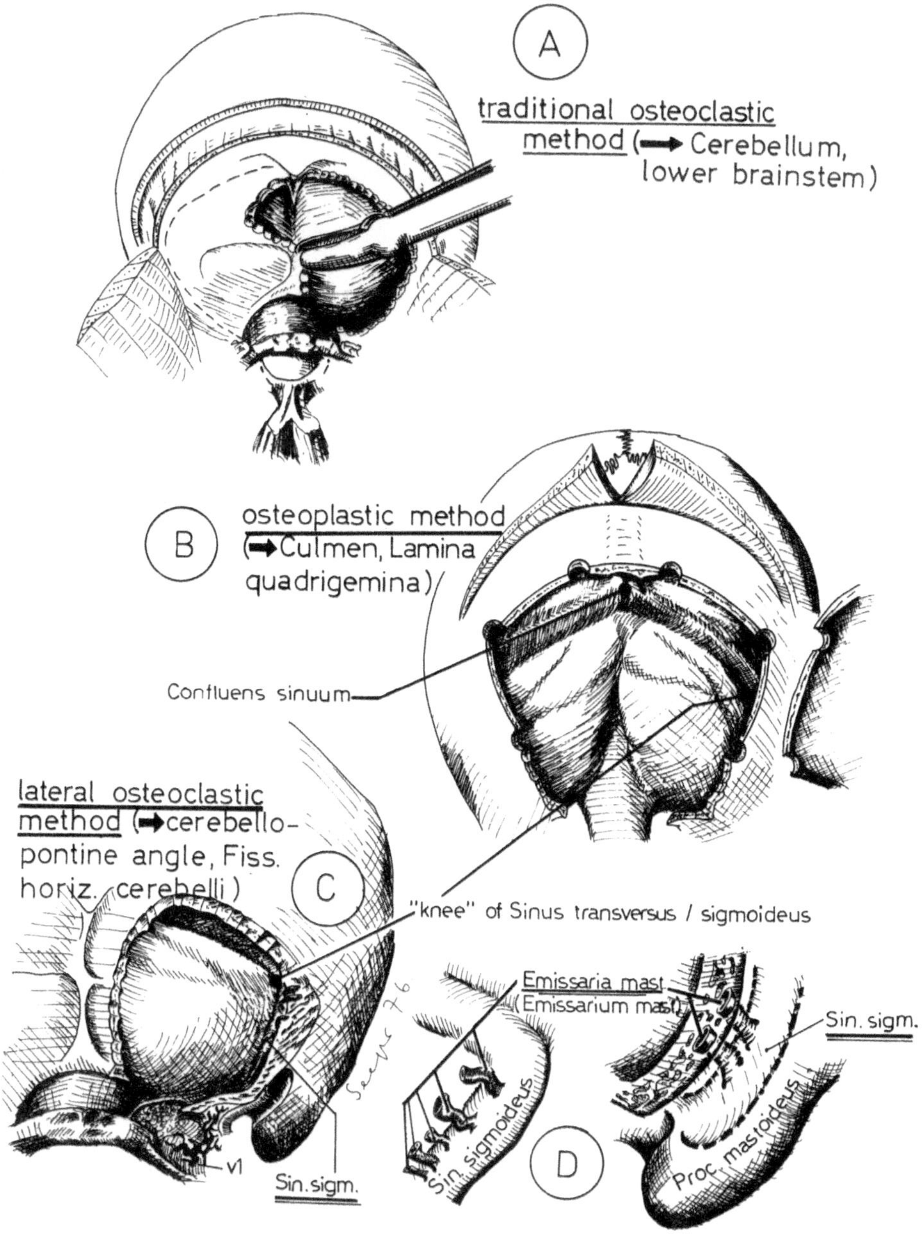
A
traditional osteoclastic method (➡ Cerebellum, lower brainstem)
B
osteoplastic method (➡Culmen, Lamina quadrigemina)
Confluens sinuum
lateral osteoclastic method (➡cerebello-pontine angle, Fiss. horiz. cerebelli)
C
"knee" of Sinus transversus / sigmoideus
v1
Sin.sigm.
Emissaria mast.
(Emissarium mast.)
Sin. sigm.
Sin. sigmoideus
D
Proc. mastoideus

Fig. 234. Straight-line approach to the ventral surface of Medulla oblongata without luxation of Medulla oblongata
Upper picture: With traditional method not possible
Lower picture: Method of Fig. 235: Straight-line approach without luxation of Medulla oblongata to the ventral surface is possible

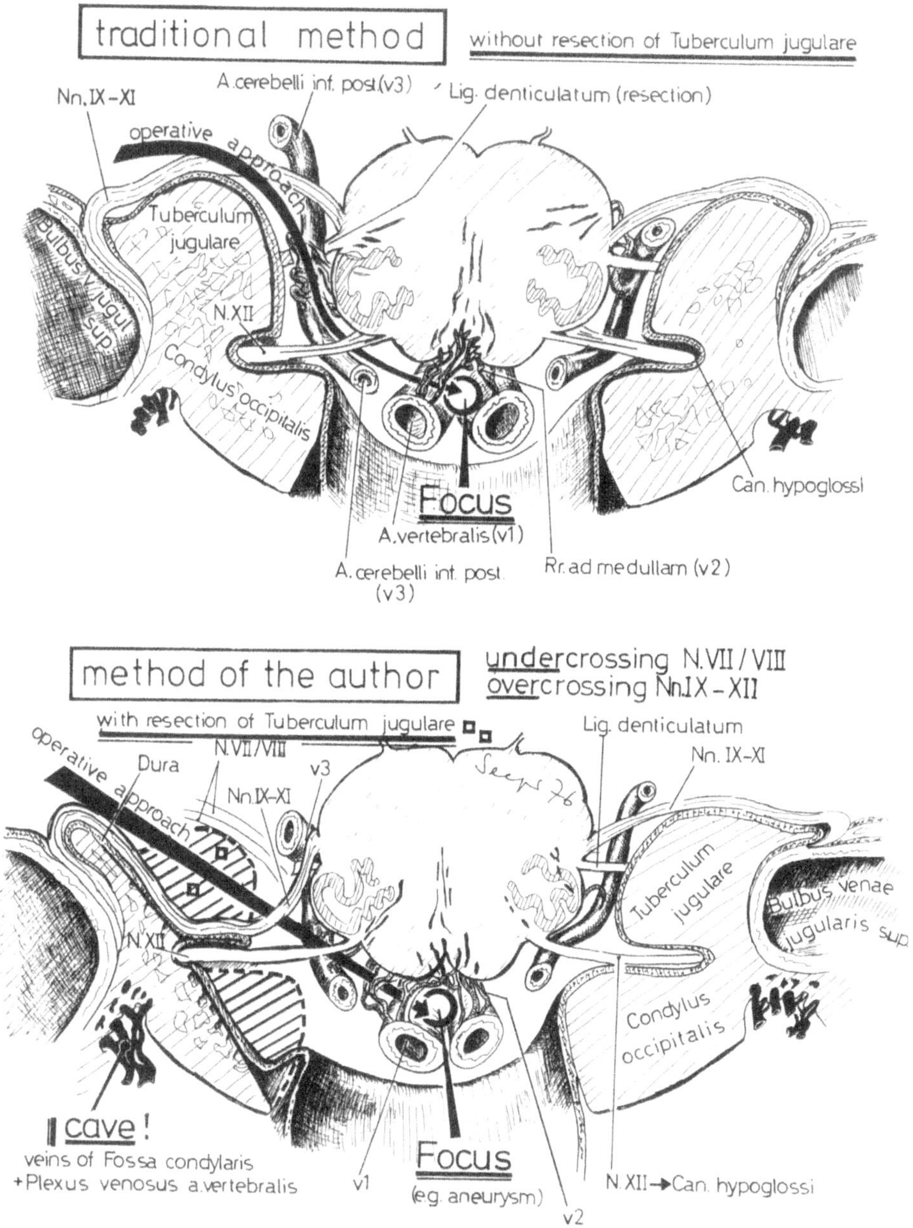
traditional method
without resection of Tuberculum jugulare
Nn. IX–XI
A. cerebelli inf. post.(v3)
Lig. denticulatum (resection)
operative approach
Tuberculum jugulare
Bulbus v. jugul. sup.
N. XII
Condylus occipitalis
Can. hypoglossi
Focus
A. vertebralis (v1)
A. cerebelli inf. post. (v3)
Rr. ad medullam (v2)
method of the author
undercrossing N. VII / VIII
overcrossing Nn. IX – XII
with resection of Tuberculum jugulare
Lig. denticulatum
Nn. IX–XI
operative approach
Dura
N. VII / VIII
v3
Nn. IX–XI
N. XII
Tuberculum jugulare
Bulbus venae jugularis sup.
Condylus occipitalis
cave !
veins of Fossa condylaris
+ Plexus venosus a. vertebralis
v1
Focus
(e.g. aneurysm)
v2
N. XII → Can. hypoglossi

Fig. 235. Approach to the ventral surface of Medulla oblongata (method of the author)
A-C Anatomical preparation
A Resection of Condylus occipitalis (medial portion). Oblique view from left caudal direction
B View from above
C Dorsal view into Foramen occip. magnum
C' Neurosurgical preparation, same view as *C*

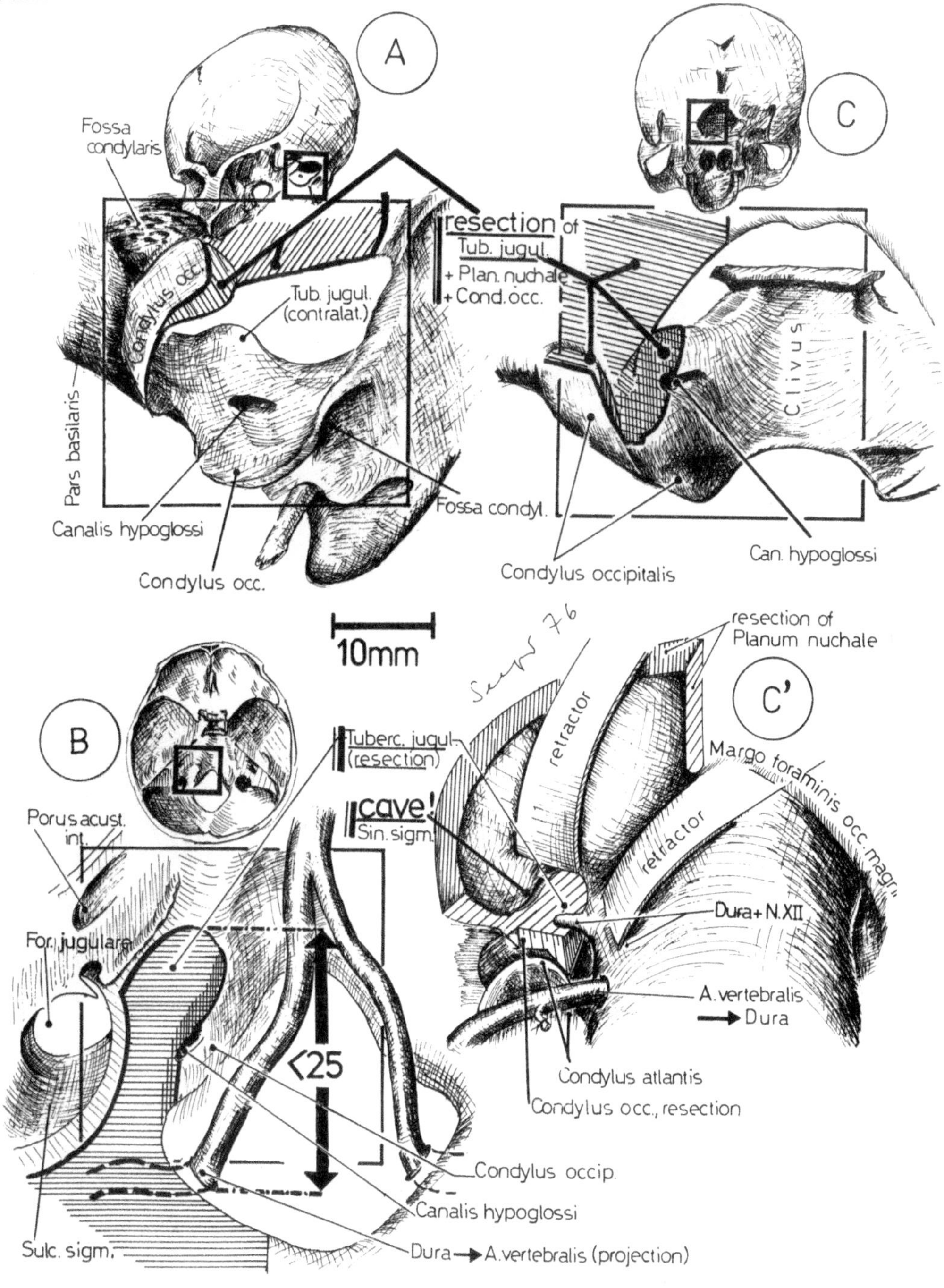
A
Fossa condylaris
resection of
Tub. jugul.
+ Plan. nuchale
+ Cond. occ.
Condylus occ.
Tub. jugul. (contralat.)
Pars basilaris
Canalis hypoglossi
Condylus occ.
Fossa condyl.
C
Clivus
Condylus occipitalis
Can. hypoglossi
10mm
B
Porus acust. int.
For. jugulare
Tuberc. jugul. (resection)
cave! Sin. sigm.
<25
Condylus occip.
Canalis hypoglossi
Sulc. sigm.
Dura → A. vertebralis (projection)
C'
resection of Planum nuchale
retractor
retractor
Margo foraminis occ. magn.
Dura + N. XII
A. vertebralis → Dura
Condylus atlantis
Condylus occ., resection

Fig. 236. Schematic representation of position o
Nucleus dentatus (arrow)

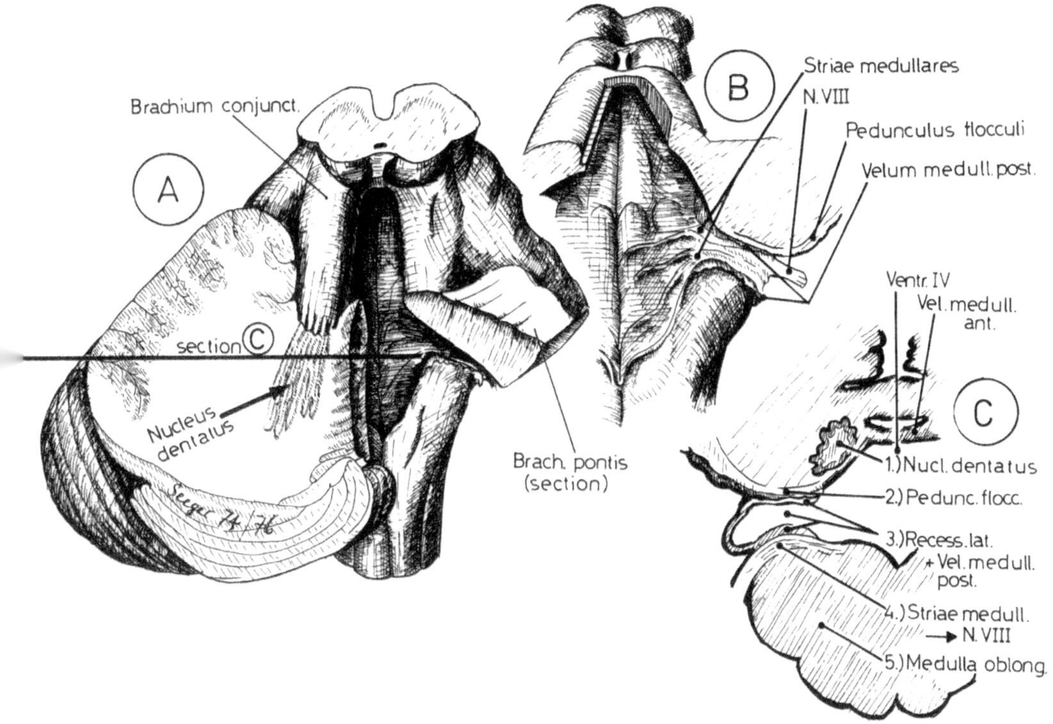
Brachium conjunct.
A
section C
Nucleus dentatus
Seeger 74/76
Brach. pontis (section)
B
Striae medullares
N. VIII
Pedunculus flocculi
Velum medull. post.
Ventr. IV
Vel. medull. ant.
C
1.) Nucl. dentatus
2.) Pedunc. flocc.
3.) Recess. lat. + Vel. medull. post.
4.) Striae medull. → N. VIII
5.) Medulla oblong.

Fig. 237. Suboccipital site

A Anatomical representation of relationships between the sinus and superficial brain vessels. Sinus variant (Sinus occipitalis) with lacunae

B Excessive resection of Cerebellum. Variants of A. cerebelli inferior ant. (*b4.1.1*) must also be conserved far peripherally, if branches in the flocculus region go off to Brachium pontis

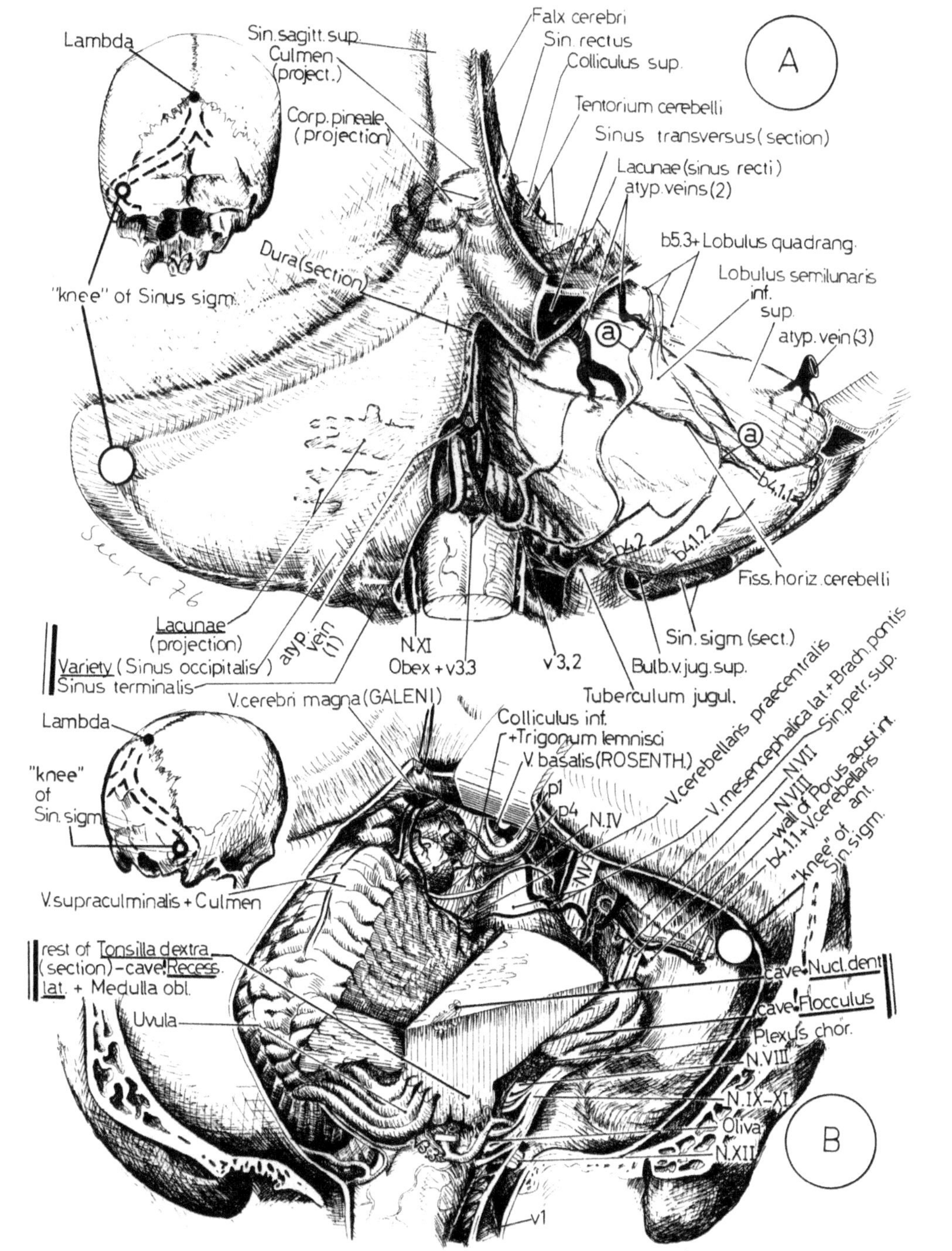
A
Lambda
Sin. sagitt. sup.
Culmen (project.)
Corp. pineale (projection)
Falx cerebri
Sin. rectus
Colliculus sup.
Tentorium cerebelli
Sinus transversus (section)
Lacunae (sinus recti)
atyp. veins (2)
b5.3+ Lobulus quadrang.
Lobulus semilunaris
inf.
sup.
atyp. vein (3)
"knee" of Sinus sigm.
Dura (section)
a
a
b4.1.1
b4.2
b4.1.2
Fiss. horiz. cerebelli
Lacunae (projection)
Variety (Sinus occipitalis)
Sinus terminalis
atyp. vein (1)
N.XI
Obex + v3.3
v3.2
Sin. sigm. (sect.)
Bulb. v. jug. sup.
Tuberculum jugul.
B
Lambda
"knee" of Sin. sigm.
V. cerebri magna (GALENI)
Colliculus inf. + Trigonum lemnisci
V. basalis (ROSENTH.)
p1
p4
N.IV
N.V
V. cerebellaris praecentralis
V. mesencephalica lat. + Brach. pontis
Sin. petr. sup.
N.VII
N.VIII
wall of Porus acust. int.
b4.1.1 + V. cerebellaris ant.
"knee" of Sin. sigm.
V. supraculminalis + Culmen
rest of Tonsilla dextra (section) - cave! Recess. lat. + Medulla obl.
Uvula
cave! Nucl. dent.
cave! Flocculus
Plexus chor.
N.VIII
N.IX-XI
Oliva
N.XII
v1

Fig. 238. Distances and possibilities of resection. Measurements in millimetres (mm)

A Endangering of Brachium pontis at resection of Lobulus semilunaris superior and inferior

B and *C* Endangering of Nucleus dentatus and perforating vessels in region of tonsil at resection of Lobulus biventer

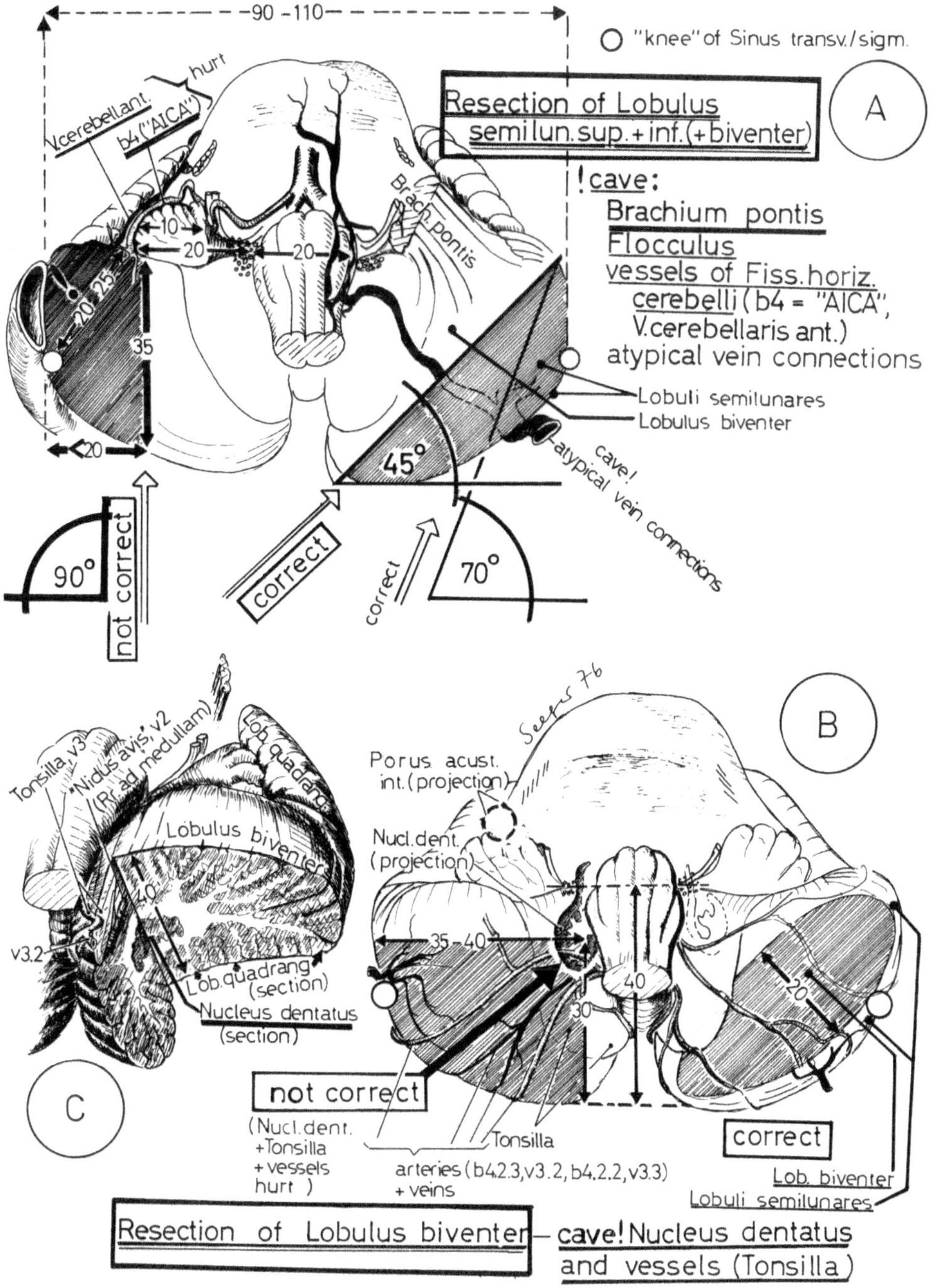

90 - 110
"knee" of Sinus transv./sigm.
Resection of Lobulus semilun. sup. + inf. (+ biventer)
A
! cave:
Brachium pontis
Flocculus
vessels of Fiss. horiz. cerebelli (b4 = "AICA", V. cerebellaris ant.)
atypical vein connections
Lobuli semilunares
Lobulus biventer
cave! atypical vein connections
hurt
V. cerebell. ant.
b4 ("AICA")
Brach. pontis
10
20
20
20
25
35
20
45°
90°
not correct
correct
correct
70°
B
Porus acust. int. (projection)
Nucl. dent. (projection)
35 - 40
40
30
20
not correct
(Nucl. dent. + Tonsilla + vessels hurt)
Tonsilla
arteries (b4.2.3, v3.2, b4.2.2, v3.3) + veins
correct
Lob. biventer
Lobuli semilunares
Tonsilla, v3
"Nidus avis", v2 (Rr. ad medullam)
Lob. quadrang.
Lobulus biventer
40
v3.2
Lob. quadrang. (section)
Nucleus dentatus (section)
C
Resection of Lobulus biventer – cave! Nucleus dentatus and vessels (Tonsilla)

Fig. 239. Distances at the base of brain and skull. Measurements in millimetres (mm)

A Basal brain structures

B Basal bony and dural structures

C Positional relationships between Lobulus quadrangularis and simplex, also Flocculus and internal auditory meatus

* Pons-Medulla border, Lobulus quadrangularis – Flocculus-point and Porus acusticus internus lie almost in a frontal plane

** Pons projects slightly into the clivus groove

*** Medulla oblongata projects deeply into the clivus groove

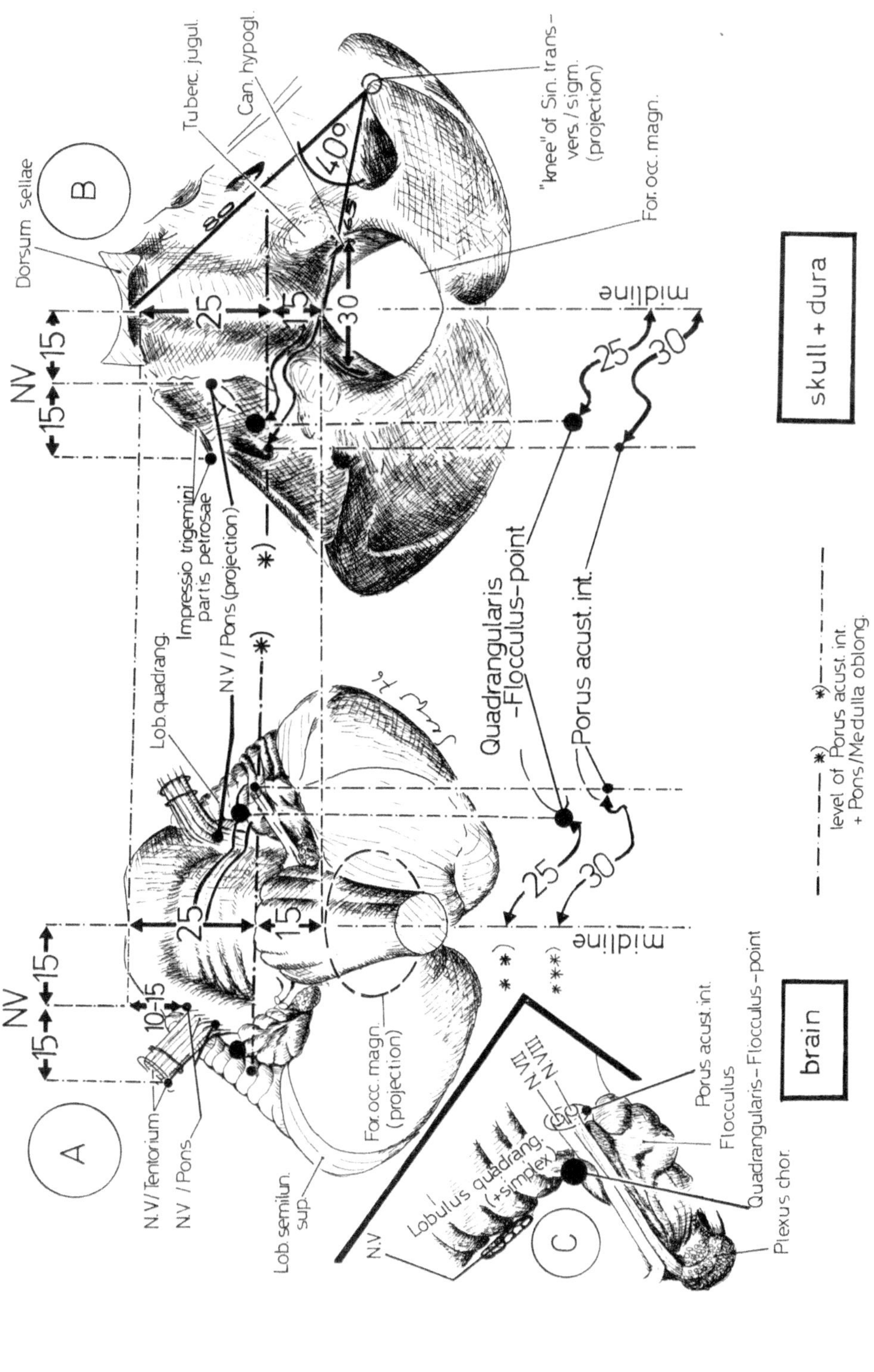
A
B
C
Dorsum sellae
Tuberc. jugul.
Can. hypogl.
40°
80
45
"knee" of Sin. trans-vers./sigm. (projection)
For. occ. magn.
midline
NV
15
25
15
30
Impressio trigemini partis petrosae
N.V / Pons (projection)
Lob. quadrang.
Quadrangularis -Flocculus-point
Porus acust. int.
skull + dura
level of Porus acust. int. + Pons/Medulla oblong.
N.V/Tentorium
N.V / Pons
10-15
Lob. semilun. sup.
For. occ. magn. (projection)
brain
N.V
Lobulus quadrang. (+simplex)
N.VII
N.VIII
Porus acust. int.
Flocculus
Quadrangularis-Flocculus-point
Plexus chor.

Fig. 240. Distances between infratentorial median structures. Median section of Cerebellum and lower brainstem
Measurements in millimetres (mm)

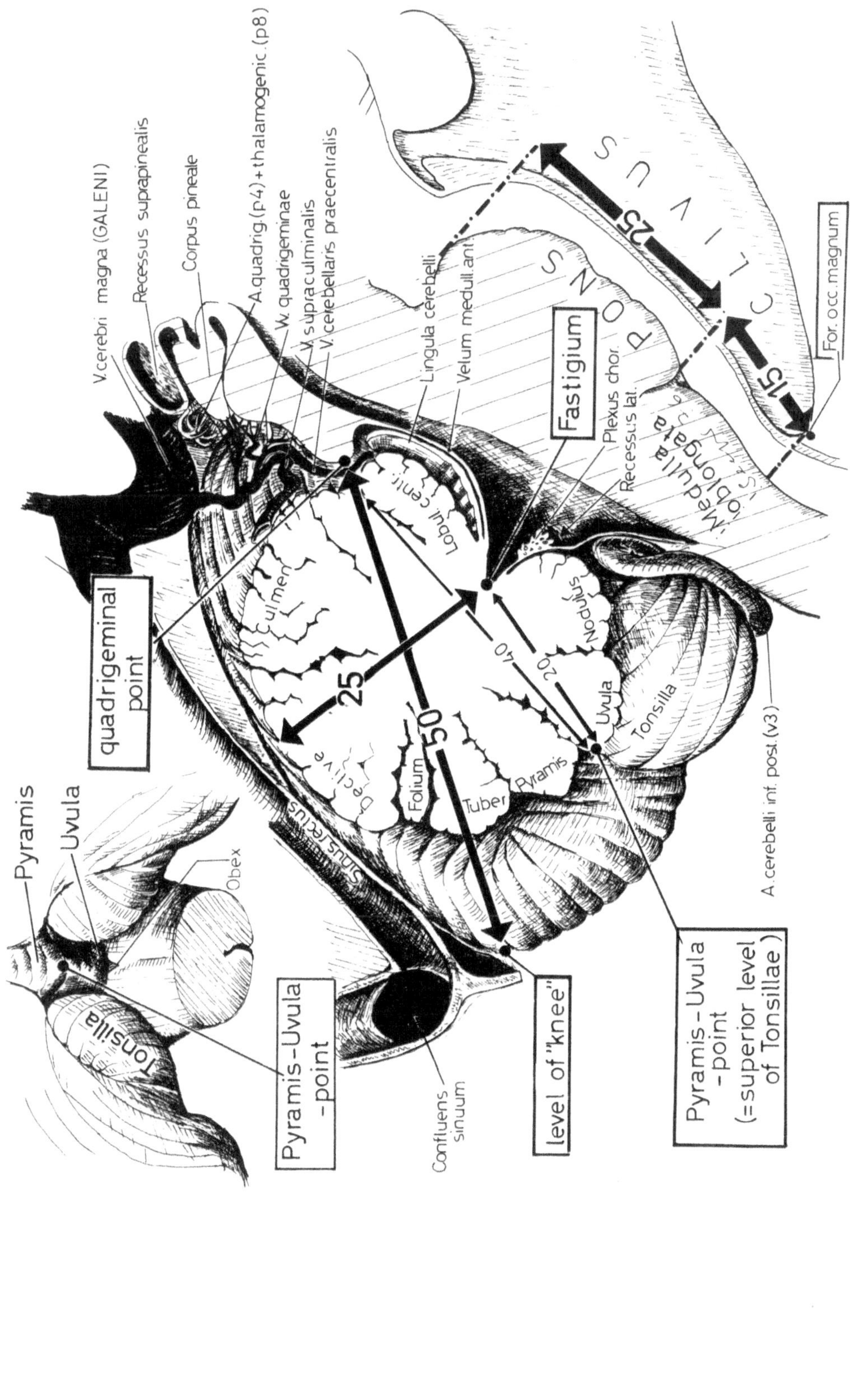
V.cerebri magna (GALENI)
Recessus suprapinealis
Corpus pineale
A.quadrig.(p4)+thalamogenic.(p8)
W. quadrigeminae
V. supraculminalis
V. cerebellaris praecentralis
Lingula cerebelli
Velum medull.ant.
Fastigium
Plexus chor.
Recessus lat.
Medulla oblongata
PONS
CLIVUS
25
15
For. occ. magnum
Lobul. centr.
Culmen
Nodulus
Uvula
Tonsilla
A.cerebelli inf. post.(v3)
quadrigeminal point
25
50
40
20
Declive
Folium
Tuber
Pyramis
Sinus rectus
Pyramis
Uvula
Obex
Tonsilla
Pyramis-Uvula -point
Confluens sinuum
level of "knee"
Pyramis-Uvula -point (=superior level of Tonsillae)

Fig. 241. Positional relationships of significance in processes at pontine angle. Measurements in millimetres (mm)

A At right bony base of skull and at left dura-covered base, with cranial nerves and vessels

B Ventral base of brain: Lobulus quadrangularis has been removed in order to show the extension of Brachium pontis before entry into Lobulus biventer.

C Operation site at cerebellopontine angle. Stretching of cranial nerves due to spatula retraction of Cerebellum (view from behind left)

* Dangerous spatula compression of V. mesencephalica lateralis and A. cerebelli inferior ant.

D Exit of perforating vessels from A. cerebelli inferior ant. to Brachium pontis between Flocculus, Lobulus quadrangularis, and Lobulus biventer. Arachnoidea removed and Flocculus drawn aside (view from basal direction, left)

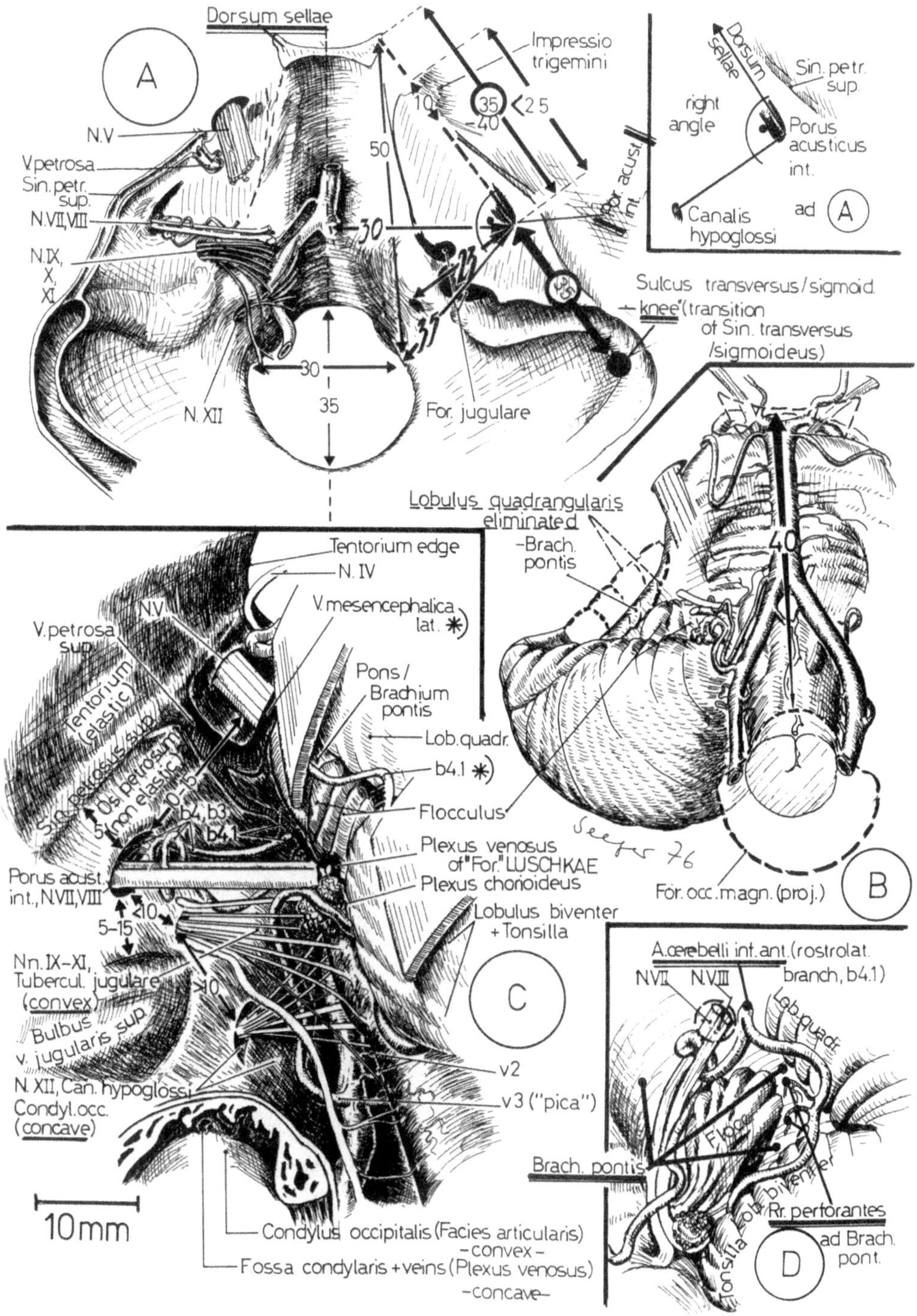

A
Dorsum sellae
Impressio trigemini
35
<25
40
10
50
30
23
35
45
N.V
V.petrosa
Sin. petr. sup.
N.VII,VIII
N.IX, X, XI
N. XII
For. jugulare
Sulcus transversus/sigmoid.
knee (transition of Sin. transversus /sigmoideus)
Dorsum sellae
Sin. petr. sup.
right angle
Porus acusticus int.
por. acust. int.
Canalis hypoglossi
ad A
Lobulus quadrangularis eliminated
Brach. pontis
40
For. occ. magn. (proj.)
B
Tentorium edge
N. IV
V. mesencephalica lat. ✱
N.V
V. petrosa sup.
Tentorium (elastic)
Sin. petrosus sup.
Os petrosum (non elastic)
Pons / Brachium pontis
Lob. quadr.
b4.1 ✱
b4, b3
b4.1
Flocculus
Plexus venosus of "For." LUSCHKAE
Plexus chorioideus
Porus acust. int., N.VII,VIII
<10
5–15
0–5
5
Lobulus biventer + Tonsilla
Nn. IX–XI, Tubercul. jugulare (convex)
Bulbus v. jugularis sup.
>10
C
v2
v3 ("pica")
N. XII, Can. hypoglossi
Condyl. occ. (concave)
10mm
Condylus occipitalis (Facies articularis) -convex-
Fossa condylaris + veins (Plexus venosus) -concave-
A. cerebelli inf. ant. (rostrolat. branch, b4.1)
N.VII
N.VIII
Lob. quadr.
Flocc.
Brach. pontis
Lob. biventer
Tonsilla
Rr. perforantes ad Brach. pont.
D

Fig. 242. Positional relationships of N. facialis and stato-acusticus to Porus and Fundus of Meatus acusticus internus (according to Rhoton, modified)

A View from behind above

B After removal of N. vestibularis superior. Risk of haemorrhage from A. petrosa during drilling of auditory meatus

C Auditory meatus drilled open further, N. vestibularis superior, inferior and cochleae resected. N. intermedius (N. i.) visualized

D N. facialis and A. cerebelli inferior ant., rostrolateral branch (*b4.1*) preserved. Note the variants of N. intermedius in *C* and *D*. Aa. auditivae internae may arise independently from A. basilaris or A. cerebelli superior

E Bony Fundus of Meatus acusticus internus

F Fundus with nerve stumps. Note also the separate dural penetration sites of nerves IX to XI

FIG. 242

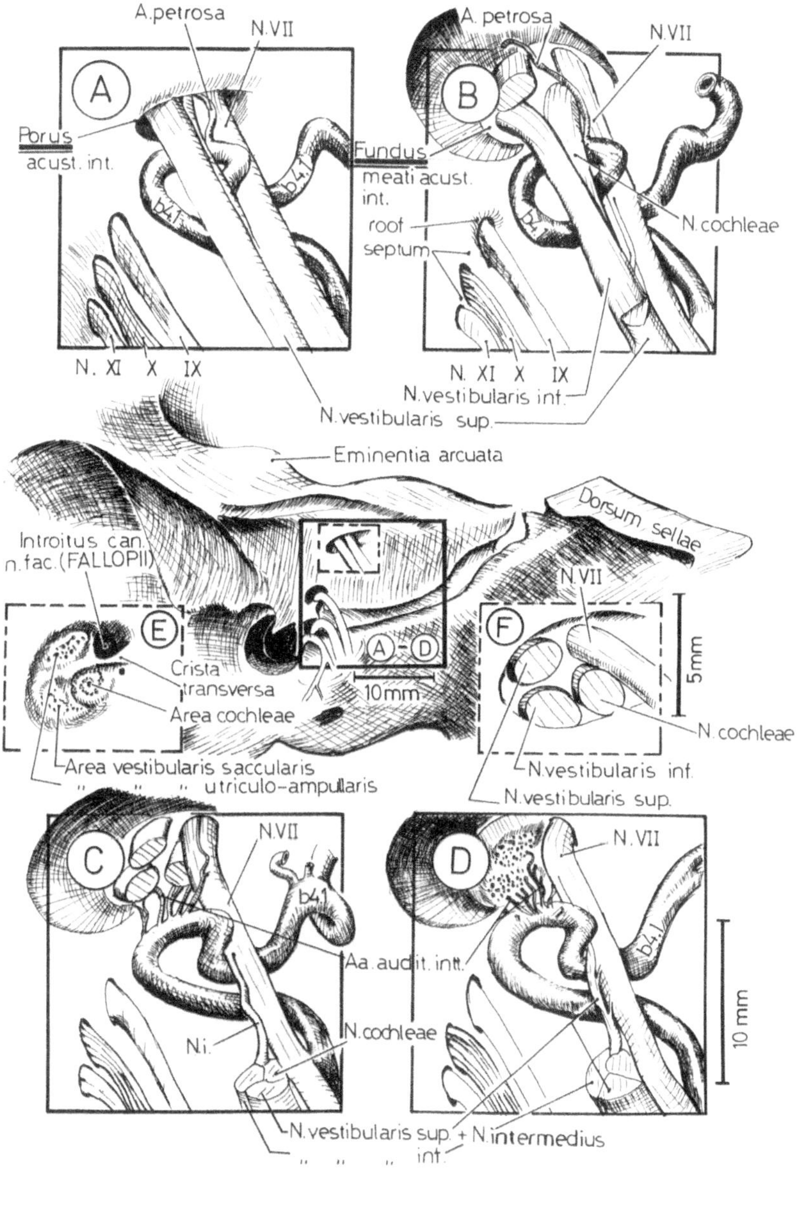
A.petrosa
N.VII
A
Porus
acust. int.
b41
N. XI X IX
A. petrosa
N.VII
B
Fundus
meati acust.
int.
roof
septum
N.cochleae
N. XI X IX
N.vestibularis inf.
N.vestibularis sup.
Eminentia arcuata
Dorsum sellae
Introitus can.
n.fac.(FALLOPII)
E
Crista
transversa
Area cochleae
Area vestibularis saccularis
" " " utriculo-ampullaris
A-D
10mm
F
N.VII
5mm
N.cochleae
N.vestibularis inf.
N.vestibularis sup.
C
N.VII
b41
Aa.audit.intt.
N.i.
N.cochleae
D
N.VII
b41
10 mm
N.vestibularis sup. + N.intermedius
" " " int.

Fig. 243. Variants of Sinus petrosus inferior and its relations to cranial nerves IX to XI and to Foramen jugulare (according to Rhoton, modified)
Risk of damage to veins, particularly at *D*. When internal auditory meatus is distended, close relationship to inferior border of auditory meatus

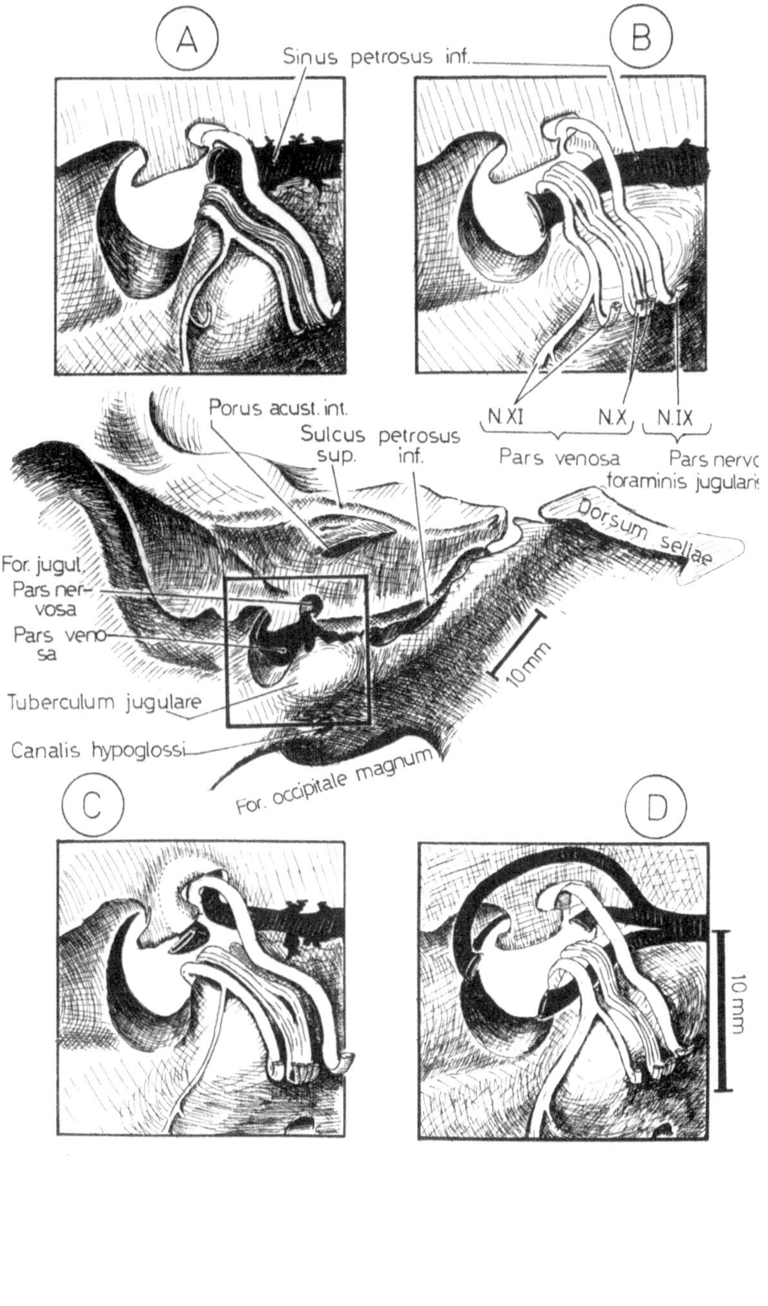
A
B
C
D
Sinus petrosus inf.
Porus acust. int.
Sulcus petrosus
sup.
inf.
N.XI
N.X
N.IX
Pars venosa
Pars nervc
foraminis jugularis
Dorsum sellae
For. jugul.
Pars ner-
vosa
Pars veno-
sa
Tuberculum jugulare
Canalis hypoglossi
For. occipitale magnum
10 mm
10 mm

Fig. 244. Oblique view of Cerebellum *A* and the bony base of the skull *B*. Distance measurements in vicinity of cerebellopontine angle in millimetres (mm)

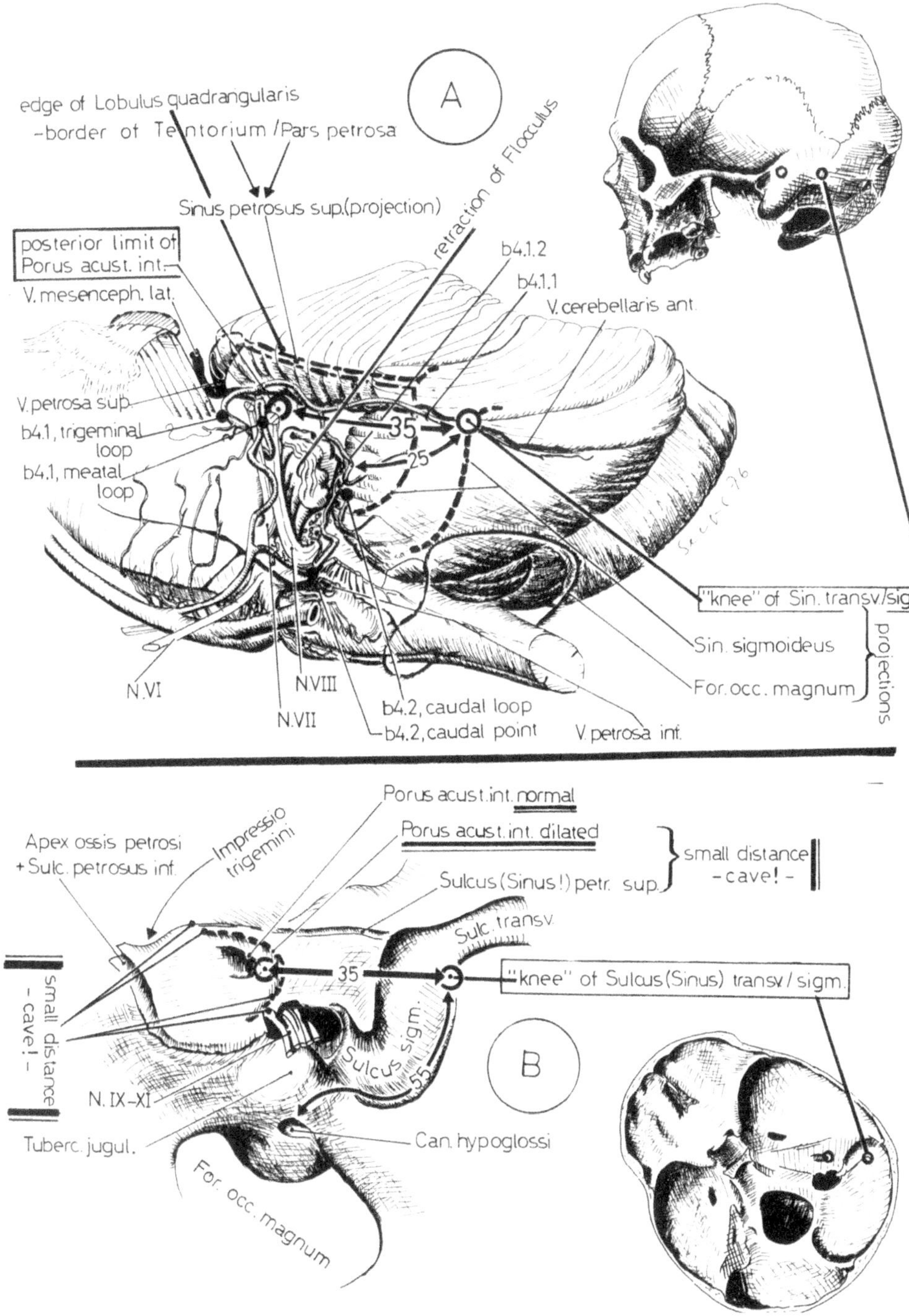
A
edge of Lobulus quadrangularis
-border of Tentorium /Pars petrosa
Sinus petrosus sup.(projection)
retraction of Flocculus
posterior limit of Porus acust. int.
V. mesenceph. lat.
b4.1.2
b4.1.1
V. cerebellaris ant.
V. petrosa sup.
b4.1, trigeminal loop
b4.1, meatal loop
35
25
"knee" of Sin. transv./sigm.
Sin. sigmoideus
For. occ. magnum
projections
N.VI
N.VIII
N.VII
b4.2, caudal loop
b4.2, caudal point
V. petrosa inf.
B
Porus acust. int. normal
Porus acust. int. dilated
Apex ossis petrosi
+ Sulc. petrosus inf.
Impressio trigemini
Sulcus (Sinus!) petr. sup.
small distance
- cave! -
Sulc. transv.
35
"knee" of Sulcus (Sinus) transv / sigm.
small distance
- cave! -
Sulcus sigm.
55
N. IX-XI
Tuberc. jugul.
Can. hypoglossi
For. occ. magnum

Fig. 245. Bony structures in vicinity of cerebel-lopontine angle
A Frequency of varying distances of A. cerebell inferior ant. from Meatus acusticus internus
B Positional relationships of A. cerebelli inferior ant. to the caudal cranial nerves (for variants see Figs. 248 to 251)

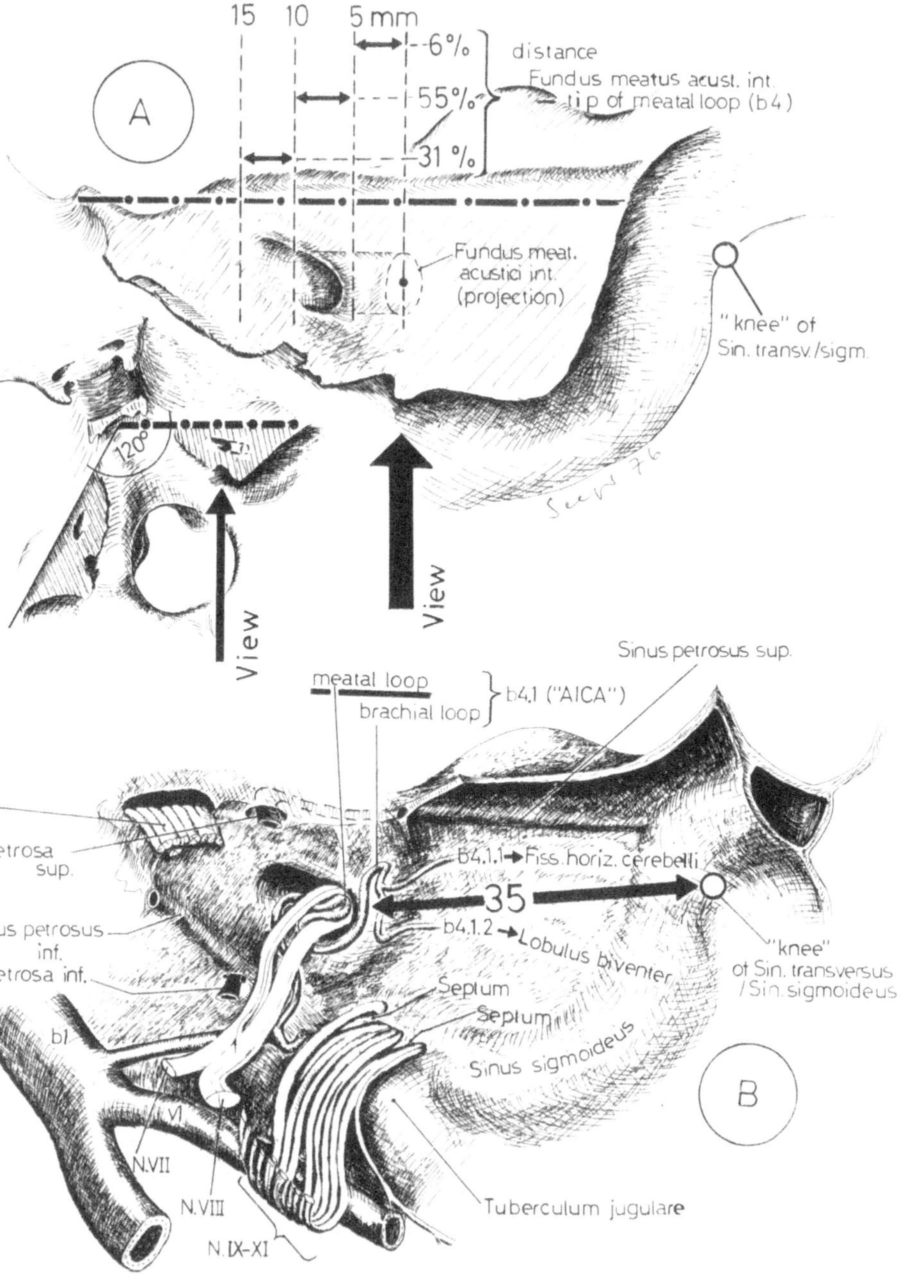
15
10
5 mm
6%
55%
31%
distance
Fundus meatus acust. int.
tip of meatal loop (b4)
A
Fundus meat. acustici int. (projection)
"knee" of Sin. transv./sigm.
120°
View
View
Sinus petrosus sup.
meatal loop
brachial loop
b4.1 ("AICA")
N.V.
V. petrosa sup.
b4.1.1 → Fiss. horiz. cerebelli
35
Sinus petrosus inf.
b4.1.2 → Lobulus biventer
"knee" of Sin. transversus / Sin. sigmoideus
V. petrosa inf.
Septum
Septum
b1
Sinus sigmoideus
B
VI
N.VII
N.VIII
N.IX-XI
Tuberculum jugulare

Fig. 246. Altered positional relationships between Sinus petrosus sup. – Nn. VI/VIII and Nn. IX/XI in the presence of Meatus acusticus int. due to tumour

A Normal findings

B Enlargement of internal auditory meatus due to tumour

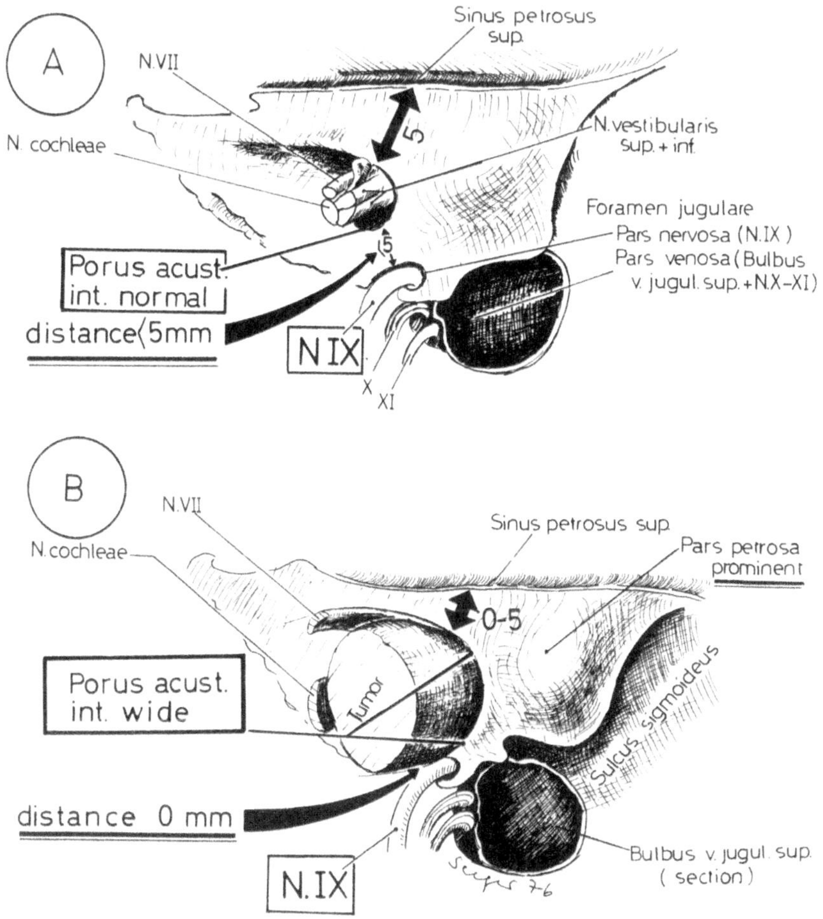
A
N.VII
N. cochleae
Sinus petrosus sup.
5
N. vestibularis sup. + inf.
Foramen jugulare
Pars nervosa (N.IX)
Pars venosa (Bulbus v. jugul. sup. + N.X–XI)
Porus acust. int. normal
distance ‹5mm
N IX
X
XI
B
N.VII
N.cochleae
Sinus petrosus sup.
Pars petrosa prominent
0-5
Tumor
Sulcus sigmoideus
Porus acust. int. wide
distance 0 mm
N.IX
Bulbus v. jugul. sup. (section)

Fig. 247. Distance measurements of brain structures in the vicinity of the cerebellopontine angle in millimetres (mm)
A General view
B Region of cerebellopontine angle with Flocculus lifted to show Brachium pontis between Flocculus and Lobulus biventer. Arachnoidea and Recessus lateralis opened
C The same site with vessels sketched in
* Rami perforantes of A. cerebelli inferior ant. (rostrolateral and caudal-medial branch) to Brachium pontis. For *b4.2.1* arterial nomenclature, see catalogue of arteries, pages 3–4

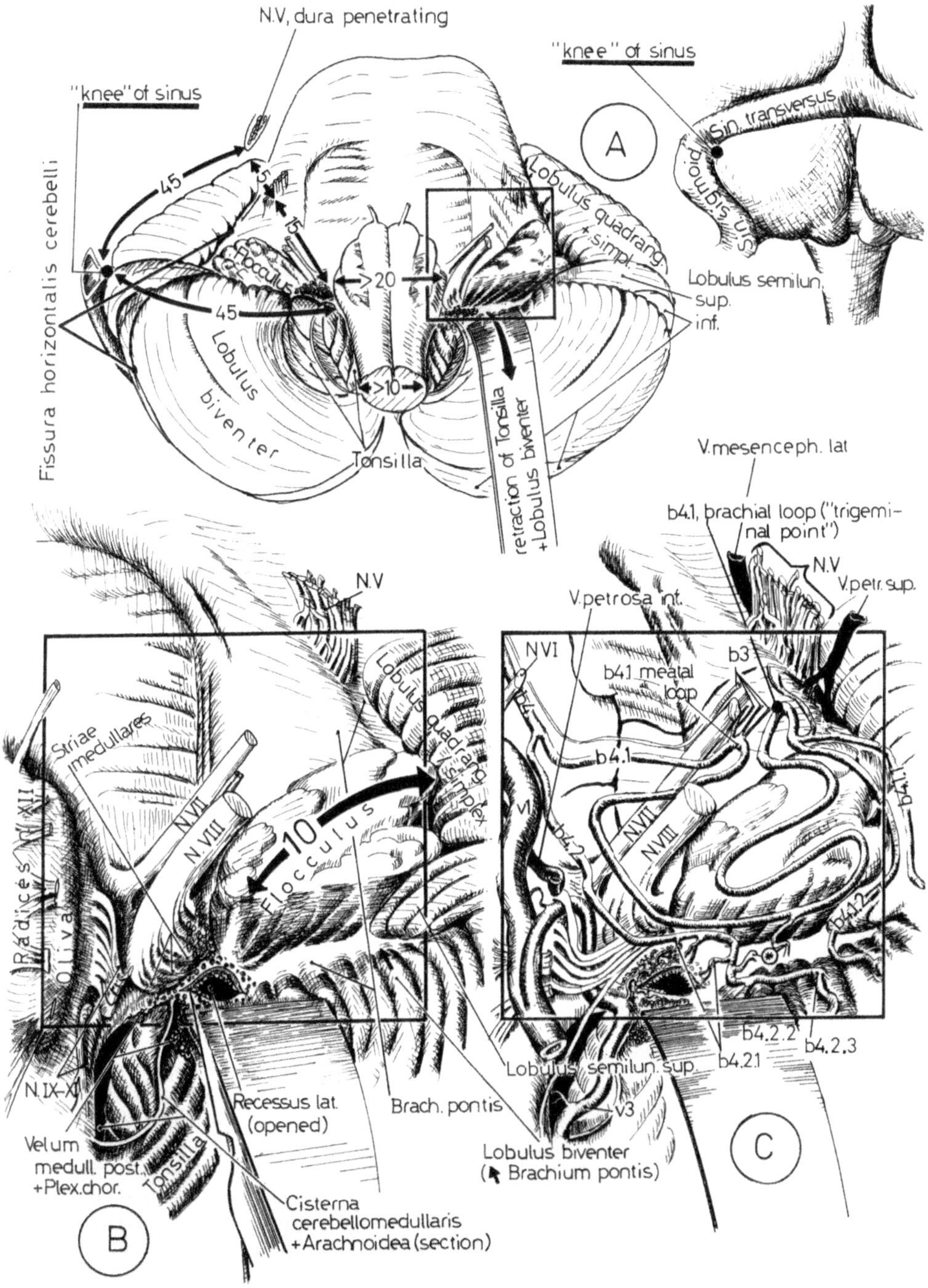

N.V, dura penetrating
"knee" of sinus
"knee" of sinus
A
Sin. transversus
Sin. sigmoid.
Fissura horizontalis cerebelli
45
5
15
Flocculus
20
45
Lobulus quadrang. + simpl.
Lobulus semilun.
sup.
inf.
Lobulus biventer
10
Tonsilla
retraction of Tonsilla + Lobulus biventer
V.mesenceph. lat
b4.1, brachial loop ("trigeminal point")
N.V
N.V
V.petr. sup.
V.petrosa int.
NVI
b4.1 meatal loop
b3
b4.1
b4.1
N.VII
N.VIII
V1
b4.2
b4.2.2
b4.2.1
b4.2.3
Lobulus semilun. sup.
V3
C
Striae medullares
Lobulus quadrang. + simplex
Radices N. XII
Oliva
N.VII
N.VIII
10
Flocculus
N.IX-XI
Velum medull. post. + Plex. chor.
Tonsilla
Recessus lat. (opened)
Brach. pontis
Lobulus biventer (➘ Brachium pontis)
Cisterna cerebellomedullaris + Arachnoidea (section)
B

Fig. 248. Region of cerebellopontine angle, obliqu
view
A General view. A. basilaris lifted in order t
show the perforating arteries to the pons-medull
region. Lobulus quadrangularis retracted in order t
bring the quadrigeminal region into view
B Schematic representation of positional relation
ships between Flocculus, N. stato-acusticus/facialis
Plexus chorioideus, Brachium pontis, and Medull
oblongata
C Variations of Flocculus and Nn. VII/VIII

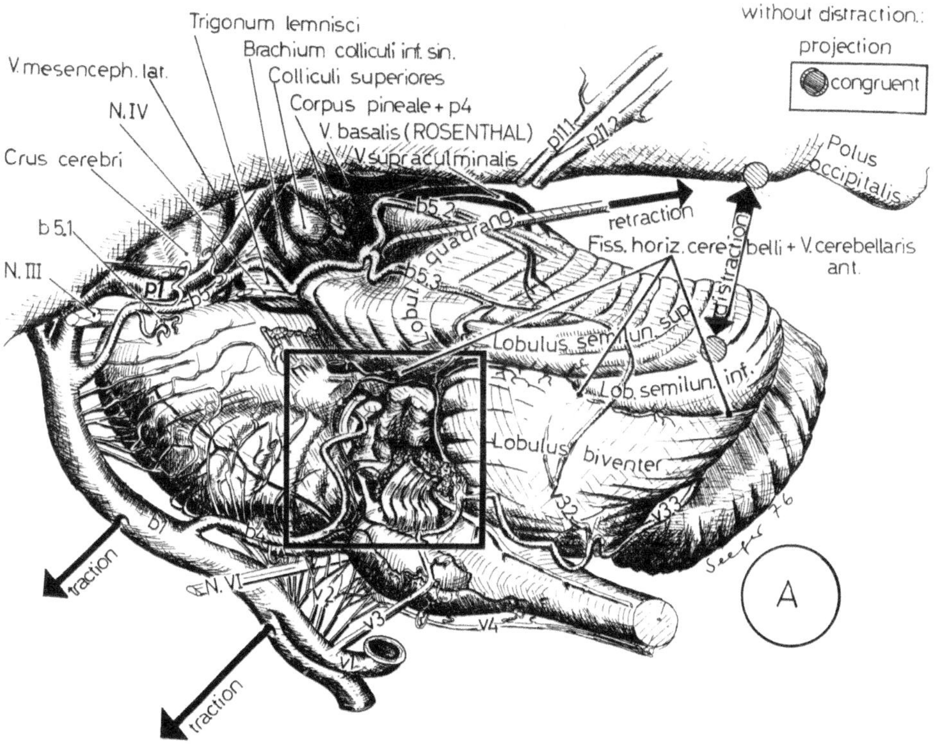
Trigonum lemnisci
Brachium colliculi inf. sin.
V. mesenceph. lat.
Colliculi superiores
N. IV
Corpus pineale + p4
V. basalis (ROSENTHAL)
Crus cerebri
V. supraculminalis
p11.1
p11.2
without distraction:
projection
congruent
Polus occipitalis
b 5.1
b5.2
retraction
N. III
Lobulus quadrang.
Fiss. horiz. cerebelli + V. cerebellaris ant.
distraction
p1
b5.3
Lobulus semilun. sup.
Lob. semilun. inf.
Lobulus biventer
b1
b4
v3.2
v3.3
traction
N. VI
v2
v3
v4
v1
traction
A

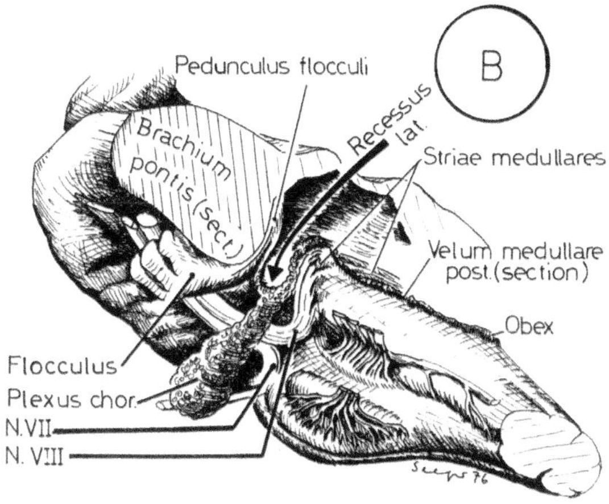
Pedunculus flocculi
B
Recessus lat.
Brachium pontis (sect.)
Striae medullares
Velum medullare post. (section)
Obex
Flocculus
Plexus chor.
N. VII
N. VIII

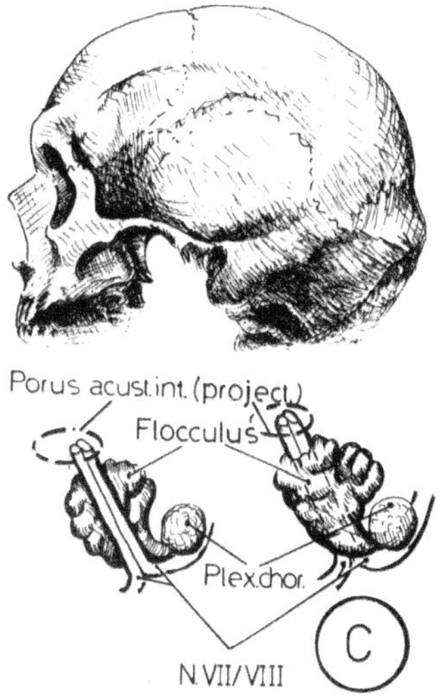
Porus acust. int. (project.)
Flocculus
Plex. chor.
N. VII/VIII
C

Fig. 249. Enlargement of part of Fig. 248 *A*. In this preparation the anastomoses of all cerebellar arteries in the region of Plexus chorioideus can be recognized. An outer ring of arteries around the flocculus also connects all cerebellar arteries (variant)

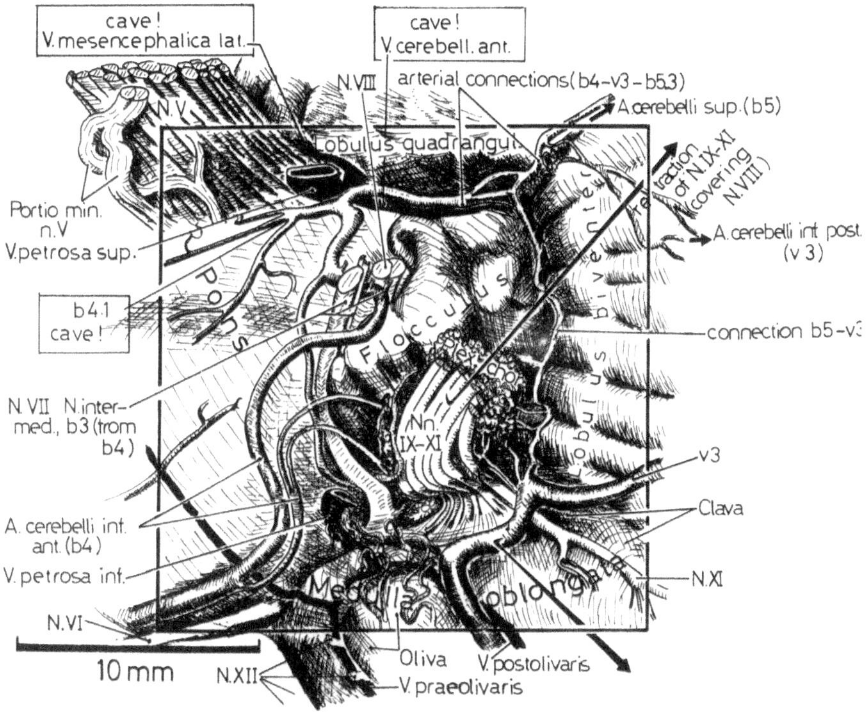
cave!
V. mesencephalica lat.
cave!
V. cerebell. ant.
N.VIII
arterial connections (b4-v3-b5.3)
A. cerebelli sup. (b5)
N.V
Lobulus quadrangul
retraction of N.IX-XI (covering N.VIII)
A. cerebelli inf. post. (v 3)
Portio min. n.V
V. petrosa sup.
Pons
Flocculus
b4.1 cave!
connection b5-v3
Lobulus biventer
Plex. chor.
N. VII N. inter-med., b3 (from b4)
Nn. IX-XI
v3
Clava
A. cerebelli inf. ant. (b4)
V. petrosa inf.
N.XI
Medulla oblongata
N.VI
10 mm
Oliva
V. postolivaris
N.XII
V. praeolivaris

Fig. 250. Ventrolateral aspect of Pons, oblique view
A General view
B Section with variant of A. cerebelli superior drawn in (arrow)
N.i. N. intermedius

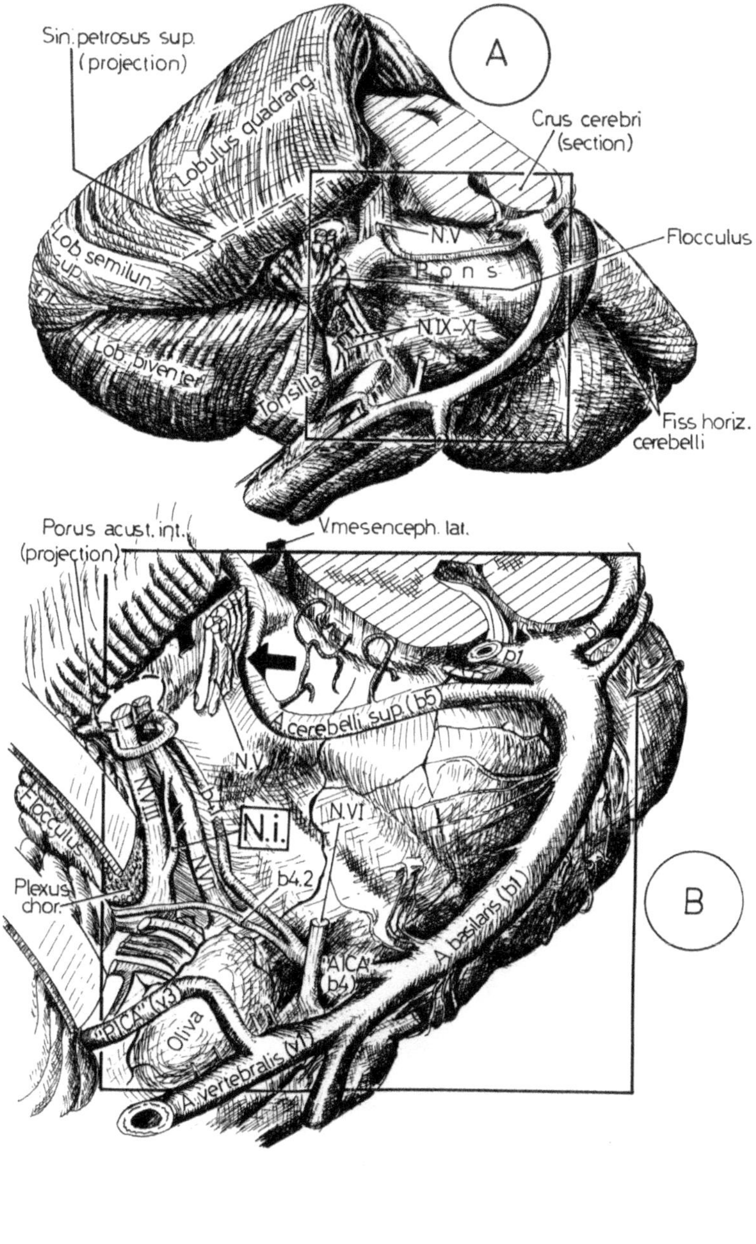
A
Sin. petrosus sup.
(projection)
Lobulus quadrang.
Crus cerebri
(section)
Lob. semilun.
sup.
inf.
N.V
Flocculus
Pons
N.IX–XI
Lob. biventer
Tonsilla
Fiss. horiz.
cerebelli
Porus acust. int.
(projection)
V. mesenceph. lat.
p1
A. cerebelli sup. (b5)
N.V
N.VII
N.VIII
N.i.
N.VI
Flocculus
Plexus
chor.
b4.2
"AICA"
b4
A. basilaris (b1)
"PICA" (v3)
Oliva
A. vertebralis (v1)
B

Fig. 251. Section corresponding to Fig. 250 A
C Variant of A. cerebelli inferior ant. (arrow)
D Variant of A. vertebralis (arrow)
N.i. N. intermedius

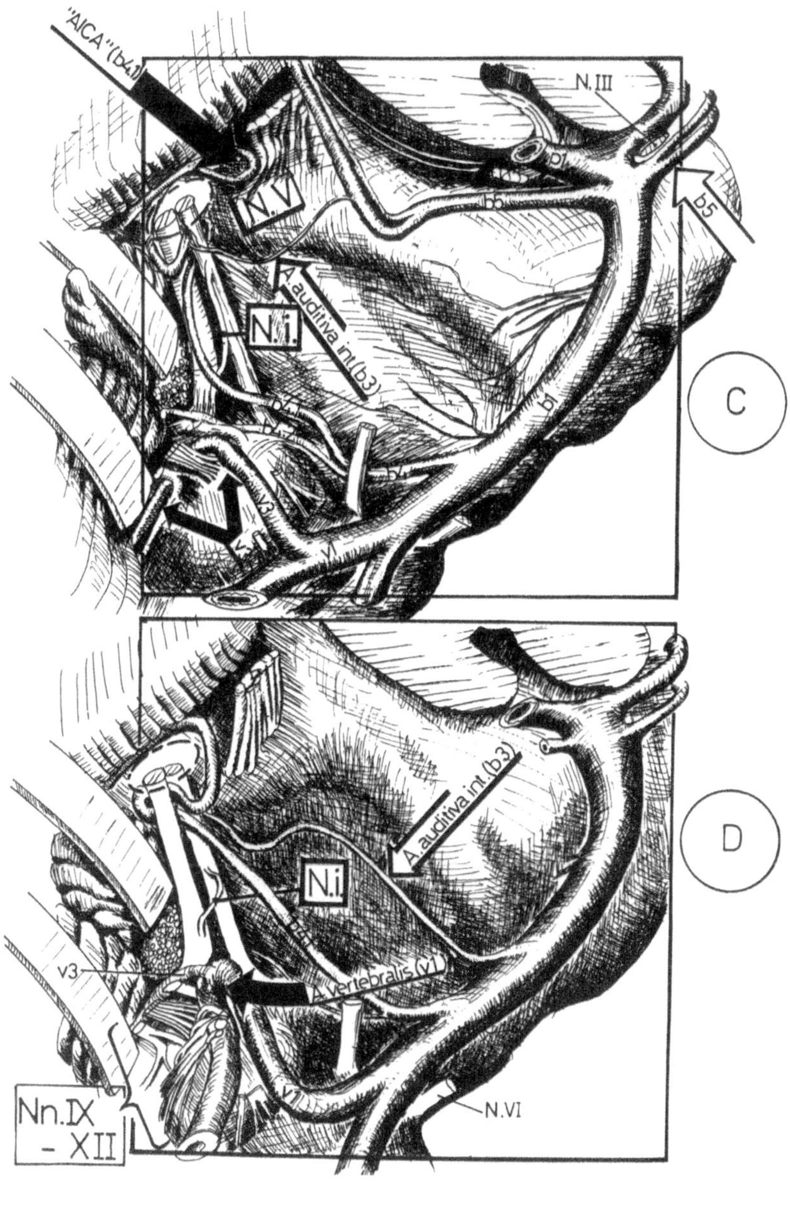
"AICA"(b4.1)
N.V
N.III
p1
b5
A.auditiva int.(b3)
N.i.
b1
C
v3
v1
D
A.auditiva int.(b3)
N.i
v3
A.vertebralis (v)
Nn.IX - XII
N.VI

Fig. 252. Considerably enlarged structures caudally and basally to cerebellopontine angle
A Bony structures with vessels and nerves drawn in without the dura
B Vicinity of Medulla oblongata

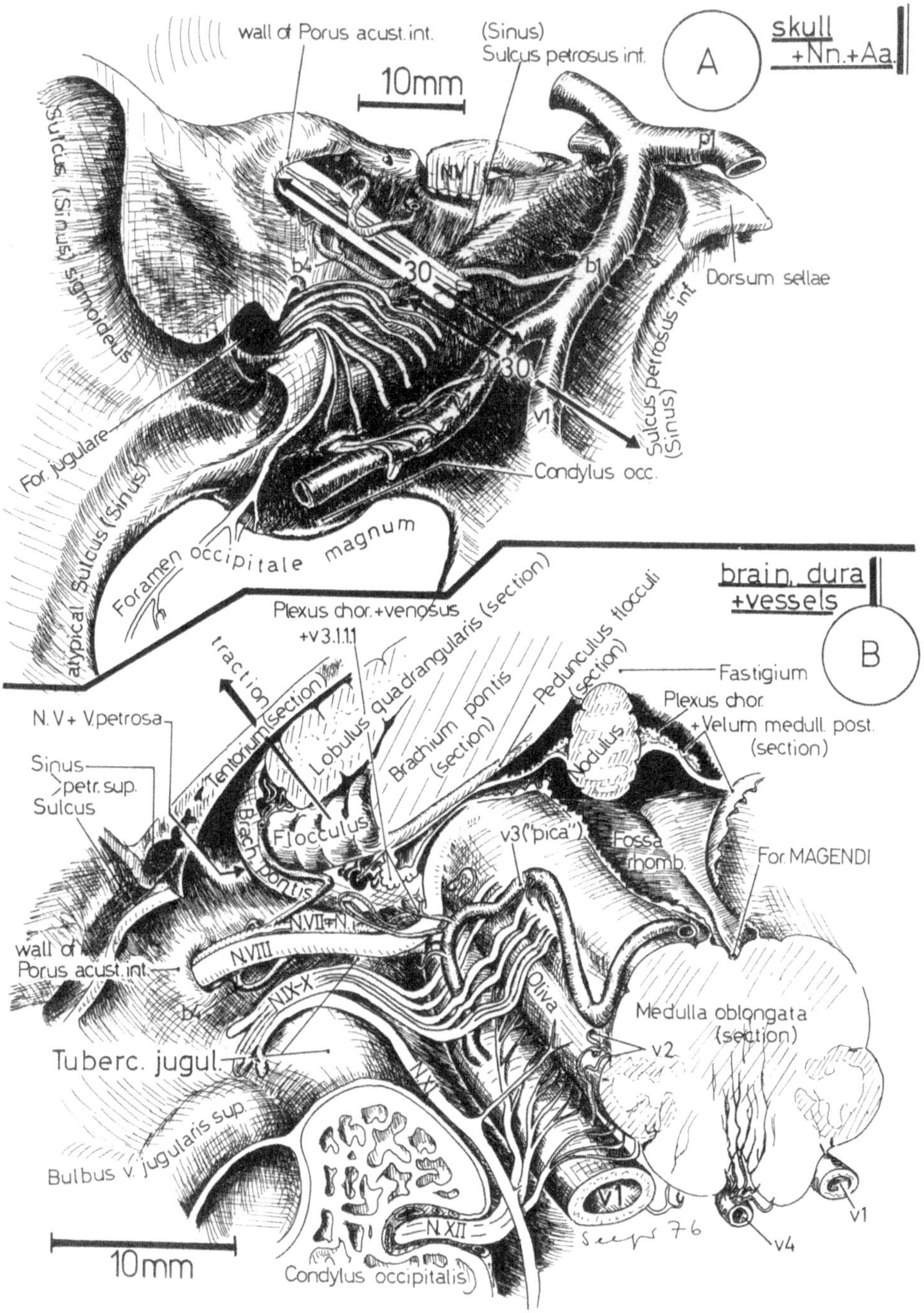
wall of Porus acust. int.
(Sinus)
Sulcus petrosus inf.
10mm
A
skull
+Nn.+Aa.
Sulcus (Sinus) sigmoideus
b4
30
30
b1
P1
Dorsum sellae
Sulcus petrosus inf. (Sinus)
v1
For. jugulare
Condylus occ.
atypical Sulcus (Sinus)
Foramen occipitale magnum
brain, dura
+vessels
B
Plexus chor.+venosus
+v 3.1.1.1
Lobulus quadrangularis (section)
Pedunculus flocculi (section)
Fastigium
traction
Tentorium (section)
Brachium pontis (section)
Plexus chor.
+Velum medull. post. (section)
N. V+ V.petrosa
Sinus
petr. sup.
Sulcus
Nodulus
Flocculus
Brach. pontis
v3 ("pica")
Fossa rhomb.
For. MAGENDI
N.VII+N.I
wall of Porus acust. int.
N.VIII
N.IX-X
b4
Oliva
Medulla oblongata (section)
v2
Tuberc. jugul.
N.XI
Bulbus v. jugularis sup.
v1
v1
v4
N.XII
10mm
Condylus occipitalis

Fig. 253. Medulla oblongata and its vicinity, dorsal view. The right cerebellar tonsil is dissected and everted at the transition to Brachium pontis. For nomenclature of arteries see arterial catalogue, pages 3–4

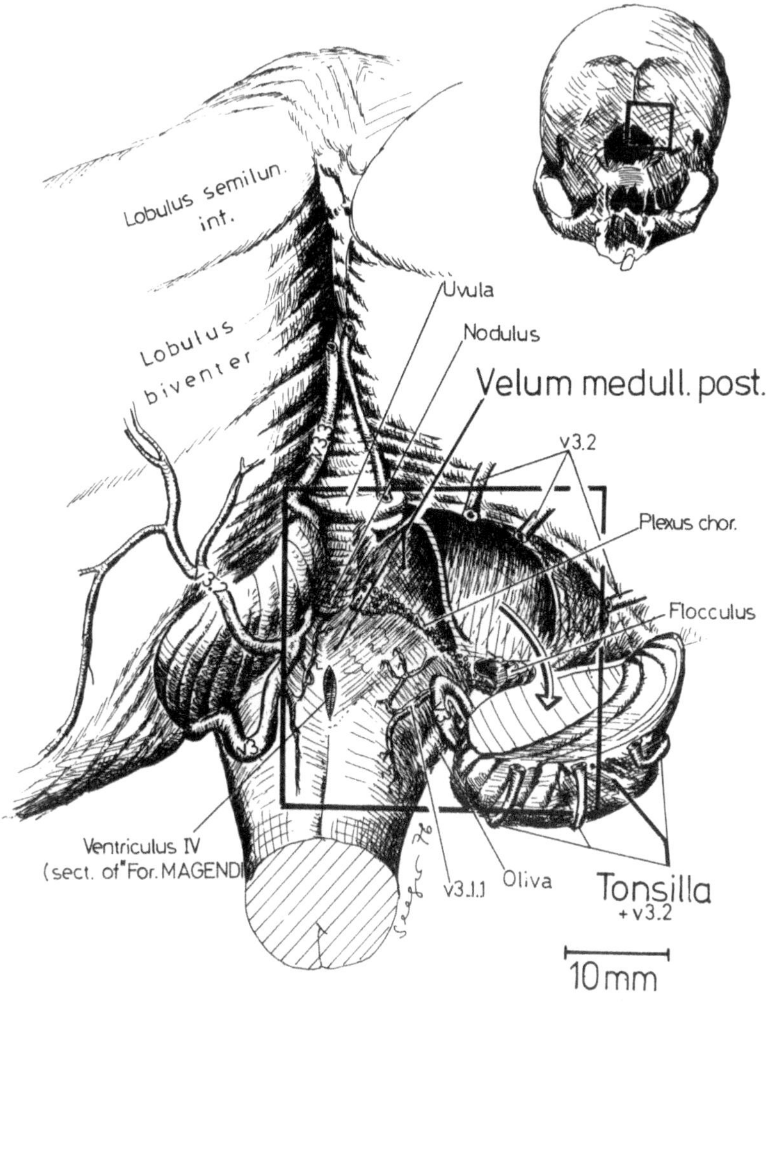
Lobulus semilun. int.
Lobulus biventer
Uvula
Nodulus
Velum medull. post.
v3.2
Plexus chor.
Flocculus
Ventriculus IV
(sect. of "For. MAGENDI)
v3.1.1
Oliva
Tonsilla
+ v3.2
10 mm

Fig. 254. Positional relationships of right cerebellar tonsil
A View from dorsal direction
B View from above

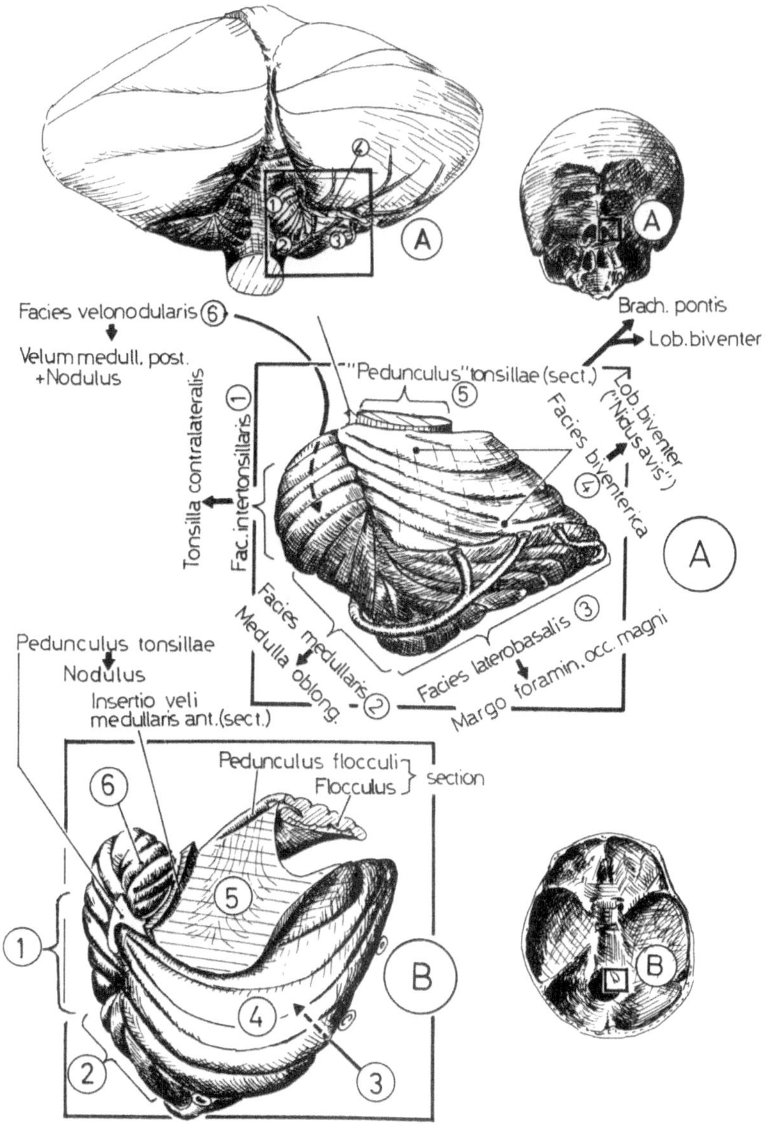
A
A
Facies velonodularis ⑥
Velum medull. post.
+Nodulus
Brach. pontis
Lob. biventer
"Pedunculus" tonsillae (sect.)
⑤
Lob. biventer
("Nidus avis")
Facies biventerica ④
Tonsilla contralateralis
Fac. intertonsillaris ①
A
Facies medullaris ②
Medulla oblong.
Facies laterobasalis ③
Margo foramin. occ. magni
Pedunculus tonsillae
Nodulus
Insertio veli
medullaris ant. (sect.)
Pedunculus flocculi
Flocculus
section
6
5
1
B
4
2
3
B

Fig. 255.
A Cerebellar tonsil from basal direction
B Bed of cerebellar tonsil in Velum medullare post. For nomenclature see Fig. 254

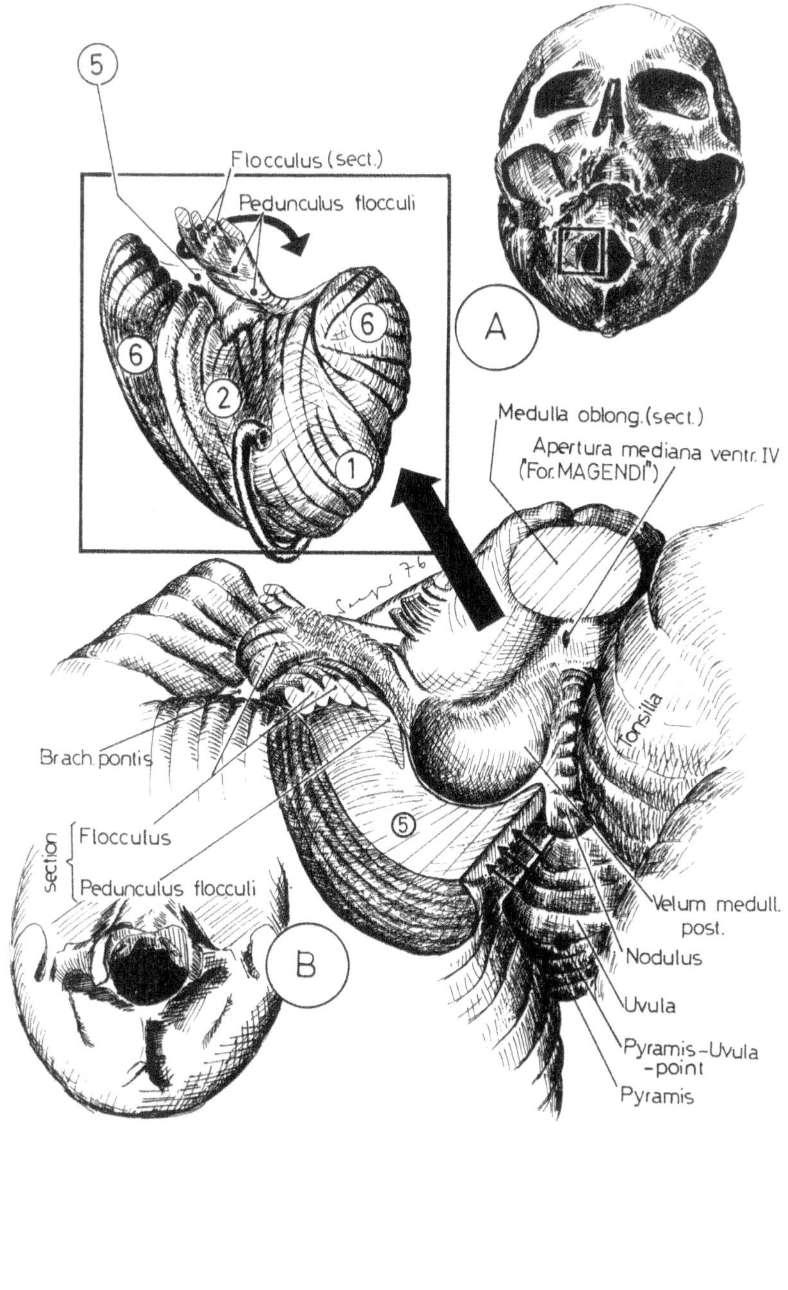
5
Flocculus (sect.)
Pedunculus flocculi
6
6
2
1
A
Medulla oblong. (sect.)
Apertura mediana ventr. IV
("For. MAGENDI")
Tonsilla
Brach. pontis
section
Flocculus
Pedunculus flocculi
5
B
Velum medull. post.
Nodulus
Uvula
Pyramis-Uvula -point
Pyramis

Fig. 256. Oblique view of Medulla oblongata and its vicinity after removal of right cerebellar tonsil

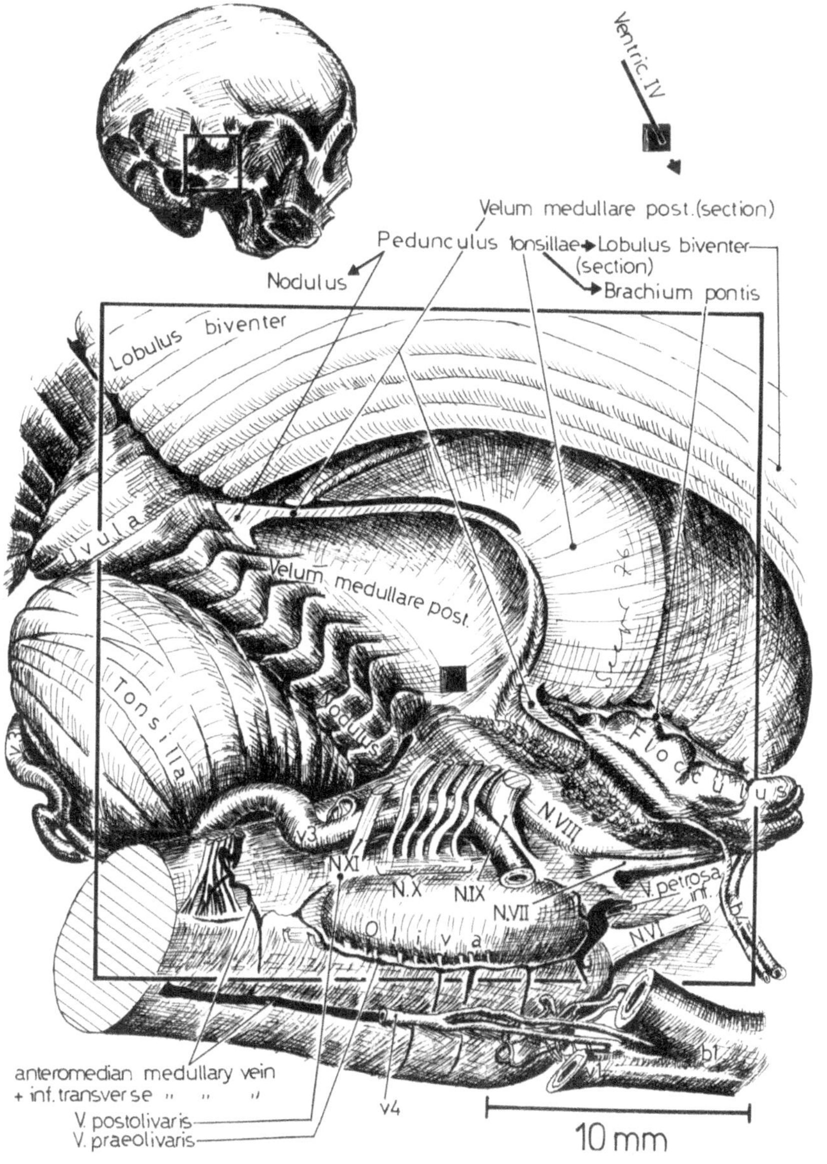
Ventric. IV
Velum medullare post. (section)
Pedunculus tonsillae
Lobulus biventer
(section)
Brachium pontis
Nodulus
Lobulus biventer
Uvula
Velum medullare post.
Tonsilla
Nodulus
Flocculus
N.VIII
v3
N.XI
N.X
N.IX
N.VII
V. petrosa inf.
N.VI
Oliva
b1
v1
v4
anteromedian medullary vein
+ inf. transverse " " "
V. postolivaris
V. praeolivaris
10 mm

Fig. 257. View into 4th ventricle after removal of Cerebellum with preservation of the Nodulus/Uvula complex and the left cerebellar tonsil as well as parts of Velum medullare ant. and post.

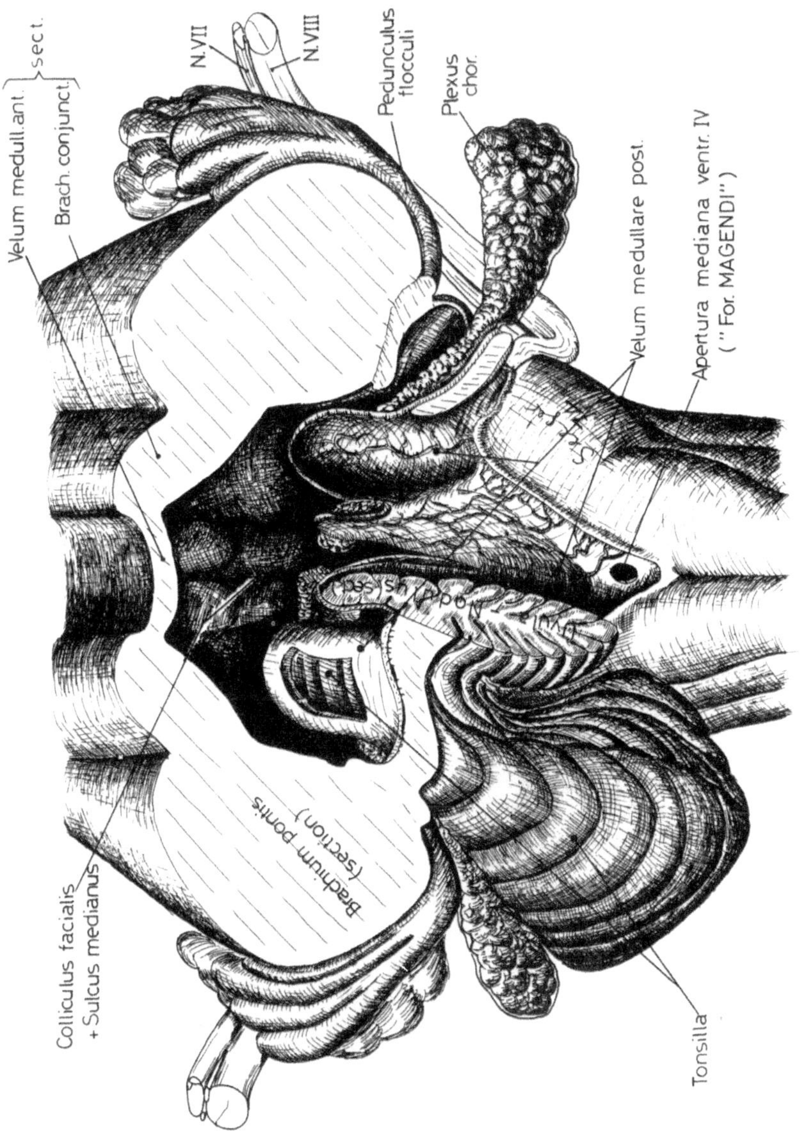
Velum medull. ant.
Brach. conjunct.
sect.
N.VII
N.VIII
Pedunculus flocculi
Plexus chor.
Velum medullare post.
Apertura mediana ventr. IV
("For. MAGENDI")
Colliculus facialis
+ Sulcus medianus
Brachium pontis
(section)
Tonsilla

Fig. 258. Preparation of Fig. 257 with arteries drawn in. For nomenclature of arteries, see arterial catalogue, pages 3–4

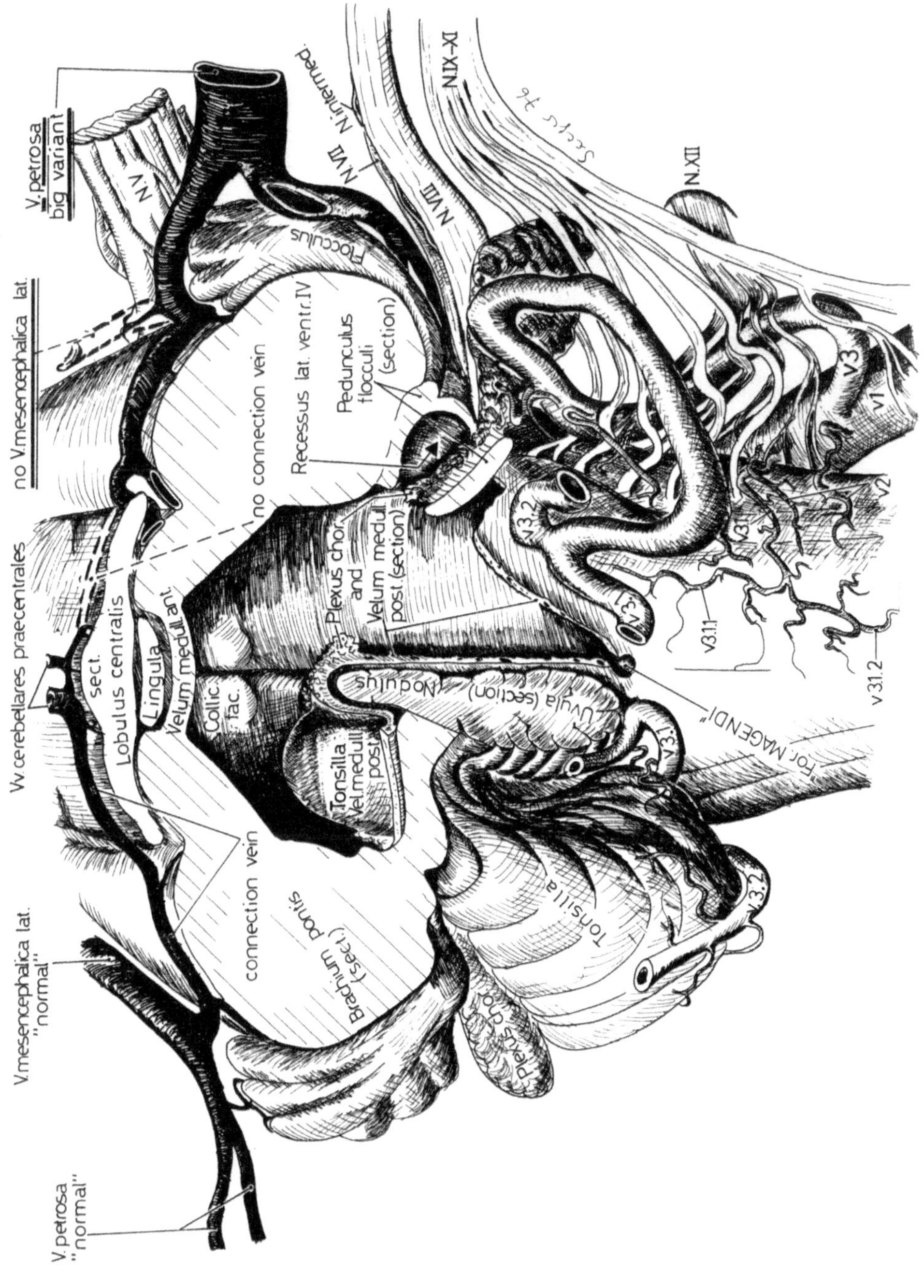
V.petrosa
big variant
no V.mesencephalica lat.
Vv.cerebellares praecentrales
V.mesencephalica lat.
"normal"
V.petrosa
"normal"
N.V
Flocculus
N.VII
N.intermed.
N.VIII
N.IX-XI
N.XII
Recessus lat. ventr.IV
Pedunculus
flocculi
(section)
no connection vein
Plexus chor.
and
Velum medull.
post.(section)
sect.
Lobulus centralis
Lingula
Velum medull. ant.
Collic.
fac.
Nodulus
Uvula (section)
Tonsilla
Vel.medull.
post.
connection vein
Brachium pontis
(sect.)
Tonsilla
Plexus chor.
"For. MAGENDI"
v3.1.1
v3.1.2
v3.1
v3.2
v3
v1
v2

Subject Index

Filmset by Ferd. Berger & Söhne OHG, A-3580 Horn
Reproduction of illustrations by Beissner & Co., A-1060 Wien
Printing by Novographic, Ing. W. Schmid, A-1230 Wien

GPSR Compliance

The European Union's (EU) General Product Safety Regulation (GPSR) is a set of rules that requires consumer products to be safe and our obligations to ensure this.

If you have any concerns about our products, you can contact us on ProductSafety@springernature.com

In case Publisher is established outside the EU, the EU authorized representative is:

Springer Nature Customer Service Center GmbH
Europaplatz 3
69115 Heidelberg, Germany

Batch number: 10726298

Printed by Printforce, the Netherlands